PRECIS

AN UPDATE IN OBSTETRICS AND GYNECOLOGY

Primary and Preventive Care

Fourth Edition

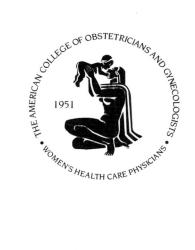

Precis: An Update in Obstetrics and Gynecology represents the knowledge and experience of experts in the field and does not necessarily reflect policy of the American College of Obstetricians and Gynecologists (ACOG). This publication describes methods and techniques of clinical practice that are accepted and used by recognized authorities. The recommendations do not dictate an exclusive course of treatment or of practice. Variations taking into account the needs of the individual patient, resources, and limitations unique to the institution or type of practice may be appropriate.

Medicine is an ever-changing field. As new research and clinical experience emerge, changes in treatment and drug therapy are required. Every effort has been made to ensure that the drug dosage schedules contained herein are accurate and in accordance with standards accepted at the time of publication. Readers are advised, however, to check the product information literature of each drug they plan to administer to be certain that there have been no changes in the dosage recommended or in the contraindications for administration. This recommendation is of particular importance for new or infrequently used drugs.

Lists of web sites provided throughout this volume were prepared by ACOG Resource Center librarians from other sources and are provided for information only. Referral to these web sites does not imply ACOG endorsement. The lists are not meant to be comprehensive; the exclusion of a Web site does not reflect the quality of that site. Please note that web sites and URLs are subject to change without warning. Web sites were verified on June 13, 2008.

Library of Congress Cataloging-in-Publication Data

Precis: an update in obstetrics and gynecology. Primary and preventive care. — 4th ed.
    p. ; cm.
title: Primary and preventive care
    Includes bibliographical references and index.
    ISBN 978-1-934946-80-0 (pbk.: alk. paper)
    1. Obstetrics—Outlines, syllabi, etc. 2. Gynecology—Outlines, syllabi, etc. 3. Women—Diseases—Outlines, syllabi, etc. 4. Primary care (Medicine)—Outlines, syllabi, etc. I. American College of Obstetricians and Gynecologists. II. Title: Primary and preventive care.
    [DNLM: 1. Genital diseases, Female—prevention & control. 2. Evidence-Based Medicine. 3. Pregnancy Complications—prevention & control. 4. Primary Health Care. 5. Women's Health. WP 140 P922 2009]
RC112.P753 2009
618—dc22

                    2008052661

The American College of Obstetricians and Gynecologists
409 12th Street, SW
PO Box 96920
Washington, DC 20090-6920
www.acog.org

12345/32109

Contents

Contributors

Editorial Committee

Thomas E. Nolan, MD, Chair

Paul D. Blumenthal, MD

Susan Johnson, MD

Neil Murphy, MD

Jeffrey F. Peipert, MD, PhD

Thomas C. Peng, MD

Herbert B. Peterson, MD

Sharon T. Phelan, MD

Advisory Committee

Donald R. Coustan, MD, Chair

Jonathan Berek, MD

Roger P. Smith, MD

Authors

Raul Artal, MD

Robert L. Barbieri, MD

Rosemary Basson, MD

Paul D. Blumenthal, MD

D. Ware Branch, MD

George A. Bray, MD

Linda Brubaker, MD

Thomas Buchanan, MD

Catherine M. Champagne, PhD

Philip D. Darney, MD

Tracy Gaudet, MD

Paul A. Gluck, MD

Pratima Gupta, MD

Keith A. Hansen, MD

Katherine J. Hladky, MD

Allan J. Jacobs, MD, JD

Siri L. Kjos, MD

Nicole Marshall, MD

Cathy L. Melvin, MD, PhD

J. V. (Ian) Nixon, MD

Thomas E. Nolan, MD

Jeffrey F. Peipert, MD, PhD

Herbert B. Peterson, MD

Sharon T. Phelan, MD

Rachel A. Rabinowitz, MD

William F. Rayburn, MD

Jeanne M. Schilder, MD

Stephen D. Silberstein, MD

Roger P. Smith, MD

Harise Stein, MD

Zachary N. Stowe, MD

Gerald S. Zavorsky, PhD

STAFF

Sterling B. Williams, MD, MS
Vice President of Education

Thomas Dineen
Director of Publications

Deirdre Allen, MPS
Editorial Director

Nikoleta Dineen
Senior Editor

Mark D. Grazette
Senior Graphic Designer

Preface

Education is a lifelong process. In no field is this process more important than in medicine. As scientific advances unfold, new techniques and technologies emerge, knowledge expands, and the art and science of medicine undergo dynamic change. Progress in medicine is ongoing, and so too must be the continuing medical education of those who practice it.

Precis: An Update in Obstetrics and Gynecology is intended to meet the continuing education needs of obstetricians and gynecologists. It is a broad, yet concise, overview of information relevant to the specialty. As in earlier editions, the emphasis is on innovations in clinical practice, presented within the context of traditional approaches that retain their applicability to patient care.

Precis is an educational resource to be used in preparation for the cognitive assessment of clinical knowledge, regardless of the form of the assessment—formal or informal, structured or independent. It is one of the recognized vehicles useful in preparing for certification and accreditation processes, and it is designed to complement those evaluations while serving as a general review of the field.

Each year, one volume of this five-volume set is revised. This process provides continual updates that are critical to the practice of obstetrics and gynecology, and it echoes the dynamic nature of the field. The focus is on new and emerging techniques, presented from a balanced perspective of clinical value and cost-effectiveness in practice. Hence, discussion of traditional medical practice is limited. The information has been organized to unify coverage of topics into a single volume so that each volume can stand on its own merit.

This fourth edition of *Precis: Primary and Preventive Care* reflects current thinking on optimal practice. The information is intended to be a useful tool to assist practicing obstetrician–gynecologists in maintaining current knowledge in a rapidly changing field and to prepare them better for the role of primary care practitioner for women.

Some information from the previous edition continues to be of value and, thus, has been retained and woven into the new structure. The efforts of authors contributing to previous editions, as well as the work of those authors providing new material, must be recognized with gratitude. Collectively, they represent the expertise of the specialty. With such a breadth of representation, differences of opinion are inevitable and have been respected.

Other *Precis* volumes are *Oncology*, Third Edition; *Obstetrics*, Third Edition; *Gynecology*, Third Edition, and *Reproductive Endocrinology*, Third Edition. Each is an educational tool for review, reference, and evaluation. *Precis* establishes a broad scientific basis for the delivery of quality health care for women. Rather than being a statement of the American College of Obstetricians and Gynecologists (ACOG) policy, *Precis* serves as an intellectual approach to education. An effort has been made, however, to achieve consistency within *Precis* and with other ACOG recommendations. Variations in patient care, based on individual needs and resources, are encouraged as an integral part of the practice of medicine.

—THE EDITORS

PRECIS

AN UPDATE IN OBSTETRICS AND GYNECOLOGY

Primary and Preventive Care

Fourth Edition

Introduction

Precis: Primary and Preventive Care, Fourth Edition, reflects the expanding role of health care providers in optimizing women's health and preventing disease. The previous edition was revised with the goal of identifying areas that underwent dramatic changes and helping readers to navigate through those changes. One such area is patient safety, and an entire new section has been devoted to it. In other cases, current information was retained, and areas that have not undergone substantial transformation have been omitted.

Basic approaches to prevention and general treatment guidelines also are included, with the caveat that because they often change, practitioners should consult sources to ensure that they are familiar with the most recent recommendations, particularly those of the American College of Obstetricians and Gynecologists. To aid in finding additional resources, sections on information retrieval and evaluation of evidence-based medical literature have been updated. Resource boxes for individual sections will lead readers to helpful web sites.

Some sections cover topics that are traditionally part of office practice and have a major prevention component, such as fertility control, sexuality and sexual dysfunction, and violence against women. The last portion includes domestic violence, mistreatment of elders, and rape and sexual assault of adults and children—topics that cannot be ignored and areas in which obstetrician–gynecologists can make an important difference.

Common medical disorders are addressed within the context of screening and initial management that are well in the realm of practicing obstetrician–gynecologists. Obesity, a major cause of chronic disease, and the metabolic syndrome are addressed in sections on nutrition and weight management, hypertension, dyslipidemia, and diabetes mellitus. Other sections cover mood disorders, headache, fibromyalgia, chronic fatigue syndrome, thyroid diseases, and coagulopathies. Coverage of gastrointestinal disorders has been expanded to include the newest information on peptic ulcer disease, irritable bowel syndrome, rectal incontinence, colorectal cancer, and Crohn disease. There has been no attempt to provide an in-depth discussion of disease management; rather, the emphasis is on advances in screening and early detection. It is hoped that this approach to prevention, counseling, screening, and early detection and intervention will aid obstetrician–gynecologists in their goal of providing comprehensive health care for women.

—THOMAS E. NOLAN, MD
Chair, Editorial Committee

Information Management and Communication

Paul A. Gluck and Roger P. Smith

Information Management

Physicians are immersed in information; they obtain it, process it, modify it, and dispense it. Today, the tools that are available to perform these tasks have changed dramatically, although the tasks themselves have not. Practicing obstetrician–gynecologists must be able to access and manage an ever-growing amount of information. Whether accessing current, accurate, and authoritative information on patient care guidelines, educational materials to help patients understand their conditions, or electronic medical systems to provide and guide care directly, the possession, management, and distribution of information are critical to safe, effective care.

Information Retrieval

The Internet has become a "library card to the world" (1, 2). Information repositories around the world are open to everyone, and advanced search engines make finding the information in these repositories so simple that many take it for granted. But some care must be exercised. Almost anyone can become connected to the Internet and add or retrieve information with no constraints on content, opinion, or quality (3). It is important to discriminate between trustworthy, reliable sources and the unreliable ones. The most reliable sites are the ones for which authorship is known and trusted. Institutions, recognized organizations, and government agencies are the most reliable. However, even

---

Resources

Communication

Agency for Healthcare Research and Quality
http://www.ahrq.gov

Centers for Disease Control and Prevention
http://www.cdc.gov

Institute for Healthcare Improvement
http://www.ihi.org/ihi

The Joint Commission
http://www.jointcommission.org

National Center for Patient Safety
http://www.patientsafety.gov

National Library of Medicine
http://www.nlm.nih.gov

National Patient Safety Foundation
http://www.npsf.org

---

their sites can, and do, change with time, making it vital to check frequently for updated information and for sites that maintain current information.

Many professional organizations or disease-specific web sites have links to related sites that are assessed for quality. Organizations often have internal search features. Finally, because evidence-based medicine is becoming the standard for current medical practice (see "Principles of Evidence-Based Medicine"), online resources providing clinical research information are gaining wide popularity (Boxes 1 and 2).

Information (Clinical and Practice) Management

No longer just the province of the business office, information management is now critical to practice marketing, delivery of care, and patient safety. One example is the use of computer algorithms to monitor care, assist in diagnosis, and prompt for safety issues. These systems are referred to as expert systems. Expert systems are not intended to serve as computerized surrogates for physicians. Rather, they are designed to assist physicians in clinical decisions regarding diagnosis and treatment. When used in combination with good (human) clinical judgment, they can be an effective clinical tool. At the same time, they can serve as a teaching aid, helping us to understand the thought process involved in clinical decision making. Neural networks offer the possibility of developing an expert system when the exact relationships between factors are either unknown or unknowable.

MARKETING AND MANAGING A PRACTICE

Many practices have found the Internet, with its high-speed connectivity, ease of use, and image capability, an ideal way to promote, manage, or develop a practice (4). At the most basic, the concrete application can provide pictures of the practice, information about office hours or policies, useful telephone or other contact information, and links to patient information about topics of interest. Some practices have extended their Internet presence to include patient-driven appointment scheduling, password-protected access to laboratory results, and even computer-generated telephone follow-up (5).

In some locations, consultation by e-mail is permissible and billable. However, before adding this capability to a practice's offerings, local regulations and insurer policies should be checked. (There have been questions raised about "practicing without a license" if the patient

3

Box 1

Description of Selected Web Resources for Clinicians

Web Site of the American College of Obstetricians and Gynecologists (http://www.acog.org)

The web site of the American College of Obstetricians and Gynecologists (ACOG) covers topics of interest to practicing obstetrician–gynecologists. It has a strong search engine and provides members with access to full-text documents. Web site members' page lists sites of interest under the Online Resources heading. One example is the ACOG members-only section where members can enter complex search terms to retrieve information from current ACOG publications or the full text of *Obstetrics and Gynecology* (1989–present).

Government-Maintained Web Sites

Centers for Disease Control and Prevention (http://www.cdc.gov)
Whether faced with difficult-to-treat care or just a request for travel-related health precautions, this site can be invaluable to practitioners.

MEDLINEplus (http://medlineplus.gov)
This web resource is maintained by the National Library of Medicine. It is a source of good health information for patients and health care practitioners.

ClinicalTrials.gov (http://clinicaltrials.gov)
The National Institutes of Health, through the National Library of Medicine, has developed this web site for information about ongoing clinical trials. The site's mission is to provide physicians, patients, family members, and members of the public with current information about clinical research studies.

Web Resources for Evidence-Based Medicine

The Cochrane Library (http://www.cochrane.org)
This is a particularly good resource for the clinician to help sort out information of significance from a background flurry of information. *Cochrane Reviews*, the primary output of the Cochrane Collaboration, are published electronically in successive issues of the *Cochrane Database of Systematic Reviews*. These are available by subscription on the Internet or CD-ROM. The abstracts of *Cochrane Reviews* are available without charge and can be browsed or searched on the Internet.

ScHARR (www.shef.ac.uk/scharr)
The Internet site ScHARR is hosted by the School of Health and Related Research in Sheffield, England, that is devoted to applying research data to develop evidence-based medical practice. The School of Health and Related Research is one of the four schools in the faculty of medicine at the University of Sheffield. The easy-to-navigate ScHARR web site has an extensive list of links and resources for finding, appraising, and implementing current health-related research findings. Resources for software, journals, databases, and organizations are well represented, easy to find, accurate, and current.

---

who receives care lives across a state line and the physician does not have a license in that state. Great care must also be taken to remain compliant with the privacy rules of the U.S. Health Insurance Portability and Accountability Act, or HIPAA.)

Some practices have taken advantage of the ease of word processing and desktop publishing and created newsletters, informational fliers, patient education program announcements, and similar materials. These materials may be printed or distributed electronically to promote the practice to patients and others.

One of the strengths of electronic database systems is the ability to retain and process information in ways that may not have been apparent at the time the data were collected. Database management systems have the capacity to manage large volumes of data with multiple cross-indexes. Most programs also can exchange data with other programs, such as word processors and list

makers. In a gynecologic practice, these programs are useful in a wide variety of administrative tasks, including tasks related to patient files, inventory lists, reference indexes, registries, systematic reviews, risk analysis, and outcomes assessment (6–11). Examples of this type of application in women's health care range from using databases to establish mammography registries to assessing the outcomes of urogynecologic surgeries (12, 13).

ELECTRONIC MEDICAL RECORDS

Electronic medical records hold a number of opportunities for improved efficiency and safety in patient care (14, 15). The idea of computerized medical records is not new. However, despite the universal use of computers in hospitals, the implementation of a computerized medical record has been disappointing, and computer-

---

Box 2

Searching in PubMed

The National Library of Medicine's free search engine PubMed allows topics to be searched as medical subject headings (MeSH) or text words or both. It has many useful features:

- It will "explode" MeSH terms to include more specific terms in the search unless otherwise specified. For example, if the user enters *Filovirus*, the system will search for *Filovirus* and add the more specific terms *Ebola virus* and *Marburg virus*.

- It can change requests presented in unqualified terms to valid MeSH headings.

- The upper-case Boolean operators AND, OR, or NOT can be used to refine the search process. Construction of the request will determine the search results. The following search statements will not retrieve the same information:

  —Common cold AND vitamin C OR zinc

  —Common cold OR vitamin C AND zinc

  In the first statement, the citations for the common cold will be compared with those for vitamin C, and those with references to both will be added to citations referring to zinc, even if the zinc citations are not about either of the other two topics. In the second search, citations will be retrieved that refer to either the common cold or vitamin C. These citations will then be compared to a list of citations for zinc, and only those in both groups will be in the results; eg, those citations that are about zinc AND either the cold or vitamin C. This is a seemingly subtle but very important difference.

- The order in which PubMed processes a search statement can be changed by enclosing individual concepts in parentheses. The terms inside parentheses will be processed as a unit and then incorporated into the overall strategy; eg, common cold AND (vitamin C OR zinc).

- Search results are displayed with the most recent listed first.

- Search results may be viewed online, printed, or downloaded as a text file.

- The PubMed abstract indicates whether full-text access is provided by the publisher, perhaps for a fee.

For reasons of cost, low demand, publication age, copyright restrictions, and other barriers that may prevent access, not all articles are available electronically. If the full text of an article cannot be obtained online, a copy can be requested through a local medical library. One way to request copies of articles through the Internet via search results in PubMed is to establish a Loansome Doc agreement with the library. Requests will be routed automatically through the National Library of Medicine's interlibrary loan system (DOCLINE) and copies will be sent by mail, fax, or e-mail. Local medical librarians can help in setting up a Loansome Doc account and introducing other library services, such as librarian-performed searches and training in using the Internet, evidence-based medicine resources, and MEDLINE. For those who do not have a local medical library, the National Network of Libraries of Medicine home page (http://nnlm.gov/members) provides help in finding one. For advanced techniques on searching PubMed, try the PubMed Tutorial (http://www.nlm.nih.gov/bsd/disted/pubmed.html).

---

ized medical records account for only a small percentage of medical records (16, 17). Developing a computerized record is not simple and requires extensive advance preparation to ensure efficiency and privacy.

This form of patient record has the allure of standardization of information, ready access from multiple locations, ease of storage, and enhanced capabilities (eg, digital photos) not available in a paper record (18). The lack of standards for content and user interface, poor performance of some of the initially available products, associated equipment, and conversion costs have constrained the rapid adoption of this technology (19, 20). Although standards have emerged for how these types of data are stored and transferred between various systems, the user interface, clinical content, and other aspects have not enjoyed the same consensus. A number of commercial suppliers have made available electronic prenatal systems, but similar systems for gynecologic or primary care management are fewer.

Enhancing Patient Safety Through Effective Communication

In the context of medical care, communication occurs on two levels—between health care providers and between a health care provider and the patient and the family. Miscommunication on either of these levels appreciably affects health outcomes and increases the potential for patient harm. The Veterans Administration National Center for Patient Safety database of more than 12,000 root case analyses of adverse events identified communication failures in 70–80% of cases (21). According to the Joint Commission (formerly the Joint Commission on Accreditation of Healthcare Organizations), communication errors were present in 65% of sentinel events from 1996 to 2005. The number was unchanged in the analysis of sentinel events reported in 2006 (21).

The errors in the transfer of information from one health care provider to another can seriously jeopardize patient safety; thus, from routine morning rounds to handoffs between partners, reliably communicating information is vital (22). This communication can be verbal, paper-based, or electronic (23). The key is the information transferred, not the medium or method of information management. The critical nature of this form of information management has been recognized by the emergence of team rounds, the repeating verbal orders, and the preoperative "time out" (24). Electronic information management can assist in this cause by ensuring that all providers have instant access to the same information (eg, laboratory reports, imaging, and electronic medical records); in the case of electronic order entry, electronic information management can avert potential errors (25).

The possibility of patient-carried medical records in the form of smart cards has been raised. These plastic identification cards carry an electronic chip that retains critical information in computer-readable digital forms. Used like a credit card, these devices could contain the contents of the patient's medical record, results of recent laboratory and imaging studies, medication history, and other pertinent information. The role that these cards may have in a future of paperless records has been debated and is far from clear (26, 27).

Communication errors are especially problematic during transitions in care from one unit to another or from one provider to another in the hospital, as well as during transitions from an inpatient to an ambulatory environment. Most commonly, discontinuity occurs between the hospital and primary care physicians as a result of communication errors (28). There also is an appreciable lack of care coordination among providers of ambulatory care. Important clinical information was missing in 13% of visits to primary care physicians; it included laboratory data (45%), radiology reports (28%), current medications (26%), and pathology reports (15%) (29). Furthermore, in a patient survey, 23% of respondents reported that important clinical information was not available at the time of their office visit; in 18% of respondents, duplicate tests were ordered (30). These information gaps resulted in delay in care, duplication of tests, or both. At times, physicians were forced to make important clinical decisions with incomplete information, increasing the risk of patient harm.

At the time of discharge, one half of patients experienced a medication error. One third of patients were given either the wrong medication or the wrong dose. As a result, 19–23% of patients experienced an adverse event, with a readmission rate of 14% (28). Safety was

further compromised with 11% of patients being unaware of which symptoms would require evaluation and 27% of patients being unsure of whom to see for follow-up care (30).

Finally, problems with health literacy create additional communication gaps between providers and patients. As defined by the Institute of Medicine, "health literacy is the degree to which individuals have the capacity to obtain, process, and understand basic health information and services needed to make appropriate decisions regarding their health" (31). Medical information often is written at a 12th-grade level even though most Americans read at an 8th- to 9th-grade level (32). As many as 90 million American adults have difficulty functioning in our health care system because of low literacy. Even the most educated individuals may at times be unable to process information and make appropriate health care decisions. The consequences of this problem can be catastrophic. After controlling for other factors, such as demographics, socioeconomic status, and baseline health, individuals with inadequate health literacy had a 52% increased risk of dying from cardiovascular disease (33). Health literacy, as an independent variable, directly relates to compliance with appropriate mammography and cervical cytology screening intervals. Poor health literacy is frequently not recognized, leading to the misperception that the patient understands the recommendation of the health care provider.

Effective Communication

The principles of effective communication apply to communication among health care professionals, as well as between providers and patients. Closed-loop communication is important to ensure that the message, whether written or oral, has been received and understood correctly by the recipient. In this form of communication, the sender initiates communication, the receiver confirms that the communication has been heard and repeats the content, and the sender verifies the accuracy of that content (34). Closed-loop communication also provides the recipient an opportunity to clarify any ambiguities in the content or the intent of the message. The message itself should be clear, complete, brief, and timely (35).

Barriers in Communication

Several barriers impede the flow and understanding of medical communication between providers and patients, as well as among providers. Recognizing and ameliorating these barriers is important to achieve clear, effective communication.

During the medical interaction, the patient may be intimidated by the authority of the medical provider. Fear of appearing "stupid" in the face of this authority figure may prevent the patient from asking for additional explanations. The fact that a discussion is taking place in the examination room with the patient wearing a flimsy paper gown further adds to the patient's vulnerability. Medical jargon may seem like a foreign language to the patient. Language itself, especially for individuals of limited English proficiency, poses another barrier. The content of the message itself may interfere with comprehension. It often is said that once patients are told of a bad diagnosis, such as cancer, they hear and remember very little of the rest of the conversation. Patients also have difficulty understanding multiple, complex, often interrelated medical problems, especially if they are presented all at one time. Finally, stressors occurring in the patient's personal life or concerns about family members may be unknown to the provider but distracting to the patient.

Communication between providers may be face to face, but it increasingly takes place by telephone or by pager, and often interrupts or is interrupted by other tasks. These communications are frequently inefficient, incomplete, and not heard as intended; and they are at times inaccurate, leading to a significant increase in patient harm (29). Additional barriers to effective communication include 1) professional silos; 2) lack of assertiveness; 3) organizational hierarchy; 4) lack of mutual respect; 5) lack of situational awareness; 6) lack of care coordination; and (7) use of acronyms, abbreviations, and incomplete sentences (21).

Communication Strategies for Health Care Providers

Poor communication by health care providers often results in error and harm, regardless of the provider's clinical skill and commitment to patients (21). Five important communication techniques facilitate the accurate transmission and reception of the message: situation–background–assessment–recommendation (SBAR); callout; timeout; check-back; and handoff (35).

SITUATION – BACKGROUND – ASSESSMENT – RECOMMENDATION

Situation–background–assessment–recommendation is structured verbal communication that conveys critical information. This strategy is timely, unambiguous, and requires an immediate response (Box 3).

The following example illustrates an SBAR communication from the nurse in the postpartum unit to the obstetrician on call:

Situation	"Mrs. Smith has a blood pressure of 90/50, a pulse rate of 120, and heavy vaginal bleeding."
Background	"She had an uneventful spontaneous vaginal delivery by your partner early this morning with repair of a second-degree laceration. The placenta was delivered intact."

Box 3	
Situation – Background – Assessment – Recommendation	
Situation	The change in clinical status that requires immediate attention
Background	The clinical context
Assessment	The speaker's evaluation of the problem
Recommendation	The speaker's suggested clinical action in response to the problem

Assessment	"I suspect that she could have uterine atony. I have been massaging the uterine fundus but see little improvement in the bleeding."
Recommendation	"I would like to start oxytocin intravenously and send blood sample for a complete blood count and type and crossmatch for two units of packed cells. I feel that you should come in to assess the patient. Are you available?"

The information is clear, concise, and timely and solicits an immediate response.

CALLOUT

Callout is a strategy used during an emergency in which all team members participate. It is a method of communicating critical information to one another. It ensures that all members of the team are aware of the situation, assigns individual responsibilities, elicits input, and helps other team members anticipate additional actions. The following example illustrates the use of callout in the operating room during an emergency cesarean delivery performed because of nonreassuring fetal status with persistent bradycardia:

Attending physician: "Has the newborn intensive care unit been notified?"

Nurse: "Newborn intensive care unit notified. The neonatologist is coming."

Attending physician: "The patient has increased bleeding. What is the blood pressure and pulse rate?"

Anesthesiologist: "Blood pressure 110/70, pulse rate 84."

Attending physician: "Is blood available for transfusion?"

Nurse: "Blood bank has a specimen and is crossmatching two units of packed cells."

TIMEOUT

Timeout is a component of the Joint Commission's Universal Protocol (36) and the World Health Organization's Safe Surgery Save Lives program (37). It is designed to ensure that the correct patient, site, position, and procedure are identified before any invasive procedure is initiated. The timeout is initiated by a designated member of the health care team. In the operating room, it ideally should occur before the induction of general anesthesia.

During the timeout there must be explicit verbal agreement among the members of the health care team (surgeon, anesthesia professional, circulating nurse, and scrub nurse) regarding the patient's identification, planned procedure, operative site, and consent form. Other activities in the operating room should be suspended until the timeout is completed. There is consensus from the Joint Commission and the World Health Organization regarding the components of the timeout in the operating room (Box 4). There should be documentation in the medical record that the timeout was accomplished with agreement of the health care team. Any disagreements must be resolved before the procedure can continue.

CHECK-BACK

Check-back is closed-loop communication during which a message is sent, repeated by the recipient, and then confirmed by the sender before any action is initiated. This method is used in aviation for communication between the flight crew and the control tower, as well as between the pilot and the copilot. The following example illustrates the check-back process in closed-loop communication:

Attending physician: "Add 20 units of oxytocin to the intravenous infusion."

Nurse: "Twenty units of oxytocin to the current intravenous infusion?"

Attending physician: "Correct, 20 units of oxytocin."

HANDOFF

Handoff is defined as the transfer of patient information and knowledge, along with authority and responsibility, from one health care provider or team to another on a temporary or permanent basis. This fragmented care increases the risk of miscommunication. Properly conducted handoffs are the most critical element in improving safety in maternity care, which typically requires coordination of several health care providers (38). Specific details must become part of standard procedure for these handoffs to occur safely; these details include where, when, who, how, and what (38, 39):

Where The physical setting should be private to preserve patient confidentiality and be free from distractions and interruptions. Having a well-lit area and a desk or counter with writing space to take notes also is helpful.

When There must be a dedicated time for handoffs. Handoffs should occur with each change of provider, change of patient location, or change in the patient's health status.

Box 4

Timeout Checklist

The following components of the safety protocol must be identified before any major surgical procedure is performed:

1. Correct patient identity
2. Correct surgical site (marked if appropriate)
3. Accurate consent form
4. Correct procedure planned
5. Relevant images and laboratory results available in the operating room
6. Appropriate antibiotic prophylaxis given
7. Necessary equipment available in the operating room

Who All individuals assuming care of the patient must attend. Ideally, if teams are part of the culture, these handoffs should be multidisciplinary. Otherwise, there can be individual handoff sessions for physicians, nurses, anesthesia providers, and management.

How Handoffs are best accomplished face to face. Hierarchy should be minimized; everyone should be comfortable to ask questions. The use of closed-loop communication assures everyone that the information is clearly understood. There must be tools, such as a notebook or a computer, to record critical information and pending tasks. Patient charts, either paper or electronic, should be available. Unacknowledged communications, such as e-mail or voice mail, are not acceptable for handoffs.

What A standardized list of elements should be presented during the transitions. At a minimum, there should be the following components: 1) the name, age, and location of the patient; 2) the chief complaint and diagnosis; 3) the current clinical situation; 4) critical laboratory findings and precautions; 5) other important medical conditions, current medications, and allergies; 6) actions that are needed for the patient and their urgency; 7) the individuals responsible for these actions; 8) the plan; and 9) the contingencies for unexpected problems.

This information must be complete, but at the same time concise and relevant. Computer support has been shown to facilitate handoffs, not only improving the efficiency but also increasing the accuracy (39). Documentation should note that the handoff has occurred and identify the current responsible individuals for the patient's care. A useful approach to organizing handoffs is SBAR strategy.

Communication With Patients

An estimated 39–43% of Americans have low levels of literacy skills, and an estimated 55% cannot use numbers to accomplish everyday tasks (40). In addition, an appreciable number of foreign-born Americans have limited English proficiency. These populations are especially susceptible to problems with health literacy. However, problems with health literacy can affect people from all socioeconomic levels, age groups, and cultures. An estimated 90 million adults in the United States are limited in their ability to read, process, and understand basic medical information (40). The economic burden of low health literacy in these patients is estimated to be $106 billion to $238 billion (41).

RECOGNIZING PATIENTS WITH LOW HEALTH LITERACY

Although there are tools to recognize patients with limited health literacy, few practitioners have the time to use them routinely. However, there are several clues that suggest limited health literacy. One example is the patient who takes an inordinate amount of time to fill out the basic registration forms. Probably it is safest to use a "universal precaution" approach and assume that all patients may not understand medical information. Providers should use strategies to clearly transmit complex medical information and confirm the patient's comprehension:

1. *Create an atmosphere conducive to communication.* Encourage patients to bring a written list of questions or problems to the appointment. Provide blank paper in the waiting area for this purpose. Many patients will be too nervous to remember all their questions, especially if the discussion occurs in the examination room when they are wearing only a flimsy paper gown. Discussion of complex issues or bad news ideally occurs in the consulting room, with the patient fully clothed and a close friend or family member at the patient's side. If you sit down during discussions, wherever they occur, it sends a clear message to the patient that you are receptive to her message and are not rushing out the door.

2. *Be an active listener.* Let the patient tell her story without interruption. Avoid the temptation to fixate on a diagnosis or interrupt with questions before the patient completes her story. Do not interrupt the patient visit with phone calls or other distractions unless there is an emergency.

3. *Clearly transmit your message with the assumption that the patient may have problems with health literacy.* Use plain language instead of technical language, acronyms, or medical jargon. For example, use *high blood pressure* instead of *hypertension* and *eye damage from diabetes* instead of *diabetic retinopathy*. Visual aids, such as drawings, illustrations, or videos, help reinforce the verbal message. You may wish to develop your own printed materials for common conditions. In addition, commercially available printed materials also can help explain various diagnoses and treatments. If they are used, it is best to review the material with the patient to highlight the critical messages. If videos are used, it is best to speak with the patient after she has viewed the material to answer any questions. Giving the patient printed material to take home and review at her leisure also reinforces the message (40).

4. *Confirm the patient's comprehension.* Never ask the patient if she understands. Many patients may feel too embarrassed to admit their lack of comprehension and respond "yes." However, you have no way to know if the patient misunderstood the information. Thus, probe for understanding by asking open-ended questions that begin with "what" or "how." Also, there is a technique known as "teach back" that you can use to confirm comprehension. Ask the patient how she would explain her diagnosis, treatment, or both to a friend or to tell you in her own words what she should do, and why (32).

INFORMED CONSENT

Informed consent is a process, not just a signed form. The provider must communicate and confirm that the patient understands the diagnosis, the proposed procedure, common complications, and any alternatives. Communication is a two-way street. "Ask Me 3" is an elegant, simple, and validated tool that has been developed by experts in health literacy at the Partnership for Clear Health Communication (Box 5). In addition, the

---

Box 5

Ask Me 3

This tool empowers patients to actively participate in this process. Through buttons, posters, and printed brochures this program encourages patients to ask and health care providers to answer three simple questions at each medical encounter:

1. What is my problem? (The diagnosis)
2. What do I need to do? (The treatment)
3. Why is it important for me to do this? (Compliance)

Ask Me 3 material has been translated into several languages in conjunction with the World Health Organization's Alliance for Patient Safety. Health literacy information and Ask Me 3 material are available as a free download from the Partnership for Clear Health Communication at the National Patient Safety Foundation web site (www.npsf.org/askme3/PCHC).

consent form should be written in simple language, not medical jargon. This is particularly important regarding the name of the procedure to which the patient is consenting. Misunderstanding during the informed consent process may lead to patient disappointment or anger in the event of an unexpected outcome, thus increasing the likelihood of litigation (40).

DISCLOSURE OF ADVERSE EVENTS OR ERRORS

Disclosure of adverse events is an ethical imperative. In the event of an adverse outcome, patients deserve an honest and compassionate explanation of the cause or causes. In addition, patients want to know what measures will be taken to prevent similar problems from affecting others (42). A perceived barrier to disclosure is the fear of increased litigation. However, experience at a number of institutions has shown the opposite to be true. At one hospital, after implementation of a hospital-wide policy for full disclosure, there was an overall reduction in malpractice payouts (although the frequency of claims increased) (42).

The disclosure of error should take into account many of the same considerations important for good communication. In addition, disclosure is complicated by the patient's emotions and the health care provider's fear of litigation. The following are some specific considerations of the process:

Where   The discussion should occur in a quiet, confidential setting.

When   Disclosure should begin as soon as possible after the medical error leading to harm is recognized. Often, all the facts surrounding the incident are not known at that time. In those circumstances, the patient and her family should be told what is known, what additional investigation will take place, and when they can anticipate further communication.

Who   Depending on the circumstances, attendees at the initial discussion may include the patient and her family or friends. Hospitals usually have a specific policy about which professionals (ie, risk managers, a lawyer, or a chief nursing officer) should attend the disclosure conference. Ideally, the attending obstetrician–gynecologist should be present and provide the initial disclosure.

What   It is important not to speculate but only to communicate the facts as best as they are understood at the time. Usually all the reasons for the adverse outcome are not known until a root cause analysis is completed. Arrangements for follow-up contact should be confirmed.

How   Proper demeanor is critical during these difficult discussions. The medical personnel must be empathetic and sincere. An apology is an expression of remorse and responsibility. In most cases an apology will facilitate the emotional healing of the patient and the provider. An explicit apology, however, has very specific legal implications based on prevailing state law. Even though an apology is desirable, it may not be recommended, depending on the locale. Consult your legal department regarding laws in your jurisdiction.

Transparency and honesty are central to professionalism and the patient–physician relationship. Disclosure of adverse events, although often difficult, is essential.

References

1. Godlee F, Horton R, Smith R. Global information flow [editorial]. BMJ 2000;321:776–7.

2. Smith RP. The internet for physicians. 3rd ed. New York (NY): Springer–Verlag; 2001.

3. Jadad AR, Gagliardi A. Rating health information on the Internet: navigating to knowledge or to Babel? JAMA 1998;279:611–4.

4. Rigby M, Roberts R, Williams J, Clark J, Savill A, Lervy B, et al. Integrated record keeping as an essential aspect of a primary care led health service. BMJ 1998;317:579–82.

5. Dini EF, Linkins RW, Chaney M. Effectiveness of computer-generated telephone messages in increasing clinic visits. Arch Pediatr Adolesc Med 1995;149:902–5.

6. Shafer RW. Rationale and uses of a public HIV drug-resistance database. J Infect Dis 2006;194 Suppl 1:S51–8.

7. Harrington DJ, Redman CW, Moulden M, Greenwood CE. The long-term outcome in surviving infants with Apgar zero at 10 minutes: a systematic review of the literature and hospital-based cohort. Am J Obstet Gynecol 2007;196:463.e1,463.e5.

8. Jones R, Latinovic R, Charlton J, Gulliford MC. Alarm symptoms in early diagnosis of cancer in primary care: cohort study using General Practice Research Database. BMJ 2007;334:1040.

9. Konety BR, Sadetsky N, Carroll PR, CaPSURE Investigators. Recovery of urinary continence following radical prostatectomy: the impact of prostate volume— analysis of data from the CaPSURE Database. J Urol 2007;177:1423–5; discussion 1425–6.

10. Payen D, Sablotzki A, Barie PS, Ramsay G, Lowry S, Williams M, et al. International integrated database for the evaluation of severe sepsis and drotrecogin alfa (activated) therapy: analysis of efficacy and safety data in a large surgical cohort. Surgery 2007;141:548–61.

11. Hahn PF, Lee MJ, Gazelle GS, Forman BH, Mueller PR. A simplified HyperCard data base for patient management in an interventional practice: experience with more than 4000 cases. AJR Am J Roentgenol 1994;162:1443–6.

12. Clark R, Geller B, Peluso N, McVety D, Worden JK. Development of a community mammography registry: experience in the breast screening program project. Radiology 1995;196:811–5.

13. Schraffordt Koops SE, Bisseling TM, Heintz AP, Vervest HA. The effectiveness of tension-free vaginal tape (TVT) and quality of life measured in women with previous urogynecologic surgery: analysis from The Netherlands TVT database. Am J Obstet Gynecol 2006;195:439–44.

14. Sullivan F, Wyatt JC. How informatics tools help deal with patients' problems. BMJ 2005;331:955–7.

15. Ventres W, Shah A. How do EHRs affect the physician-patient relationship? Am Fam Physician 2007;75:1385, 1390.

16. Institute of Medicine. The computer-based patient record: an essential technology for health care. Revised ed. Washington, DC: National Academy Press; 1997.

17. Ornstein S, Bearden A. Patient perspectives on computer-based medical records. J Fam Pract 1994;38:606–10.

18. Torrecillas DR, Soler-Gonzalez J, Rodriguez-Rosich A. Digital photography in the generalist's office. CMAJ 2006;175:1519–21.

19. Pescovitz D. To your online health. Sci Am 1999;281:60.

20. Hippisley-Cox J, Pringle M, Cater R, Wynn A, Hammersley V, Coupland C, et al. The electronic patient record in primary care—regression or progression? A cross sectional study [published erratum appears in BMJ 2003;327:483]. BMJ 2003;326:1439–43.

21. Falzette L, Carmack A, Robinson L, Murphy J, Dunn E. Medical team training: improving communication in healthcare. Pat Safe Qual Healthc 2007;4(5):18–20. Available at: http://www.psqh.com/sepoct07/medical-team.html. Retrieved November 14, 2008.

22. Glasziou P. Managing the evidence flood. Surg Clin North Am 2006;86:193–9, xi.

23. Van Eaton EG, Horvath KD, Lober WB, Rossini AJ, Pellegrini CA. A randomized, controlled trial evaluating the impact of a computerized rounding and sign-out system on continuity of care and resident work hours. J Am Coll Surg 2005;200:538–45.

24. Williams RG, Silverman R, Schwind C, Fortune JB, Sutyak J, Horvath KD, et al. Surgeon information transfer and communication: factors affecting quality and efficiency of inpatient care. Ann Surg 2007;245:159–69.

25. Lehmann CU, Kim GR. Computerized provider order entry and patient safety. Pediatr Clin North Am 2006;53:1169–84.

26. Krysztoforski J. Are patient smart cards the right way to go? Yes. Hosp Health Netw 1994;68:10.

27. Evers WM. Are patient smart cards the right way to go? No. Hosp Health Netw 1994;68:10.

28. Kripalani S, Jackson AT, Schnipper JL, Coleman EA. Promoting effective transitions of care at hospital discharge: a review of key issues for hospitalists. J Hosp Med 2007;2:314–23.

29. Smith PC, Araya-Guerra R, Bublitz C, Parnes B, Dickinson LM, Van Vorst R, et al. Missing clinical information during primary care visits. JAMA 2005;293:565–71.

30. The Commonwealth Fund. 2005 international health policy survey of sicker adults. New York (NY): The Commonwealth Fund; 2005. Available at: http://www.commonwealthfund.org/surveys/surveys_show.htm?doc_id = 313115. Retrieved November 6, 2008.

31. Selden CR, Zorn M, Ratzan S, Parker RM, compilers. Health literacy. Bethesda (MD): National Library of Medicine; 2000. Available at: http://www.nlm.nih.gov/archive// 20061214/pubs/cbm/hliteracy.pdf. Retrieved November 6, 2008.

32. National Patient Safety Foundation, The Partnership for Clear Health Communication. AskMe3. North Adams (MA): NPSF, PCHC; 2003. Available at: http://www.npsf.org/askme3. Retrieved November 6, 2008.

33. Baker DW, Wolf MS, Feinglass J, Thompson JA, Gazmararian JA, Huang J. Health literacy and mortality among elderly persons. Arch Intern Med 2007;167:1503–9.

34. Pratt SD, Sachs BP. Perspectives on safety: team training: classroom training vs. high-fidelity situation. Rockville (MD): AHRQ; 2006. Available at: http://www.webmm.ahrq.gov/perspective.aspx?perspectiveID = 21. Retrieved November 6, 2008.

35. Agency for Healthcare Research and Quality. TeamSTEPPS: national implementation. Rockville (MD): AHRQ; 2006. Available at: http://teamstepps.ahrq.gov. Retrieved November 6, 2008.

36. The Joint Commission. Speak up: the universal protocol. Oakbrook Terrace (IL): The Joint Commission; 2008. Available at: http://www.jointcommission.org/NR/rdonlyres/E3C600EB-043B-4E86-B04E-CA4A89AD5433/0/universal_protocol.pdf. Retrieved December 29, 2008.

37. World Health Organization. Safe surgery saves lives. Geneva: WHO; 2008. Available at: http://www.who.int/patientsafety/safesurgery/tools_resources/SSSL_Checklist_finalJun08.pdf. Retrieved November 6, 2008.

38. Communication strategies for patient handoffs. ACOG Committee Opinion No. 367. American College of Obstetricians and Gynecologists. Obstet Gynecol 2007; 109:1503–5.

39. Solet DJ, Norvell JM, Rutan GH, Frankel RM. Lost in translation: challenges and opportunities in physician-to-physician communication during patient handoffs. Acad Med 2005;80:1094–9.

40. The Joint Commission. What did the doctor say? Improving health literacy to protect patient safety. Oakbrook Terrace (IL): The Joint Commission; 2007. Available at: http://www.jointcommission.org/NR/rdonlyres/D5248B2E-E7E6-4121-8874-99C7B4888301/0/improving_health_literacy.pdf. Retrieved November 6, 2008.

41. Friedland R. New estimates of the high costs of inadequate health literacy. In: Proceedings of Pfizer Conference "Promoting Health Literacy: A Call to Action"; 1998 Oct 7–8; Washington, DC. Washington (DC): Pfizer, Inc; 1998. p. 6–10.

42. Weiss PM, Miranda F. Transparency, apology and disclosure of adverse outcomes. Obstet Gynecol Clin North Am 2008;35:53–62, viii.

Legal and Ethical Issues*

Allan J. Jacobs

A variety of legal and regulatory issues affect office practice. Many of these issues have ethical dimensions as well. Readers are referred to the publications of the American College of Obstetricians and Gynecologists Committee on Ethics (available at www.acog.org/from_home/publications/ethics) and the *Code of Professional Ethics* (available at www.acog.org/from_home/acogcode.pdf) to read about these topics.

Medical Liability

A physician who causes harm to a patient may be liable for medical malpractice. This is a type of tort. If a patient sues a physician for medical liability, the patient must allege the following four elements:

1. The physician owed the patient a duty of care.
2. The physician breached that duty.
3. The breach of duty caused the patient's injury.
4. The patient suffered damages as a result of that injury.

It is the patient's burden to prove the last three of these elements. The duty of care is established by law. The court then will determine whether the patient has met this burden. A physician who is found liable by the court must pay damages to the patient.

A physician's duty of care often is defined as the duty to "exercise such reasonable care, skill, and diligence as other similarly situated health care providers in the same general line of practice ordinarily have and exercise in a like case" (1). The patient usually will need to present an expert witness to establish whether the medical standard of care has not been met (2). The physi-

cian also will present an expert witness to prove that the physician met the standard. The patient must prove each element of the case by a preponderance of evidence, which means that it is more likely (ie, 51%) than not that the physician breached that duty and caused her injury and that she suffered damages. Damages may be economic, such as lost income, costs of care, or monetary value of housework. They also may be noneconomic, compensating a patient for the pain and suffering she incurred. Some states have caps on damage awards for pain and suffering (3).

Physicians who are sued learn of the lawsuits from a summons and should immediately call their medical professional liability insurance carriers (see Box 6). If a physician is employed by a hospital, the contact usually is the hospital's risk manager. An uninsured physician should immediately retain a lawyer. Failure to answer the summons within a specified time may result in an automatic judgment for the plaintiff. Preparation of the answer requires considerable legal work, which is best done promptly. Also, physicians should not discuss the matter with anyone but their lawyers. Even fellow defendants may have opposing interests as the case develops. For example, a situation may point to one defendant or the other—but not both—being liable.

It is ethical for physicians to testify as expert witnesses, either for defendants or plaintiffs, in lawsuits in which they are not personally involved. They must testify "solely in accordance with their judgment on the merits of the case," and must not "misrepresent the standard of care relevant to the case" (4, 5). Furthermore, excessive fees or fees that are dependent on the outcome of the case are unethical.

Physicians are liable for activities that they know are likely to hurt patients or that disregard patient safety; eg, refusing to see a patient who needs prompt care. Such acts go beyond negligence and may not be covered by malpractice insurance, especially if punitive damages (damages in excess of harm to patients) are involved (6). Furthermore, a physician who harms others intentionally or recklessly may be reported for unprofessional behavior or criminal charges (7). Finally, performing without consent any procedure that entails contact with

---

*This chapter does not define a standard of care, nor should be interpreted as legal advice. Physicians should consult their personal attorneys about legal requirements in their jurisdictions and for legal advice on particular matters. The American College of Obstetricians and Gynecologists makes no representations or warranties, expressed or implied, regarding the accuracy of the information contained in this chapter and disclaims any liability or responsibility for any consequences resulting from, or otherwise related to, any use of, or reliance on, this chapter.

the patient could constitute the intentional tort of battery (8). Strategies for reducing medical professional liability are listed in Box 7.

Licensures

The states grant physicians permission to practice medicine by issuing a medical license. Requirements for obtaining and maintaining a medical license generally include the following:

- Completion of medical school and some approved postgraduate training

---

Box 6

Medical Professional Liability Insurance

Medical professional liability insurance can be written as occurrence policy or claims-made policies. An occurrence policy insures a physician against claims arising from events that happen during the period that the policy is in effect (usually 1 year) regardless of when the claim is filed, even if the physician is no longer covered by that policy. A claims-made policy insures against claims filed against a doctor during the period of coverage arising from events that happen during the period of coverage. Such a policy is cheaper than an occurrence policy, but has some major disadvantages. Physicians who wish to be covered for past practice need to continue coverage, even if they move, switch insurance companies, or retire. Physicians who terminate claims-made insurance must either expect to pay legal fees and possible judgments using their personal assets, or must buy "tail" coverage, which is a policy that covers these subsequent lawsuits. A tail is paid in a lump sum; this may cost up to several hundred thousand dollars in areas with high rates of lawsuits. Physicians who cannot afford to purchase tail coverage may have difficulty in relocating or retiring.

Medical professional liability insurance typically does not cover every incident for which a physician may be sued. It usually does not cover sexual misconduct, punitive damages, and criminal or grossly negligent acts. Furthermore, it covers only medical acts. If a patient slips on a wet floor in the doctor's office and falls, the doctor will be covered only if he has a general casualty policy.

Physicians should be aware of two conditions generally imposed in insurance policies. First, the policyholder is required to cooperate in her defense. This includes prompt reporting of claims, as well as reasonable availability for depositions and trials. Second, the policyholder often cedes to the insurance company the right to make decisions ordinarily made by defendants, such as whether to settle the case or go to trial. The company may settle a lawsuit in which the doctor's conduct was appropriate merely to avoid the cost and uncertainty of litigation.

- Engaging in continuing medical education
- Refraining from unprofessional misconduct
- Refraining from committing serious crimes

To practice within a health care facility, such as a hospital, physicians must obtain privileges from the facility and renew them biennially. Terms under which privileges are given are regulated by accrediting agencies, such as the Joint Commission (formerly the Joint Commission on Accreditation of Healthcare Organizations). These terms generally are similar to those that govern licensure. Privileges may be denied, limited, or revoked for a number of reasons, including, but not limited to, an excessive number of bad results or malpractice losses or failure to admit a sufficient number of patients. The medical license is undifferentiated, whereas hospital privileges specify those procedures physicians may perform and the type of patients they may treat. Most insurance payers require physicians to obtain privileges and credentials.

The basis for state disciplinary action against the license is based on the laws and regulations of the state. Punitive actions against physicians' medical licenses may include censure, probation, and license suspension

---

Box 7

Strategies for Reducing Medical Professional Liability

- Be courteous to patients and answer their questions in language they understand.
- Use printed materials, such as patient education pamphlets from the American College of Obstetricians and Gynecologists.
- When there is an adverse outcome, explain the reasons and the likely consequences in a sympathetic way.
- Do not hide information from patients.
- Write or dictate all records (including operative notes and discharge summaries) at the same time as service is provided.
- Avoid abbreviations. Never use abbreviations that are not on your hospital's approved list of abbreviations.
- Use leading zeroes (eg, 0.4 mg), but do not use trailing zeroes (eg, 1.0 g).
- Do not destroy or obliterate records. If they need to be amended, cross out the wrong entry with one line, write "error," and add your initial and the date.
- Do not criticize patients or other professionals on a medical record.
- Keep a copy of all prescriptions written.
- Write legibly, especially prescriptions.

---

or license revocation. Probation may include restrictions on the scope of the physician's practice or requirements for supervision. Felony convictions, substance abuse, and boundary violations (eg, sexual misconduct) also may be grounds for disciplinary action, as may a repeated pattern of negligence. Sexual contact or a romantic relationship between a physician and a current patient always is unethical, and it may be unethical between a physician and a former patient. It is wise for a physician to have a chaperone present when performing a physical examination. The request by either a patient or a physician to have a chaperone present during a physical examination should be accommodated regardless of the physician's sex (9).

The basis for hospital discipline is the hospital bylaws. The basis for discipline by a payer is the contract between the payer and the physician, combined with the rules of the payer (these rules would be incorporated into the payer–physician contract). Hospitals and payers also can discipline physicians on grounds similar to those for which the state can discipline them.

Physicians who are subject to disciplinary action are entitled to due process. Due process includes a chance to contest the proposed discipline (not always in a formal hearing). Physicians against whom disciplinary action is proposed are advised to consult an attorney experienced in these matters as well as their professional liability insurance company. Legal costs might not be covered by medical professional liability insurance.

Refusal to Treat and Termination of Care

Physicians have the right to refuse patients whose conditions are beyond their competence to treat. Also, they may limit the size of their practices to a number of patients they can safely treat. However, refusal to treat a patient based on race, sex, ethnicity, disability, or religion is illegal throughout the United States. Discrimination on the basis of sexual orientation is illegal in some states and cities. Physicians should treat all of their patients equitably, regardless of ability to pay or any other factors.

Physicians are not legally or ethically compelled to perform procedures that they consider immoral. They must, however, provide potential patients with accurate and prior notice of their personal moral commitments. In providing prior notice, physicians should not use their professional authority to argue or advocate their positions. Furthermore, these physicians have the duty to refer patients to other providers in a timely manner if they feel they cannot provide the standard reproductive services their patients request. In an emergency in which referral is not possible or might negatively affect a patient's physical or mental health, providers have an

obligation to provide medically indicated and requested care regardless of personal moral objections (10).

Physicians may terminate their professional relationships with patients. A patient is someone who a physician is treating (or has agreed to treat) or who reasonably expects treatment from a physician (eg, someone assigned to a physician's panel under an insurance plan). Legitimate reasons for terminating professional relationships include fundamental disagreements over treatment, patient noncompliance with treatment plans, disruptive patient behavior, failure to make an effort to pay for services, or limitation of practice by the physician. Box 8 lists the responsibilities of physicians who are terminating their professional relationships with patients.

Decision Making and Incompetent Patients

Patients generally have the right to make decisions related to their health care and need information about the possible courses of treatment to do so. However, not all patients are capable of making decisions for themselves. The legal ability to make decisions is termed *competence*, and the objective ability to make decisions is termed *decisional capacity*. A widely cited set of criteria to consider in determining decisional capacity includes the following:

- Demonstration of a choice
- Reasonable outcome of the choice
- Rational basis of the choice
- Ability to understand the choice
- Actual understanding of the choice (11)

Box 8

Responsibilities of Physicians Terminating Their Professional Relationships With Patients

Physicians discharging patients should do the following:

- Notify the patient in writing in advance, including the reasons for terminating the relationship.
- Provide information to help the patient find another physician who can provide the care.
- Provide care for a specified period (communicated in writing via certified mail) sufficient to allow the patient to transfer her care.
- Give special consideration to pregnant patients; pregnant patients in the third trimester should continue in the physician's care until they give birth.
- Check the contracts with health plans to determine if there are restrictions on the physician's ability to terminate the patient–physician relationship.

Causes of incapacity in adults include coma, dementia, mental retardation, and psychosis. Incapacity also can be temporary, such as is induced by medications or acute illness (12, 13). However, poor education, eccentric religious beliefs (14), or cultural patterns do not affect the competence of otherwise capable adults. The law determines the default surrogate decision maker for incompetent patients. This generally is a family member specified either by statute or by a court (15).

Surrogate decision makers may be bound by one of three standards. The first two standards apply primarily to adults, including adults who are permanently incompetent, and each state determines which standard to adopt. The third standard applies to children (16):

1. Substituted judgment that requires the surrogate to do what the incompetent patient would have done were she competent (17).

2. Pure autonomy that obliges the surrogate to implement the incompetent patient's explicit interests (18).

3. The best interests standard by which parents usually make decisions for their children and are presumed to be acting in their children's best interest. Physicians who believe that a parent's decision is not in the child's best interest, however, may petition state courts to supersede the parent's authority.

Medical Directives

Competent individuals have recourse to two mechanisms to direct medical decisions if they later become incapacitated (19). One form of advance directive is the durable power of attorney for health care, or health care proxy. This mechanism designates who will make decisions if the patient cannot, and it can appoint secondary proxies in case the first proxy is unavailable. Even healthy people should consider executing a durable power of attorney, especially people who do not want the default surrogate to serve in this role. The second mechanism is the living will. This document stipulates circumstances under which a person would want to refuse or terminate certain life-prolonging treatments. Living wills often do not contemplate all possible situations, and patients may change their minds after executing a living will. The statutory requirements and breadth of both of these documents vary considerably among states. A physician who contemplates discontinuation of treatment against the wishes of a patient's family, regardless of the presence of a living will, should seek legal and ethical consultation.

People may legally discontinue their own life-sustaining treatment. A surrogate may discontinue the treatment of another only if permitted by state law, which usually requires strong evidence that termination of care reflects the patient's desire (20). Each state may legislate whether to prohibit (21) or permit (22) physician-assisted suicide. Euthanasia is not permitted in any American jurisdiction. Palliative measures that shorten life, such as the administration of large doses of narcotics for pain relief in terminally ill patients, ordinarily are not considered euthanasia.

Research

Patients asked to participate in research are protected by a panoply of regulations. Not all research is subject to the same regulations. For example, federally conducted or funded research projects must be approved by an institutional review board and must require that patients give informed consent in order to participate. The institutional review board determines which risks, complications, and alternatives are presented to participating patients. Innovative treatment—treatment whose benefit has not been proved, but that is not being given as part of a research protocol—has more stringent requirements (23). Informed consent for investigative treatment should include disclosure of the innovative nature of the treatment and gaps in knowledge regarding possible adverse effects. Physicians should be cautious in employing innovative treatment, whose risks may outweigh the benefits compared with standard techniques. Innovations that deviate greatly from standard treatment are best applied in a formal research setting. Many other non–federal-government institutions or journals also may require compliance with federal regulations. Researchers should be familiar with the policies before conducting research and submitting their reports for publication.

Confidentiality

Confidentiality of patient health information is protected by the U.S. Health Insurance Portability and Accountability Act of 1996. The rules under this document also establish the right of patients to inspect and copy their protected health information, to receive an account of nonroutine disclosures of their information, and to request amendment or correction of their protected health information.

Confidentiality is vital in reproductive health care, where intimate and private issues frequently arise. Fear of disclosure may distress patients or jeopardize their care (24). However, disclosure without consent may be permitted or even required by law in special circumstances, such as those listed in Box 9. Disclosure generally is to the government, but if a patient poses a danger to a third person, there may be a duty of disclosure to that person (25).

Box 9

Some Circumstances in Which Disclosure is Permitted Without Written Health Insurance Portability and Accountability Act Patient Authorization

- Treatment; eg, transfer of information to a hospital to schedule a procedure
- Payment; eg, providing insurance company with diagnosis and records
- Legally sanctioned or required monitoring of care activities by institutions; eg, quality reviews or research audits
- Research, if patient is unidentifiable in reports or publications
- Communicable diseases where disclosure is required by law; eg, syphilis or tuberculosis
- Other patient activities where disclosure is required by law; eg, suspected child abuse or family violence
- Legal action; eg, disclosure of relevant patient information to a physician's lawyer if the physician is involved in a legal case
- Subpoena or other requirement of a court, as during testimony
- Verbal agreement of the patient for certain notification, payment, or care purposes; eg, informing a friend or relative about a patient's health care

---

Advertising

Physicians may legally and ethically market their practices. Such marketing should not 1) use false, misleading or deceptive language; 2) convey discriminatory attitudes toward race, ethnicity, sex, or sexual orientation; or 3) denigrate other medical practices (26).

References

1. Code of Ala. 6-5-548 (2007).
2. Dobbs DB. The law of torts. St. Paul (MN): West; 2000.
3. Tex. Civ. Prac. & Rem. Code. 74.301 (2007).
4. Patents, medicine, and the interests of patients. ACOG Committee Opinion No. 364. American College of Obstetricians and Gynecologists. Obstet Gynecol 2007;109: 1249-54.
5. American College of Obstetricians and Gynecologists. ACOG code of professional ethics of the American College of Obstetricians and Gynecologists. Washington, DC: ACOG; 2008. Available at http://www.acog.org/from_home/acogcode.pdf. Retrieved October 1, 2008.
6. Northwestern Nat'l Casualty Co. v. McNulty. 307 F.2d 432, 1962 U.S. App. LEXIS 4261 (5th Cir. Fla. 1962).
7. McCarthy KM. Doing time for clinical crime: the prosecution of incompetent physicians as an additional mechanism to assure quality health care. Seton Hall Law Rev 1997;28:569-619.
8. Perna v. Pirozzi. 92 N.J. 446, 457 A.2d 431, 1983 N.J. LEXIS 2354, 39 A.L.R.4th 1018 (1983).
9. Sexual misconduct. ACOG Committee Opinion No. 373. American College of Obstetricians and Gynecologists. Obstet Gynecol 2007;110:441-4.
10. The limits of conscientious refusal in reproductive medicine. ACOG Committee Opinion No. 385. American College of Obstetricians and Gynecologists. Obstet Gynecol 2007;110:1203-8.
11. Roth LH, Meisel A, Lidz CW. Tests of competency to consent to treatment. Am J Psychiatry 1977;134:279-84.
12. Ethical decision making in obstetrics and gynecology. ACOG Committee Opinion No. 390. American College of Obstetricians and Gynecologists. Obstet Gynecol 2007;110: 1479-87.
13. Sterilization of women, including those with mental disabilities. ACOG Committee Opinion No. 371. American College of Obstetritians and Gynecologists. Obstet Gynecol 2007;110:217-20.
14. Fosmire v. Nicoleau. 75 N.Y.2d 218, 551 N.Y.S. 2d 876, 551 N.E.2d 77, 1990 N.Y. Lexis 91 (1990).
15. Furrow BR, Greaney TL, Johnson SH, Just TS, Schwartz RL. Health law. 6th ed. St. Paul (MN): West; 2008.
16. Beauchamp TL, Childress JF. Principles of biomedical ethics. 6th ed. New York (NY): Oxford University Press; 2009.
17. Superintendent of Belchertown State School v. Saikewicz. 373 Mass. 728, 370 N.E.2d 417, 1977 Mass. LEXIS 1129 (1977).
18. Woods v. Commonwealth. 142 S.W.3d 24, 2004 Ky. LEXIS 187 (Ky. 2004).
19. Cantor NL. Twenty-five years after Quinlan: a review of the jurisprudence of death and dying. J Law Med Ethics 2001;29:182-96.
20. Cruzan v. Director, Missouri Dep't of Health. 497 U.S. 261, 110 S. Ct. 2841, 111 L. Ed. 2d 224, 1990 U.S. Lexis 3301, 58 U.S.L.W. 4916 (1990).
21. Washington v. Glucksberg. 521 U.S. 702, 117 S. Ct. 2258, 138 L.Ed. 2d 772, 1997 U.S. LEXIS 4039, 65 U.S.L.W. 4669, 97 C.D.O.S. 5008, 97 Daily Journal D.A.R. 8150, 11 Fla. L. Weekly Fed. S 190 (1997).
22. Gonzales v. Oregon. 546 U.S. 243, 126 S. Ct. 904, 163 L. Ed. 2d 748, 2006 U.S. LEXIS 767, 74 U.S.L.W. 4068, 19 Fla. L. Weekly Fed. S 49 (2006).
23. Innovative practice: ethical guidelines. ACOG Committee Opinion No. 352. American College of Obstetricians and Gynecologists. Obstet Gynecol 2006;108:1589-95.
24. Stamford Hosp. v. Vega. 236 Conn. 646, 674 A.2d 821, 1996 Conn. LEXIS 88 (1996).
25. Tarasoff v. Regents of University of Cal. 17 Cal. 3d 425, 131 Cal. Rptr. 14, 551 P.2d 334, 1976 Cal. LEXIS 297, 83 A.L.R.3d 1166 (1976).
26. Ethical ways for physicians to market a practice. ACOG Committee Opinion No. 341. American College of Obstetricians and Gynecologists. Obstet Gynecol 2006;108: 239-42.

Principles of Evidence-Based Medicine

Jeffrey F. Peipert and Katherine J. Hladky

The purpose of this overview is to review and describe the research methodologies used in the medical literature. These methodologies serve as the scientific basis of evidence-based medicine. Given the limitations of space, this review is far from comprehensive. For a more complete overview, the reader is encouraged to obtain a series of articles published in *The Lancet* (1–11). This epidemiology series provides a readable but more detailed overview, a discussion of various research designs, and articles specifically focusing on randomized trials (7–11).

Epidemiologic Studies

Clinical research can be broadly subdivided into two categories—experimental and observational—based on whether or not the investigator assigns the exposures (Fig. 1). Experimental studies can be divided into randomized and nonrandomized trials. Observational studies can be divided into analytic studies (studies with a comparison group) and descriptive studies. Analytic observational studies include cohort studies, case–control studies, and cross-sectional studies. In cohort studies, groups are compared based on an exposure of interest and subjects tracked forward in time for the outcome of interest. In case–control studies, groups are chosen based on the outcome of interest and are traced back to the exposure. Cross-sectional studies are analogous to a snapshot in time; the researcher observes the exposure and the outcome at one time point. Descriptive studies, by definition, have no comparison group. They include case reports and case-series reports. In descriptive studies, investigators cannot evaluate associations or make causal implications. These reports often are interesting clinical vignettes but have limited scientific merit.

Not all research methods are created equal (Fig. 2). The randomized clinical trial is the least likely to be subject to serious biases. Cohort, case–control, and cross-sectional studies are common observational analytic studies. In fact, observational studies dominate the

women's health literature (12). Observational studies are more susceptible than are experimental designs to many types of bias that can distort the researcher's results and conclusions.

The choice of research methodology is very important. The reader must first consider the question of whether the study design is appropriate for the specific research question. Descriptive studies are appropriate to describe a highly unusual case or collection of cases. These studies may provide valuable information about the frequency, natural history, or possible determinants of a condition and thus may generate hypotheses. However, descriptive studies cannot test hypotheses on causality or association. Analytic observational studies are particularly appropriate in assessing an association or relationship between an exposure and an outcome

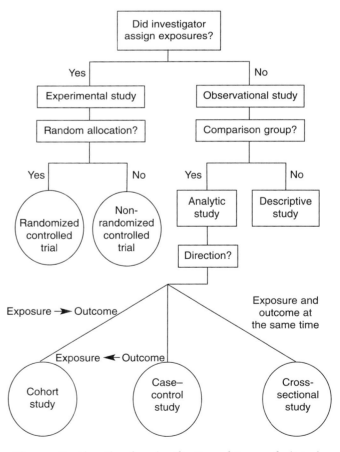

Figure 1. Algorithm for classification of types of clinical research. (Reprinted from The Lancet, Vol 359, Grimes DA, Schulz KF. An overview of clinical research: the lay of the land, page 58, Copyright 2002, with permission from Elsevier.)

Resources

Principles of Evidence-Based Medicine

Centre for Health Evidence
http://www.cche.net
Cochrane Collaboration
http://www.cochrane.org

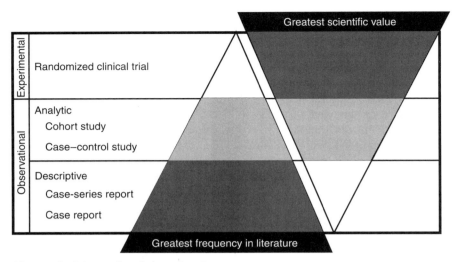

Figure 2. A hierarchy of clinical studies.

when a randomized trial is not feasible or ethical. Cohort studies proceed in a logical sequence in which the exposure precedes the outcome of interest. Cohort studies, however, may require very large sample sizes, especially for outcomes of interest that are rare. A case–control study is a more efficient design with which to address an association between a rare outcome and an exposure of interest, and this type of design may be more feasible when many years are required to develop the outcome of interest. Case–control studies may be counterintuitive to clinicians, because the population under study is selected on the basis of the outcome (ie, these studies "begin at the end") (13).

The randomized trial is the methodology of choice when a researcher or clinician is interested in the effectiveness of a particular therapy or wishes to provide the highest level of evidence for an association. When properly done, the randomized trial approximates the controlled experiment of basic science. The hallmark of this study design is the assignment of participants to exposures based purely on chance. A randomized trial reduces the likelihood of bias when it is properly implemented (with sufficient sample size). Thus, differences in outcomes can be attributed to the exposure or to the arm of a trial rather than to differences in baseline characteristics of the participants.

Randomized Clinical Trials

The randomized clinical trial is the standard by which all other methodologies are evaluated. The major advantages of a randomized clinical trial compared with an observational study are its ability to avoid selection bias and its strength of causal inference. The randomized clinical trial is the best design for controlling the influence of known and unknown confounding variables.

In a randomized clinical trial, participants are randomly assigned to an exposure of interest. Performing a randomized clinical trial involves five basic steps:

1. Assemble the study population.
2. Evaluate baseline characteristics.
3. Randomly assign participants to two or more study groups.
4. Apply an intervention or placebo, preferably in a blinded fashion.
5. Monitor the groups and measure outcome variables (blindly, if possible).

Embedded in these five steps are other methodologic issues that should be considered in a properly performed randomized clinical trial. Inclusion and exclusion criteria that are appropriate to the research question must be determined carefully. Subjects with a contraindication to the intervention must be excluded. When measuring baseline characteristics, the researcher should consider important predictors of the outcome and confounding variables. In addition, an adequate sample size should be determined, and plans for recruitment should be consistent with these calculations.

As an illustration of the five steps listed previously, consider the following example. In a report published in the *American Journal of Preventive Medicine*, the U.S. Preventive Services Task Force gave screening young women for *Chlamydia trachomatis* infection an "A" recommendation (see Table 1) (14). One of the most important studies supporting this recommendation was a large randomized trial of screening in a health maintenance organization in Seattle (15). This trial evaluated the effectiveness of screening and treating unmarried, asymptomatic women (aged 18–34 years) for *C trachomatis*. The study population selected for this trial was believed

Table 1. Standard Recommendation Language of the U.S. Preventive Services Task Force

Recommendation	Language*
A	The USPSTF strongly recommends that clinicians routinely provide [the service] to eligible patients. (The USPSTF found good evidence that [the service] improves important health outcomes and concludes that benefits substantially outweigh harms.)
B	The USPSTF recommends that clinicians routinely provide [the service] to eligible patients. (The USPSTF found at least fair evidence that [the service] improves important health outcomes and concludes that benefits outweigh harms.)
C	The USPSTF makes no recommendation for or against routine provision of [the service]. (The USPSTF found at least fair evidence that [the service] can improve health outcomes but concludes that the balance of the benefits and harms is too close to justify a general recommendation.)
D	The USPSTF recommends against routinely providing [the service]. (The USPSTF found at least fair evidence that [the service] is ineffective or that harms outweigh benefits.)
I	The USPSTF concludes the evidence is insufficient to recommend for or against routinely providing [the service]. (Evidence that [the service] is effective is lacking, of poor quality, or conflicting and the balance of benefits and harms cannot be determined.)

*All statements specify the population for which the recommendation is intended and are followed by a rationale statement providing information about the overall grade of evidence and the net benefit from implementing the service.
Abbreviation: USPSTF indicates U.S. Preventive Services Task Force.
Reprinted from American Journal of Preventive Medicine, Vol 20, Harris RP, Helfand M, Woolf SH, Lohr KN, Mulrow CD, Teutsch SM, et al. Current methods of the US Preventive Services Task Force: a review of the process, Page 33, Copyright 2001, with permission from Elsevier.

to be at high risk based on a risk score that incorporated age, race, parity, douching, and having two or more sexual partners in the previous 12 months. Participants were then randomly assigned to two groups: those receiving routine screening and those receiving no routine screening. Baseline characteristics were evaluated to ensure that the two groups were similar at randomization. The intervention was applied, and the outcomes were carefully measured. With routine screening for *C trachomatis*, the incidence of pelvic inflammatory disease (PID) was reduced from 28 cases per 1,000 women-years to 13 cases per 1,000 women-years (relative risk [RR] = 0.44; 95% confidence interval [CI] 0.2–0.9).

In randomized trials, it is extremely important to assign patients in a truly random fashion (eg, with a random-number table or computer-generated random assignment), rather than by hospital number or day of the week. It also is important to conceal the assignment (eg, with opaque envelopes) to avoid foreknowledge of the treatment assignment. In this way, investigators are unable to manipulate the randomization to get patients into their preferred treatment groups. It has been demonstrated that trials in which inadequate or unclear allocation concealment was used yielded up to 40% larger estimates of the effect than did trials in which adequate concealment was used (16).

When properly implemented, random allocation and concealment can help avoid bias or imbalances in important baseline factors that can influence the outcome of interest. Blinding the investigator and the subject to the group assignment (the double-blind approach)

is a methodological strength. By using this method, the subject follow-up and evaluation of the outcome will be performed in a strictly objective manner, uninfluenced by group assignment. When analyzing a randomized clinical trial, one should remember the principle of "once randomized, analyze." In other words, once a patient is randomized to an intervention arm, he or she should be analyzed in that group regardless of what happens after randomization. If a patient who was randomized to a group receiving a new antibiotic experiences adverse effects and stops therapy, that patient should be analyzed in the antibiotic group, not dropped from the analysis. This is referred to as intention-to-treat analysis. A randomized clinical trial in which many of the patients have been dropped from the analysis should be scrutinized carefully. Reports of clinical trials should attempt to minimize exclusions after randomization and to perform intention-to-treat analysis.

Randomized clinical trials have many advantages. In the hierarchy of clinical research, the randomized clinical trial provides the greatest strength of causal inference and is the optimal methodology to test the efficacy of treatment programs. If performed properly, randomization protects against confounding and selection bias—error due to systematic difference in characteristics of the study participants and individuals excluded from the study. Double-blinding will help ward off problems of ascertainment bias, diagnostic suspicion bias, and detection bias (Box 10). Randomized trials with adequate sample size also are the methodology of choice for the evaluation of small or moderate effects. In

---

Box 10

Glossary of Selected Epidemiologic Terms

Accuracy: The degree to which a measurement or an estimate based on measurements represents the true value of the attribute that is being measured.

Ascertainment bias: Systematic failure to represent equally all classes of cases or persons supposed to be represented in a sample. This bias may arise because of the nature of the sources from which persons come (eg, a specialized clinic), from a diagnostic process influenced by culture, custom, or idiosyncrasy, or, for example, in genetic studies, from the statistical chance of selecting from large or small families.

Bias: Deviation of results or inferences from the truth, or processes leading to such deviation; it is any trend in the collection, analysis, interpretation, publication, or review of data that can lead to conclusions that are systematically different from the truth. Three frequently occurring types of bias include selection bias, information bias, and confounding. Selection bias is error due to systematic differences in characteristics between those who are selected for study and those who are not. Information bias, also called observational bias, is a flaw in measuring exposure or outcome data that result in different quality (accuracy) of information between comparative groups. Recall bias is an example of information bias. Confounding describes a situation in which the effects of two processes are not separated; it is the distortion of the apparent effect of an exposure on risk brought about by the association with other factors that can influence the outcome.

Case–control study: An observational study of persons with a disease of interest and a suitable control group of persons without the disease; retrospective, starting after the onset of disease and looking back at postulated causal factors.

Cohort study (longitudinal or follow-up study): An observational study of large numbers over a long period with comparison of incidence rates in groups that differ in exposure levels; usually prospective in design, staring with exposed groups and following them over time.

Confidence interval: An indication of the variability of a point estimate, such as an odds ratio or relative risk. In general, the wider the confidence interval, the less precise the point estimate. The 95% confidence interval often is used. As an example, if the 95% confidence interval does not overlap 1, then one would reject the null hypothesis.

Confounding variable (confounder): A variable that can cause or prevent the outcome of interest, is not an intermediate variable, and is associated with the factor under investigation. Unless it is possible to adjust for confounding variables, their effects cannot be distinguished from those factor(s) being studied.

Cost–benefit analysis: An economic analysis in which the costs of medical care and the benefits of reduced loss of net earnings due to preventing premature death or disability are considered.

Cost-effectiveness analysis: An economic analysis that seeks to determine the costs and effectiveness of an activity or to compare similar alternative activities to determine the relative degree to which they will obtain the desired objectives or outcomes. The preferred action or alternative is one that requires the least cost to produce a given level of effectiveness, or provides the greatest effectiveness for a given level of cost. In the health care field, outcomes are measured in terms of health status.

Cross-sectional study: An observational study of prevalent cases that examines relationships between diseases and other variables of interest.

Decision analysis: A quantitative approach to evaluating the relative values of different management options. The range of choices can be plotted on a decision tree, and at each branch, or decision node, the probabilities of each outcome that can be predicted are displayed.

Detection bias: Bias due to systematic error(s) in methods of ascertainment, diagnosis, or verification of cases in an epidemiologic study. An example is verification of diagnosis by laboratory tests in hospital cases but failure to apply the same tests to cases outside the hospital.

Incidence: The number of instances of illness commencing, or persons falling ill, during a given period in a specified population. More generally, the number of new events (eg, new cases of a disease in a defined population) within a specified period.

Meta-analysis: The process of using statistical methods to combine the results of different studies; a pooling of results from a set of randomized controlled trials, none in itself necessarily powerful enough to demonstrate statistically significant differences.

Multivariable analysis: A set of techniques used when the variation in several variables has to be studied simultaneously. In statistics, any analytic method that allows the simultaneous study of two or more independent variables.

Negative predictive value: The percentage of people with a negative test result who do not have the disease of interest.

(continued)

Box 10 *(continued)*

Glossary of Selected Epidemiologic Terms

Null hypothesis (test hypothesis): The statistical hypothesis that one variable has no association with another variable or set of variables, or that two or more population distributions do not differ from one another. In simplest terms, the null hypothesis states that the results observed in a study, experiment, or test are no different from what might have occurred as a result of the operation of chance alone.

Observational study: An epidemiologic study that does not involve any intervention, experimental or otherwise. Case–control, cohort, and cross-sectional studies are observational studies in which the investigator observes without intervention other than to record, classify, count, and statistically analyze results.

Odds ratio (cross product ratio, relative odds): The ratio of two odds. The exposure odds ratio for a set of case–control data is the ratio of the odds in favor of exposure among the cases (a/b) to the odds in favor of exposure among noncases (c/d). A 2×2 table can be used to illustrate this calculation of odds ratios. Following is an example of a 2×2 table for odds ratio calculation.*

Disease Presence	Exposed	Unexposed
Disease	a	b
No disease	c	d

*The odds ratio is ad/bc.

Positive predictive value: The percentage of people with a positive test who actually have the disease of interest.

P value: The probability that a test statistic would be as extreme or more extreme than observed if the null hypothesis were true. Investigators may arbitrarily set their own significance levels, but in most biomedical and epidemiologic work, a study result whose probability value is less than 5% ($P<.05$) or 1% ($P<.01$) is considered sufficiently unlikely to have occurred by chance and would justify the designation "statistically significant." By convention, most investigators choose $P<.05$ as statistically significant.

Power (statistical power): The ability of a study to demonstrate an association if one exists. The power of the study is determined by several factors, including the frequency of the condition under study, the magnitude of the effect, the study design, and sample size.

Precision: A measure of random error or chance; precision does not imply accuracy.

Prevalence: The number of events (eg, instances of a given disease or other condition) in a given population at a designated time; sometimes used to mean prevalence rate. When used without qualification, the term usually refers to the situation at a specified time (point prevalence).

Randomized clinical trial (randomized controlled trial): A prospective, experimental study in which subjects in a population are randomly allocated into groups, usually called study and control groups, to receive or not receive an experimental preventive or therapeutic procedure, maneuver, or intervention, and followed to assess results; the gold standard of hypothesis testing.

Relative risk: The ratio of risk of disease or death among the exposed to that of the risk among the unexposed; this usage is synonymous with risk ratio. If the relative risk is greater than 1, there is a positive association between the exposure and the disease; if it is less than 1, there is a negative association.

Sensitivity, specificity: Sensitivity is the proportion of truly diseased persons in the screened population who are identified as diseased by the screening test. Specificity is the proportion of truly nondiseased persons who are so identified by the screening test. Sensitivity and specificity calculations can be illustrated as follows:

Test Result	True Status		Total
	Diseased	Not Diseased	
Positive	a	b	a + b
Negative	c	d	c + d
Total	a + c	b + d	a + b + c + d

where

a = Diseased individuals detected by the test (true positives)

b = Nondiseased individuals positive by the test (false positives)

c = Diseased individuals not detected by the test (false negatives)

d = Nondiseased individuals negative by the test (true negatives)

Sensitivity = $a/a + c$; specificity = $d/b + d$.

In screening and diagnostic tests, the probability that a person with a positive test result is a true positive (ie, does have the condition) is referred to as the predictive value of a positive test result. The predictive value of a negative test result is the probability that a person with a negative test result does not have the condition. The predictive value of a screening test is determined by the sensitivity and specificity of the test

(continued)

Glossary of Selected Epidemiologic Terms

and by the prevalence of the condition for which the test is being used.

Positive predictive value = $a/a + b$

Negative predictive value = $d/c + d$

Predictive values also can be calculated using *Bayes' Theorem*:

Positive predictive value = [sensitivity × prevalence] ÷ [(sensitivity × prevalence) + (1−specificity) × (1−prevalence)]

Negative predictive value = [specificity × (1−prevalence)] ÷ [(specificity × (1−prevalence)) + (1−sensitivity) × (prevalence)]

Stratification: The process of or result of separating a sample into several subsamples according to specified criteria, such as age groups and socioeconomic status. The effect of confounding variables may be controlled by stratifying the analysis of results. For example, lung cancer is known to be associated with smoking. To examine the possible association between urban atmospheric pollution and lung cancer, controlling for smoking, the population

may be divided into strata according to smoking status. The association between air pollution and cancer can then be appraised separately within each stratum. Stratification is used not only to control for confounding effects but also to detect modifying effects.

Systematic error: Systematic (one-sided) variation of measurements from the true values.

Type I error: The error of rejecting a true null hypothesis (ie, declaring that a difference exists when it does not).

Type II error: The error of failing to reject a false null hypothesis (ie, declaring that a difference does not exist when in fact it does).

Validity: The degree to which the inferences drawn from a study are warranted when account is taken of the study methods, the representativeness of the study sample, and the nature of the population from which it is drawn.

Reprinted from Last JM. A dictionary of epidemiology. 4th ed. New York: Oxford University Press; 2001. By permission of Oxford University Press, Inc.

---

observational studies, bias might easily explain and account for small to moderate differences (17).

The disadvantages of a randomized trial include expense, feasibility, and ethical issues surrounding the randomization of patients to intervention or placebo. For example, patients with syphilis cannot be randomized ethically to a treatment or a no-treatment group. Another disadvantage is the possible lack of external validity; a randomized trial, when properly done, should have internal validity (ie, it should measure what it sets out to measure), but it might lack external validity. External validity is the ability to generalize the results of a trial to the overall population or to a population of interest. Doing so may not be possible because of the strict inclusion and exclusion criteria of the trial and the fact that patients who consent to participate in a randomized clinical trial may differ from nonparticipants. Finally, randomized trials often are prohibitively expensive to conduct. The cost of large trials can be tens of millions of dollars.

Observational Studies

Observational studies can be divided into analytic studies and descriptive studies. Analytic observational studies include a comparison group and include cohort (longitudinal or follow-up) studies, case–control studies, and cross-sectional studies. Descriptive observational studies include case-series reports and case reports. Descriptive studies have no comparison group. Most epidemiologic studies in the reproductive health literature are observational studies. Of articles published in the journal *Obstetrics and Gynecology* in 1996, 51% were classified as observational (18).

Cohort Studies

A cohort study differs from a randomized clinical trial in that it does not have a randomization scheme that determines which patients receive the intervention or exposure. A cohort study is carried out by assembling a group of individuals who have been exposed to an intervention and comparing this group with a control group of patients who have not been exposed. These two groups are monitored over time and evaluated for a specific outcome of interest. An excellent example in the reproductive health literature is the Nurses' Health Study, one of the most comprehensive cohort studies ever performed (19, 20). Thousands of nurses have been monitored over time with comprehensive interviews and medical record reviews to evaluate various risk factors (eg, oral contraceptive use and estrogen therapy) and the development of disease (eg, cancer and cardiovascular disease).

Cohort studies are more subject to systematic (nonrandom) error than are randomized clinical trials and, thus, are weaker than randomized clinical trials in establishing causation. Because a clinician's decision to recommend a specific therapy and a patient's choice to accept therapy are clearly nonrandom decisions, the strength that the two groups are equal at baseline (provided by random allocation in a randomized trial) is lost. For example, women who take oral contraceptives may have very different baseline characteristics than women who use other forms of contraception or no contraception, and these characteristics may be related to the outcome of interest. In cohort studies, women receiving an intervention may be cared for or evaluated differently from women who do not receive the intervention. For example, a woman taking oral contraceptives is more likely to be seen by a physician regularly than a woman who has had a tubal sterilization. As a result, there is an increased chance of detecting an abnormality in the woman taking oral contraceptives. This type of bias is called *detection bias*.

In all epidemiologic studies, it is extremely important for investigators to identify and control for confounding variables (ie, factors associated with the intervention or exposure and the outcome of interest) (Box 11, Fig. 3). Cohort studies can attempt to control for confounding variables and differences in baseline characteristics through stratification and multivariable analysis. However, it is impossible to control for unknown or unmeasured confounding variables. Because of the major sources of bias just described, associations should be interpreted with caution because small or modest effect sizes may be due to residual confounding or bias.

By definition, randomized trials are prospective in design; they start with groups exposed to an intervention and monitor them over time for the outcome of interest. Cohort studies also proceed forward in time, from exposure to outcome, but they may be carried out either prospectively or retrospectively. If patients are

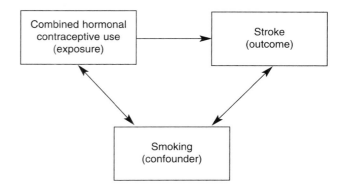

Figure 3. Example of confounding. Cigarette smoking may be associated with combined hormonal contraceptive use (exposure) and the outcome of interest (stroke). An analysis should control for the effect of smoking on the outcome of interest.

enrolled in a cohort study, grouped on the basis of their exposure, and then monitored longitudinally, the study is clearly prospective. However, it also is possible to look back in time (retrospectively) to assemble a group of patients who were and were not exposed at some time in the past and to monitor them to the present time. This type of cohort study is called a *retrospective cohort study*. In prospective and retrospective cohort studies, the study moves in the same direction: forward in time. However, data gathering may be prospective (forward in time) or retrospective (backward in time). Prospective cohort studies often require large sample sizes (for uncommon and rare outcomes) and long periods of follow-up. Thus, these studies can be very expensive and time-consuming. The case–control study can overcome some of these logistical obstacles.

CASE–CONTROL STUDIES

It has been said that a case–control study "begins at the end" (Fig. 4) (13). Cohort studies and randomized clinical trials begin with patients exposed to an intervention or risk factor and monitor these patients for the development of the outcome. Case–control studies select patients on the basis of whether they have the outcome of interest. The outcome could be a disease, if the investigation is evaluating risk factors for the disease, or it may be an ultimate outcome, such as alive or dead in a study of cancer prognosis. Cases, or patients with the outcome, are compared with controls, or individuals without the outcome, to determine whether there is an association between an exposure and the outcome of interest. Therefore, the design in a case–control study is, by definition, retrospective. As a result of the process of selecting individuals based on the outcome or disease, case–control studies typically study only one outcome, but they may evaluate several exposures.

The major advantage of case–control studies is that they are highly efficient. Often they require the fewest

---

Box 11

What Is a Confounding Variable?

Confounding comes from the Latin word *confundere*, to mix together; thus, some authorities refer to confounding as a "mixing of effects." A confounding variable is a variable that can cause or prevent the outcome of interest, is not the causal pathway as an intermediate variable, and also is associated with the factor under investigation. Consider the relationship between oral contraceptives and cervical neoplasia. A woman's sexual history (eg, onset of intercourse or new partners) may be a confounding variable in this relationship. Sexual history is related to the outcome (cervical neoplasia) and also may be related to the exposure (oral contraceptives).

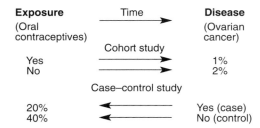

Figure 4. Examples of cohort and case-control studies of the relation between oral contraceptives and ovarian cancer.

patients to demonstrate an association and can be done in less time and with less money than other studies, especially when the disease in question is rare or takes years to develop (eg, cancer or cardiovascular disease). Consider the following example of a case-control study. Women with hereditary ovarian cancer and a pathogenic mutation in either *BRCA1* or *BRCA2* were compared with a group of controls without ovarian cancer. The investigators assessed the patients' past exposure to oral contraceptives and noted that oral contraceptive use was associated with a 50% reduction in the risk of ovarian cancer (21). If this study was done as a cohort study or randomized trial, it would take decades to evaluate the development of ovarian cancer in a cohort of women taking oral contraceptives.

Despite their advantages, case-control studies are easy to do poorly and are prone to many biases. One of the major challenges in case-control studies is choosing an appropriate control group, which is critical in these studies. For example, the Women's Health Study was a multicenter case-control study to evaluate the relationship between PID and the intrauterine device (22). Barrier contraception protects against sexually transmitted diseases and PID. Thus, the choice of control group (condom users) resulted in an inflated estimate of the relationship between the intrauterine device and PID. In general, the control group should be representative of persons who are at risk for the disease, and individuals in it should have the same opportunity for exposure as case patients. Controls should be similar to the cases in all important respects, except for not having the outcome of interest. Because the health outcome is known at the start in these studies, this knowledge may influence the measurement and interpretation of data (observer bias). In addition, subjects enrolled in these studies may have difficulty recalling medical history or exposures. If case subjects are more (or less) likely to remember an exposure than control subjects (ie, there is differential recall), then the study may be subject to recall bias. As observational studies, case-control and cohort studies are susceptible to many other types of bias. A careful reader of the literature will search for bias and uncontrolled confounding when interpreting the results of observational studies.

Studies also may be "nested," or set within an existing cohort study, such as nested case-control or nested cohort studies. In these nested studies, information previously obtained during the cohort study (eg, blood samples) is evaluated for a subset of subjects with and without the outcome of interest. Cases are subjects with the outcome or disease of interest. Control subjects are selected at random from the population without the outcome of interest (nested case-control). For example, in a nested case-control study of risk factors for uterine rupture, black women were found to have a lower risk of rupture compared with Caucasian women (23). In a nested cohort study, exposure groups are selected from within a large, established cohort.

CROSS-SECTIONAL STUDIES

Another type of observational analytic study is the cross-sectional study (also called a prevalence study or frequency survey). The cross-sectional study can be thought of as a snapshot of a group of individuals, some of whom have the disease (outcome) and exposure and some of whom do not. Individuals who have the disease of interest are considered prevalent cases. The difference between prevalence and incidence is important, because these terms often are misused in medical writing. *Incidence* refers to new cases that have developed over a specified time. *Prevalence* is the proportion of individuals in a population who have the disease at a specific time.

Using a cross-sectional study design, an investigator can evaluate associations between disease and exposure but cannot establish a temporal relationship between them. As an example, consider a hypothetical cross-sectional study of the relationship between serum prolactin levels and the use of oral contraceptives. A large group of young women are assembled, some of whom are taking oral contraceptives (exposure group) and some of whom are not. Prolactin levels are determined for all the women. The researchers may find an association between oral contraceptive use and elevated prolactin levels. However, they cannot conclude that oral contraceptive use causes elevations in prolactin levels. It is possible that women with elevated prolactin levels are more likely to have irregular bleeding and, thus, are more likely to be prescribed oral contraceptives. Because cross-sectional studies use prevalent cases rather than incident cases, a temporal relationship cannot be established, and the information provided can be misleading.

A cross-sectional study design often is used to evaluate diagnostic tests (24). To illustrate the concepts of diagnostic test performance, consider a cross-sectional study to evaluate the performance of a laboratory test for the diagnosis of PID (25). A group of women with signs and symptoms consistent with upper genital tract infection come to an emergency room to have blood drawn for the test and have a laparoscopy for the definitive diagnosis of PID. The result of the evaluation is summarized in a 2 × 2 table (Fig. 5).

Diagnostic test performance is characterized by a test's sensitivity and specificity. *Sensitivity* is the ability of a test to correctly identify patients with the disease of interest; of all the diseased patients, sensitivity is the proportion of patients who test positive (true positives/diseased = true positives/[true positives + false negatives]). *Specificity* is the ability of a test to correctly identify patients without the disease of interest (true negatives/nondiseased = true negatives/[true negatives + false positives]). For sensitivity and specificity, one must think "vertically" based on the 2 × 2 table shown in Figure 5. These test characteristics deal with the extent to which diseases are diagnosed correctly.

Receiver operating characteristic curves are another way to visualize sensitivity and specificity cutoffs for diagnostic tests. In these curves, test sensitivity is plotted on the Y axis, and (1 – specificity) on the X axis. A test that follows the diagonal line (the line between [0.0] and [1.1]) represents the flip of a coin. An ideal test will have high sensitivity and high specificity. Researchers can measure the area under the receiver-operating characteristic curve to compare two or more tests. As an example, erythrocyte sedimentation rate was compared with C-reactive protein level for the diagnosis of PID (Fig. 6). Neither test performed very well, but C-reactive protein test had a greater area under the curve (25).

Generally, clinicians are more interested in the likelihood of the disease given a positive or negative test result (the predictive values of the test). Predictive values are calculated by determining the percentage of positive (or negative) tests that correctly predict the presence (or absence) of the disease of interest. For predictive values, one must think horizontally. Positive predictive value is the percentage of women with a positive test who actually have the disease (true positives/positive tests = true positives/[true positives + false

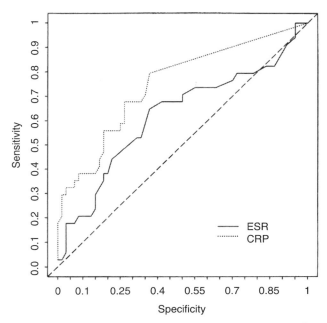

Figure 6. Receiver operating characteristic curves for C-reactive protein and erythrocyte sedimentation rate . Abbreviations: CRP indicates C-reactive protein; ESR, erythrocyte sedimentation rate. (Peipert JF, Boardman L, Hogan JW, Sung J, Mayer KH. Laboratory evaluation of acute upper genital tract infection. Obstet Gynecol 1996;87:730–6.)

positives]). The negative predictive value is the percentage of women with a negative test result who do not have the disease (true negatives/negative test results = true negatives/[true negatives + false negatives]). Predictive values depend on the prevalence of the disease in a population. For example, if a disease is extremely rare, it will be difficult to have a high positive predictive value, even if sensitivity and specificity are high. Predictive values can be calculated from the standard 2 × 2 table based on the formulas listed earlier. Predictive values also may be determined by way of Bayes' theorem (Box 10).

Likelihood ratios are an additional way to evaluate information from a diagnostic test. These calculations use sensitivity and specificity to estimate the likelihood of an outcome given a positive or negative test result. The likelihood ratio of a positive test is calculated as sensitivity/(1 – specificity), whereas the likelihood ratio for a negative test is the inverse. Large likelihood ratios (eg, higher than 10) suggest that the diagnostic test may be useful to "rule in" a disease, whereas small ratios (eg, lower than 0.1) may "rule out" a disease. Likelihood ratios also may be used to calculate the posttest probability of a disease (posttest probability = pretest probability × likelihood ratio).

DESCRIPTIVE STUDIES

Case reports and case-series reports are types of descriptive studies. These studies represent the least sophisti-

	Disease	
	Present	**Absent**
Positive	True positives (TP)	False positives (FP)
Negative	False negatives (FN)	True negatives (TN)

Figure 5. Example of a 2 × 2 table illustrating diagnostic test characteristics of sensitivity and specificity. Sensitivity is defined as TP/(TP + FN); specificity, TN/(TN + FP); positive predictive value, TP/(TP + FP); and negative predictive value, TN/(TN + FN).

cated of study designs. The purpose of descriptive studies is to assess and describe a finding in a case or group of cases. Descriptive studies are severely limited by the lack of a comparison group and by the potential bias of the investigators.

Establishing cause and effect is not possible in a descriptive study. Because they are hypothesis generating, descriptive studies may serve as the basis for future analytic studies. For example, in a case-series report of seven women who developed functional ovarian cysts while taking phasic contraceptive pills, the authors stated that "phasic contraceptive pills may be a threat to patient health and safety" (26). This report led to further investigation and refutation of these conclusions (27).

Systematic Reviews of Medical Evidence

Meta-analysis

In clinical research, meta-analysis is a commonly used tool used in the systematic review and aggregation of data from randomized controlled trials or observational studies. Obstetrics and gynecology has led other medical specialties in attempting to perform a systematic review of all randomized trials conducted in its discipline (28). One example is the *Cochrane Library*, which includes the Cochrane Database of Systematic Reviews. This electronic database began in England to review perinatal data, and it has expanded to include reviews of many areas of medicine (29). Combining data with meta-analysis can increase statistical power and the ability to evaluate treatment effects and complications in clinical trials, as well as associations between risk factors and disease in etiologic research. In addition, by combining results from several studies, generalizability may be increased. Meta-analysis is especially useful when sample sizes of individual clinical trials are too small to detect an effect or when a large trial is too costly and time-consuming to perform. For example, when investigators performed a meta-analysis to evaluate the efficacy of oral β-agonist maintenance therapy in delaying delivery and decreasing the incidence of preterm birth and its complications, they found no benefit of oral β-agonist maintenance therapy (30). A recent decision analysis to assess the use of magnesium sulfate for seizure prophylaxis in women with mild preeclampsia demonstrated that either strategy (using or not using magnesium) is acceptable because the neonatal and maternal outcomes were nearly identical (31).

A meta-analysis should adhere to specific methodological principles (28). Because the technique is a synthesis of existing studies (most commonly, randomized trials), an explicit study protocol should be developed to outline study inclusion and exclusion criteria. The researchers should provide some assessment of the combinability of the studies, including tests of homogeneity when appropriate. An evaluation and measurement of potential biases should be performed. The statistical methods used, including sensitivity analysis, should be described. Lastly, the authors should provide a discussion regarding the applicability of the results.

Decision Analysis

Decision analysis is a quantitative approach to evaluate the relative values of different management options (33). The process begins by systematically breaking down a clinical problem into its components and creating a decision tree, or algorithm, to represent the components (parameters) and decision options. Consider the problem of preventing early-onset group B streptococcal disease. A decision analysis was performed to address three different approaches to prevent early-onset neonatal group B streptococcal disease (32).

Probability values for each of the parameters in the decision tree are estimated from a review of the medical literature and expert opinion. The decision tree is then analyzed with statistical methods, and a net value for the different decision options in relation to one another is determined. A technique called *sensitivity analysis* is used to test how variations in these probabilities can affect the conclusions of the decision analysis. Factors that can be measured, such as mortality, are easier to analyze than are outcomes, such as quality of life.

Economic Analysis

The use of economic analysis has increased in recent years in the medical literature (33). For example, the issue of screening for cystic fibrosis by identifying prenatal carriers has been addressed with this technique (34). Economic analysis, including cost–benefit and cost-effectiveness analyses, is another type of systematic review. Economic analysis is similar to decision analysis but focuses on monetary cost. Once a decision analysis is performed on a specific clinical problem, data on costs of various management options are compared. A cost-effectiveness analysis compares the costs of different options to determine the best care for the least cost. Cost–benefit analysis includes some consequences of the decision options that are nonmonetary, such as years of life saved or disability avoided. For example, using a decision analytic model, investigators demonstrated that a policy of elective cesarean delivery for ultrasonographically diagnosed fetal macrosomia of nondiabetic women is economically unsound (35).

Economic analyses, however, are not without limitations. Often it is difficult to put a monetary cost or a utility on a clinical outcome, and these estimates often are highly subjective. In addition, a recent study has demonstrated that many cost-effectiveness studies reported in the obstetric and gynecologic literature have important methodological shortcomings (36). Therefore, the reader must be highly cautious in interpreting some of these findings and should have some basic knowledge about the methodological standards of these reports.

Statistics in Reproductive Research

Hypothesis Testing and Types of Error

The concept of hypothesis testing forms the basis for most statistical testing. The hypothesis of a study often is phrased in the form of a null hypothesis (H_0) that there is no difference present. Research studies should have a clear statement of their hypothesis before the research begins. A hypothetical example of a null hypothesis is as follows: There is no association between the use of low-dose oral contraceptives and the development of endometrial cancer. If one rejects the null hypothesis (H_0), then an alternative hypothesis (H_A) that some association exists is accepted. An alternative hypothesis could be the following: The use of low-dose oral contraceptives reduces the risk of developing endometrial cancer.

An association, however, may be clinically important or trivial. It is important to distinguish between statistical significance (which can be achieved with large sample sizes, regardless of the effect size) and clinical significance. Consider a study of 2,000 women who are randomized to receive antibiotic A or B to be treated for cervical *C trachomatis* infection. If the cure rate in the 1,000 women taking doxycycline is 95%, and the cure rate for the other drug is 97%, then there is a statistically significant difference ($P=.02$). However, this difference of 2% may not be considered clinically significant.

Research studies, like diagnostic tests, are not infallible. Two specific errors are of concern to epidemiologists and researchers: the type I error (α) and the type II error (β). A type I error occurs when a statistically significant difference is found in a study when there truly is no difference. The level of type I error is based on the choice of level of statistical significance. A significance value of $P<.05$ implies that the risk of type I error, or the possibility that a positive study finding was because of chance alone, is 5%. A type II error is the chance that a study finds no difference when a difference truly does exist. A study's power is its ability to detect an association when one truly exists. Type II error $=1 -$ power. Therefore, a 20% chance of a false-negative study translates to 80% power. The chance of a type II error is related inversely to sample size and to the statistical power of the study. Increasing a study's sample size can reduce the chance of a type II error (37).

Investigators should calculate the required sample size before beginning a study to avoid the problem of a type II error. Many clinical trials have described a therapy as ineffective when, in reality, the therapy may have a clinically meaningful effect but the trial was not of sufficient size to detect it (38).

Probability Values Compared With Point Estimates and Confidence Interval Estimation

Although the use of *P* values and hypothesis testing is firmly entrenched in the medical literature, confidence interval estimation and the use of point estimates are more informative for researchers and readers (39). Many authorities favor the use of point estimates (eg, RR) and their 95% CIs to the calculation of *P* values (40). A relative risk is the risk of the outcome in the exposed population relative to that in the unexposed, or control, population. A relative risk greater than 1 implies an increased risk, and a relative risk less than 1 implies a protective effect. For example, the relative risk of endometrial cancer in women who are more than 22.7 kg overweight is 10, or a 10-fold increased risk. The risk of ovarian cancer in women with pathogenic mutations in the *BRCA1* or *BRCA2* gene is reduced by 60% in women who have used combination oral contraceptives for 6 years or more relative to women who did not use oral contraceptives. When the 95% CI excludes 1, then the results are statistically significant at the $P<.05$ level. In addition, the width of the confidence interval provides some estimate of the precision of the effect size. The narrower the confidence interval, the more precise the point estimate. This concept can be represented graphically, as seen in a meta-analysis evaluating the sensitivity and specificity of liquid-based and conventional cervical cytology (Fig. 7) (41).

Measures of Association

Another form of point estimate is the odds ratio (OR), which often is confused with relative risk. The major difference between these terms is that relative risks are calculated from prospective data, such as data from a cohort study or a randomized trial, whereas ORs usually are calculated in retrospective case–control studies. Odds ratios also may be calculated from a logistic regression analysis (see later discussion) (42). The OR is the ratio of the odds of being exposed to an agent in the case group relative to the odds in the control group. In general, the odds ratio is a reasonable approximation of the relative risk when the disease under study is rare. However, many investigators are mistakenly using an OR when the outcome of interest is not rare, and doing so can lead to inaccurate estimates of the effect. The main reason RRs or ORs and their confidence intervals often are preferred is that these data provide more than just a test of significance; they also provide a measure of the magnitude of the association, its direction (ie, whether the exposure results in an increased or

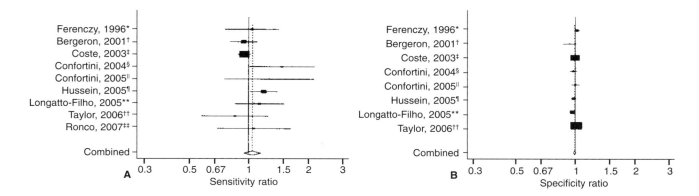

*Ferenczy A, Robitaille J, Franco EL, Arseneau J, Richart RM, Wright TC. Conventional cervical cytologic smears vs. ThinPrep smears. A paired comparison study on cervical cytology. Acta Cytol 1996;40:1136–42.

†Bergeron C, Bishop J, Lemarie A, Cas F, Ayivi J, Huynh B, et al. Accuracy of thin-layer cytology in patients undergoing cervical cone biopsy. Acta Cytol 2001;45:519–24.

‡Coste J, Cochand-Priollet B, de Cremoux P, Le Gales C, Cartier I, Molinie V, et al. Cross sectional study of conventional cervical smear, monolayer cytology, and human papillomavirus DNA testing for cervical cancer screening. BMJ 2003;326:733–6.

§Confortini M, Bulgaresi P, Cariaggi MP, Carozzi FM, Cecchini S, Cipparrone I, et al. Comparing conventional and liquid-based smears from a consecutive series of 297 subjects referred to colposcopy assessment. Cytopathology 2004;15:168–70.

ǁConfortini M, Carozzi F, Cortecchia S, Garcia MC, Sani C, Tinacci G, et al. Technical evaluation of the new thin layer device CellSlide (Menarini Diagnostics). Diagn Cytopathol 2005;33:387–93.

¶Hussein T, Desai M, Tomlinson A, Kitchener HC. The comparative diagnostic accuracy of conventional and liquid-based cytology in a colposcopic setting. BJOG 2005;112:1542–6.

**Longatto-Filho A, Pereira SM, Di Loreto C, Utagawa ML, Makabe S, Sakamoto Maeda MY, et al. DCS liquid-based system is more effective than conventional smears to diagnosis of cervical lesions: study in high-risk population with biopsy-based confirmation. Gynecol Oncol 2005;97:497–500.

††Taylor S, Kuhn L, Dupree W, Denny L, De Souza M, Wright TC Jr. Direct comparison of liquid-based and conventional cytology in a South African screening trial. Int J Cancer 2006;957–62.

‡‡Ronco G, Cuzick J, Pierotti P, Cariaggi MP, Dalla Palma P, Naldoni C, et al. Accuracy of liquid based versus conventional cytology: overall results of new technologies for cervical cancer screening: randomised controlled trial. BMJ 2007;335:28.

Figure 7. A. Relative sensitivity at cutoff high-grade squamous intraepithelial lesion or worse. **B.** Relative specificity at cutoff high-grade squamous intraepithelial lesion or worse. (Arbyn M, Bergon C, Klinkhamer P, Martin-Hirsch P, Siebers AG, Bulten J. Liquid compared with conventional cervical cytology: a systematic review and meta-analysis. Obstet Gynecol 2008;111:167–77.)

decreased risk of the disease), and some estimate of the precision of the effect. Consider a study that provides an RR of 0.7 with 95% CIs of 0.64–0.75, compared with a study with an RR of 0.7 with 95% CIs of 0.53–0.91. Both examples are statistically significant, but the first example has greater precision (because it has 10 times more patients).

A commonly used statistical tool in epidemiologic studies is mathematical modeling, such as multivariable analysis. The most common example of multivariable analysis used in the reproductive-health literature is logistic regression analysis. A confounding variable is associated with the exposure or intervention and the outcome of interest but is not in the causal pathway. Logistic regression is a statistical tool used to evaluate simultaneously the relationship of many variables (including the exposure and potential confounders) to an outcome of interest. With logistic regression, the outcome in question is dichotomous (eg, yes/no, alive/dead). The result is an adjusted estimate of the association that controls for the effect of confounding

variables. The expertise of a biostatistician or epidemiologist can be very valuable to a researcher who is interested in the technique of multivariable analysis.

Interpreting the Medical Literature

Although epidemiologic studies cannot prove causation, they can be used to determine the likelihood of causation. The following criteria should be considered when evaluating a cause-and-effect relationship:

- *Strength of the association:* The stronger the association, the more likely it is to be real.

- *Temporal relationship:* Does the cause precede the effect?

- *Consistency:* Are the study findings consistent over many reports?

- *Biologic plausibility:* Does the relationship make biologic sense?

- *Biologic gradient:* Is there a dose–response relationship?

- *Evidence:* Is there experimental evidence to support or refute the association?

A critical reader of the medical literature should be able to determine a study's methodology and recognize the scientific value of the research. When interpreting the medical literature, the reader should consider not only the methodology (eg, randomized trial or observational study) but also the quality of the study. One way to describe the quality of evidence presented is the rating system used in *Obstetrics and Gynecology*. This rating system ranges from level I to level III. Level I evidence is from a randomized controlled trial, level II evidence is from a cohort or case–control study that includes a comparison group, and level III evidence is from an uncontrolled descriptive study, including case series (43, 44).

Readers should no longer unconditionally accept the standard review or the "gospel of the expert." Opinions of authorities and reports of expert committees are no longer regarded as acceptable, high-quality medical evidence. An educated reader should evaluate the evidence available from high-quality studies in the medical literature and recognize when evidence to support a specific practice or association is weak. Several resources are available that evaluate the medical literature (see box Resources and a monograph published by the American College of Obstetricians and Gynecologists entitled *Reading the Medical Literature: Applying Evidence to Practice* available through the American College of Obstetricians and Gynecologists' Resource Center).

References

1. Grimes DA, Schulz KF. An overview of clinical research: the lay of the land. Lancet 2002;359:57–61.

2. Grimes DA, Schulz KF. Descriptive studies: what they can and cannot do. Lancet 2002;359:145–9.

3. Grimes DA, Schulz KF. Bias and causal associations in observational research. Lancet 2002;359:248–52.

4. Grimes DA, Schulz KF. Cohort studies: marching towards outcomes. Lancet 2002;359:341–5.

5. Grimes DA, Schulz KF. Uses and abuses of screening tests [published erratum appears in Lancet 2008;371:1998]. Lancet 2002;359:881–4.

6. Schulz KF, Grimes DA. Case–control studies: research in reverse. Lancet 2002;359:431–4.

7. Schulz KF, Grimes DA. Generation of allocation sequences in randomised trials: chance, not choice. Lancet 2002;359:515–9.

8. Schulz KF, Grimes DA. Allocation concealment in randomised trials: defending against deciphering. Lancet 2002;359:614–8.

9. Schulz KF, Grimes DA. Blinding in randomised trials: hiding who got what. Lancet 2002;359:696–700.

10. Schulz KF, Grimes DA. Sample size slippages in randomised trials: exclusions and the lost and wayward. Lancet 2002;359:781–5.

11. Schulz KF, Grimes DA. Unequal group sizes in randomised trials: guarding against guessing. Lancet 2002;359:966–70.

12. Funai EF, Rosenbush EJ, Lee MJ, Del Priore G. Distribution of study designs in four major US journals of obstetrics and gynecology. Gynecol Obstet Invest 2001;51:8–11.

13. Peipert JF, Grimes DA. The case-control study: a primer for the obstetrician-gynecologist. Obstet Gynecol 1994;84:140–5.

14. Nelson HD, Helfand M. Screening for chlamydial infection. Am J Prev Med 2001;20(suppl):95–107.

15. Scholes D, Stergachis A, Heidrich FE, Andrilla H, Holmes KK, Stamm WE. Prevention of pelvic inflammatory disease by screening for cervical chlamydial infection. N Engl J Med 1996;334:1362–6.

16. Schulz KF, Chalmers I, Hayes RJ, Altman DG. Empirical evidence of bias. Dimensions of methodological quality associated with estimates of treatment effects in controlled trials. JAMA 1995;273:408–12.

17. MacMahon S, Collins R. Reliable assessment of the effects of treatment on mortality and major morbidity, II: observational studies. Lancet 2001;357:455–62.

18. Funai EF. Obstetrics & Gynecology in 1996: marking the progress toward evidence-based medicine by classifying studies based on methodology. Obstet Gynecol 1997;90:1020–2.

19. Grodstein F, Manson JE, Stampfer MJ. Hormone therapy and coronary heart disease: the role of time since menopause and age at hormone initiation. J Womens Health (Larchmt) 2006;15:35–44.

20. Tworoger SS, Fairfield KM, Colditz GA, Rosner BA, Hankinson SE. Association of oral contraceptive use, other contraceptive methods, and infertility with ovarian cancer risk. Am J Epidemiol 2007;166:894–901.

21. Narod SA, Risch H, Moslehi R, Dorum A, Neuhausen S, Olsson H, et al. Oral contraceptives and the risk of hereditary ovarian cancer. Hereditary Ovarian Cancer Clinical Study Group. N Engl J Med 1998;339:424–8.

22. Burkman RT. Association between intrauterine device and pelvic inflammatory disease. Obstet Gynecol 1981;57:269–76.

23. Cahill AG, Stamilio DM, Odibo AO, Peipert J, Stevens E, Macones GA. Racial disparity of the success and complications of vaginal birth after cesarean delivery. Obstet Gynecol 2008;111:654–8.

24. Peipert JF, Sweeney PJ. Diagnostic testing in obstetrics and gynecology: a clinician's guide. Obstet Gynecol 1993;82:619–23.

25. Peipert JF, Boardman L, Hogan JW, Sung J, Mayer KH. Laboratory evaluation of acute upper genital tract infection. Obstet Gynecol 1996;87:730–6.

26. Caillouette JC, Koehler AL. Phasic contraceptive pills and functional ovarian cysts. Am J Obstet Gynecol 1987;156:1538–42.

27. Grimes DA, Godwin AJ, Rubin A, Smith JA, Lacarra M. Ovulation and follicular development associated with three low-dose oral contraceptives: a randomized controlled trial. Obstet Gynecol 1994;83:29–34.

28. Peipert JF, Bracken MB. Systematic reviews of medical evidence: the use of meta-analysis in obstetrics and gynecology. Obstet Gynecol 1997;89:628–33.

29. Starr M, Chalmers I. The evolution of The Cochrane Library, 1988–2003. Oxford: Update Software; 2003. Available at: http://www.update–software.com/history/clibhist.htm. Retrieved November 12, 2008.

30. Macones GA, Berlin M, Berlin JA. Efficacy of oral beta-agonist maintenance therapy in preterm labor: a meta-analysis. Obstet Gynecol 1995;85:313–7.

31. Cahill AG, Macones GA, Odibo AO, Stamilio DM. Magnesium for seizure prophylaxis in patients with mild preeclampsia. Obstet Gynecol 2007;110:601–7.

32. Rouse DJ, Owen J. Decision analysis. Clin Obstet Gynecol 1998;41:282–95.

33. Macones GA, Goldie SJ, Peipert JF. Cost-effectiveness analysis: an introductory guide for clinicians. Obstet Gynecol Surv 1999;54:663–72.

34. Doyle NM, Gardner MO. Prenatal cystic fibrosis screening in Mexican Americans: an economic analysis. Am J Obstet Gynecol 2003;189:769–74.

35. Rouse DJ, Owen J, Goldenberg RL, Cliver SP. The effectiveness and costs of elective cesarean delivery for fetal macrosomia diagnosed by ultrasound. JAMA 1996; 276: 1480–6.

36. Smith WJ, Blackmore CC. Economic analyses in obstetrics and gynecology: a methodologic evaluation of the literature. Obstet Gynecol 1998;91:472–8.

37. Peipert JF, Metheny WP, Schulz K. Sample size and statistical power in reproductive research. Obstet Gynecol 1995;86:302–5.

38. Freiman JA, Chalmers TC, Smith H Jr, Kuebler RR. The importance of beta, the type II error and sample size in the design and interpretation of the randomized control trial. Survey of 71 "negative" trials. N Engl J Med 1978;299: 690–4.

39. Grimes DA. The case for confidence intervals [editorial]. Obstet Gynecol 1992;80:865–6.

40. Rothman KJ. A show of confidence [editorial]. N Engl J Med 1978;299:1362–3.

41. Arbyn M, Bergeron C, Klinkhamer P, Martin-Hirsch P, Siebers AG, Bulten J. Liquid compared with conventional cervical cytology: a systematic review and meta-analysis. Obstet Gynecol 2008;111:167–77.

42. Peterson HB, Kleinbaum DG. Interpreting the literature in obstetrics and gynecology: II. Logistic regression and related issues. Obstet Gynecol 1991;78:717–20.

43. Scott JR. Adapting to the times [editorial]. Obstet Gynecol 2007;109:2–3.

44. Scott JR. Green journal refinements [editorial]. Obstet Gynecol 2007;109:1264–5.

Principles of Screening

Herbert B. Peterson

As a major provider of health care for women, the obstetrician–gynecologist has an opportunity to prevent disease and promote women's health. Most deaths among women younger than 65 years are preventable, and screening plays an important role in preventing many of these deaths. The purpose of screening is twofold:

1. *Primary prevention:* Identification and control of risk factors for disease with the intent of preventing disease before it occurs
2. *Secondary prevention:* Early diagnosis of disease to prevent or reduce morbidity and mortality once disease has occurred

Screening tests are for people who are asymptomatic and otherwise apparently free of the disease that is the reason for the test. Diagnostic tests, by contrast, are used to evaluate symptomatic people and individuals suspected of having a disease.

Annual physical examinations accompanied by an increasing battery of screening tests have become commonplace. However, because of better understanding of the cost, inefficiency, limitations, and potential hazards of that approach, periodic (rather than annual) examinations with selected screening tests are now recommended. Because screening for most diseases has little value, screening services should be restricted to those of demonstrable value. Such screening should be tailored to specific circumstances that are based on an assessment of risk factors, such as age, rather than applied to all individuals (Boxes 12–15, Table 2). Screening tests are appropriate only when effective strategies exist for early intervention in the asymptomatic individual and when such early intervention is more beneficial than treating the symptomatic individual.

Rationale for Screening

Screening tests or procedures are used to identify previously unrecognized disease or risk factors for disease. Some screening tests are offered appropriately and voluntarily as a service to the general public (eg, blood pressure measurement at shopping malls); some are

---

Resources

Principles of Screening

Centers for Disease Control and Prevention
http://www.cdc.gov

U.S. Preventive Services Task Force
http://www.ahrq.gov/clinic/uspstfix.htm

---

compulsory (eg, tests required by an insurance company as a condition of coverage); and some are provided by clinicians to prevent morbidity and mortality among patients who appear to be healthy. Screening should be considered a therapeutic intervention, and ideally, the screening policy should be based on randomized trials of the effect of screening on patient outcomes (1).

Screening to obtain an early diagnosis or early identification of a risk factor can be lifesaving; however, screening tests can have harmful as well as beneficial effects. The tests themselves can be uncomfortable and expensive (eg, sigmoidoscopy), and they can yield false-positive results that may lead to unnecessary and potentially harmful diagnostic procedures (eg, false-positive mammography that results in open breast biopsy). Even true-positive test results can lead to anxiety and harmful therapy (2). Many people must be screened and treated for a risk factor to avert a single future adverse outcome (1). True-positive test results also can identify inconsequential disease; indeed, most people found to have a risk factor at screening will be treated for inconsequential disease (1).

Screening for a disease is warranted only if the screening test can detect the disease before it would be diagnosed otherwise in symptomatic patients and if treatment is more effective or easier to administer at that point than afterward. For example, mammography is a screening test for breast cancer because it can detect disease at an early stage, when treatment is more effective than it would be in a later stage. By contrast, screening for lung cancer with chest radiography is ineffective because lung cancer lesions that can be detected radiographically are already so advanced that treatment of patients at that point is no more effective than treatment of symptomatic patients.

Several additional considerations regarding screening relate to an individual's being identified as having or not having the disease or risk factor being assessed. Genetic screening for breast cancer, for example, carries potential implications regarding insurance, employment, and emotional issues. Individuals with false-positive test results may be subject to expensive diagnostic tests and experience unnecessary alarm in the interim. For example, mammography in women aged 30 years is known to have a high false-positive rate, which has caused the abandonment of routine annual use of this test in low-risk women younger than 40 years. Women with false-negative test results may have an unwarranted delay in the diagnosis of a potentially serious problem. For some patients correctly identified as having a disease or risk factor, treatment could be ineffective or even harmful.

Box 12

Periodic Assessment: Ages 13–18 Years

Screening

History

Reason for visit

Health status: medical, menstrual, surgical, family

Dietary/nutrition assessment

Physical activity

Use of complementary and alternative medicine

Tobacco, alcohol, other drug use

Abuse/neglect

Sexual practices

Physical Examination

Height

Weight

Body mass index (BMI)

Blood pressure

Secondary sexual characteristics (Tanner staging)

Pelvic examination (when indicated by the medical history)

Skin*

Laboratory Testing

Periodic

Cervical cytology (annually beginning at approximately 3 years after initiation of sexual intercourse)

Chlamydia and gonorrhea testing (if sexually active)

High-Risk Groups*

Hemoglobin level assessment

Bacteriuria testing

Sexually transmitted disease testing

Human immunodeficiency virus (HIV) testing

Genetic testing/counseling

Rubella titer assessment

Tuberculosis skin testing

Lipid profile assessment

Fasting glucose testing

Hepatitis C virus testing

Colorectal cancer screening†

Evaluation and Counseling

Sexuality

Development

High-risk behaviors

Preventing unwanted/unintended pregnancy

—Postponing sexual involvement

—Contraceptive options, including emergency contraception

Sexually transmitted diseases

—Partner selection

—Barrier protection

Fitness and Nutrition

Dietary/nutrition assessment (including eating disorders)

Exercise: discussion of program

Folic acid supplementation (0.4 mg/d)

Calcium intake

Psychosocial Evaluation

Suicide: depressive symptoms

Interpersonal/family relationships

Sexual identity

Personal goal development

Behavioral/learning disorders

Abuse/neglect

Satisfactory school experience

Peer relationships

Date rape prevention

Cardiovascular Risk Factors

Family history

Hypertension

Dyslipidemia

Obesity

Diabetes mellitus

Health/Risk Behaviors

Hygiene (including dental); fluoride supplementation*

Injury prevention

—Safety belts and helmets

—Recreational hazards

—Firearms

—Hearing

—Occupational hazards

—School hazards

—Exercise and sports involvement

Skin exposure to ultraviolet rays

Tobacco, alcohol, other drug use

Immunizations

Periodic

Tetanus–diphtheria–pertussis booster (once between ages 11 years and 16 years)

Hepatitis B vaccine (one series for those not previously immunized)

Human papillomavirus vaccine (one series for those not previously immunized)

Meningococcal conjugate vaccine (before entry into high school for those not previously immunized)

High-Risk Groups

Influenza vaccine

Hepatitis A virus vaccine

Pneumococcal vaccine

Measles–mumps–rubella vaccine

Varicella vaccine

Leading Causes of Death

1. Accidents
2. Malignant neoplasms
3. Homicide
4. Suicide
5. Congenital anomalies
6. Diseases of the heart
7. Chronic lower respiratory diseases
8. Influenza and pneumonia
9. Septicemia
10. Pregnancy, childbirth, and puerperium

Leading Causes of Morbidity

Acne

Asthma

Chlamydia

Headache

Mental disorders, including affective and neurotic disorders

Nose, throat, ear, and upper respiratory infections

Obesity

Sexual assault

Sexually transmitted diseases

Urinary tract infections

Vaginitis

---

*See Table 2.

†Only for those with a family history of familial adenomatous polyposis or 8 years after the start of pancolitis. For a more detailed discussion of colorectal cancer screening, see Smith RA, von Eschenbach AC, Wender R, Levin B, Byers T, Rothenberger D, et al. American Cancer Society guidelines for the early detection of cancer: update of early detection guidelines for prostate, colorectal, and endometrial cancers. Also: update 2001–testing for early lung cancer detection [published erratum appears in CA Cancer J Clin 2001;51:150]. CA Cancer J Clin 2001;51:38–75; quiz 77–80.

Primary and preventive care: periodic assessments. ACOG Committee Opinion No. 357. American College of Obstetricians and Gynecologists. Obstet Gynecol 2006;108:1615–22.

Box 13

Periodic Assessment: Ages 19–39 Years

Screening

History

Reason for visit

Health status: medical, surgical, family

Dietary/nutrition assessment

Physical activity

Use of complementary and alternative medicine

Tobacco, alcohol, other drug use

Abuse/neglect

Sexual practices

Urinary and fecal incontinence

Physical Examination

Height

Weight

Body mass index (BMI)

Blood pressure

Neck: adenopathy, thyroid

Breasts

Abdomen

Pelvic examination

Skin*

Laboratory Testing

Periodic

Cervical cytology (annually beginning no later than age 21 years; every 2–3 years after three consecutive negative test results if age 30 years or older with no history of cervical intraepithelial neoplasia 2 or 3, immunosuppression, human immunodeficiency virus [HIV] infection, or diethylstilbestrol exposure in utero)[†]

Chlamydia testing (if aged 25 years or younger and sexually active)

Human immunodeficiency virus (HIV) testing[‡]

High-Risk Groups*

Hemoglobin level assessment

Bacteriuria testing

Mammography

Fasting glucose testing

Sexually transmitted disease testing

Genetic testing/counseling

Rubella titer assessment

Tuberculosis skin testing

Lipid profile assessment

Thyroid-stimulating hormone testing

Hepatitis C virus testing

Colorectal cancer screening

Bone density screening

Evaluation and Counseling

Sexuality and Reproductive Planning

High-risk behaviors

Discussion of a reproductive health plan[§]

Contraceptive options for prevention of unwanted pregnancy, including emergency contraception

Preconception and genetic counseling

Sexually transmitted diseases

–Partner selection

–Barrier protection

Sexual function

Fitness and Nutrition

Dietary/nutrition assessment

Exercise: discussion of program

Folic acid supplementation (0.4 mg/d)

Calcium intake

Psychosocial Evaluation

Interpersonal/family relationships

Intimate partner violence

Work satisfaction

Lifestyle/stress

Sleep disorders

Cardiovascular Risk Factors

Family history

Hypertension

Dyslipidemia

Obesity

Diabetes mellitus

Lifestyle

Health/Risk Behaviors

Hygiene (including dental)

Injury prevention

–Safety belts and helmets

–Occupational hazards

–Recreational hazards

–Firearms

–Hearing

–Exercise and sports involvement

Breast self-examination[||]

Chemoprophylaxis for breast cancer (for high-risk women aged 35 years or older)[¶]

Skin exposure to ultraviolet rays

Suicide: depressive symptoms

Tobacco, alcohol, other drug use

Immunizations

Periodic

Human papillomavirus vaccine (one series for those aged 26 years or less and not previously immunized)

Tetanus–diphtheria–pertussis booster (every 10 years)

*High-Risk Groups**

Measles–mumps–rubella vaccine

Hepatitis A vaccine

Hepatitis B vaccine

Influenza vaccine

Meningococcal vaccine

Pneumococcal vaccine

Varicella vaccine

Leading Causes of Death

1. Malignant neoplasms
2. Accidents
3. Diseases of the heart
4. Suicide
5. Human immunodeficiency virus (HIV) disease
6. Homicide
7. Cerebrovascular diseases
8. Diabetes mellitus
9. Chronic liver diseases and cirrhosis
10. Chronic lower respiratory diseases

Leading Causes of Morbidity

Acne	Mental disorders, including affective and neurotic disorders
Arthritis	
Asthma	
Back symptoms	Nose, throat, ear, and upper respiratory infections
Cancer	
Chlamydia	Obesity
Depression	Sexual assault/domestic violence
Diabetes mellitus	
Gynecologic disorders	Sexually transmitted diseases
Headache/migraine	Substance abuse
Hypertension	Urinary tract infections
Joint disorders	
Menstrual disorders	

*See Table 2.

[†]For a more detailed discussion of cervical cytology screening, including the use of human papillomavirus DNA testing and screening after hysterectomy, see Cervical cytology screening. ACOG Practice Bulletin No. 45. American College of Obstetricians and Gynecologists. Obstet Gynecol 2003;102:417–27.

[‡]Physicians should be aware of and follow their states' HIV screening requirements. For a more detailed discussion of HIV screening, see Branson BM, Handsfield HH, Lampe MA, Janssen RS, Taylor AW, Lyss SB, et al. Revised recommendations for HIV testing in adults, adolescents, and pregnant women in health care settings. Centers for Disease Control and Prevention. MMWR Recomm Rep 2006;55(RR-14):1–17; quiz CE1–4.

[§]For a more detailed discussion of the reproductive health plan, see The importance of preconception care in the continuum of women's health care. ACOG Committee Opinion No. 313. American College of Obstetricians and Gynecologists. Obstet Gynecol 2005;106:665–6.

[||]Despite a lack of definite data for or against breast self-examination, breast self-examination has the potential to detect palpable breast cancer and can be recommended.

[¶]For a more detailed discussion of risk assessment and chemoprevention therapy, see Selective estrogen receptor modulators. ACOG Practice Bulletin No. 39. American College of Obstetricians and Gynecologists. Obstet Gynecol 2002;100:835–43.

Primary and preventive care: periodic assessments. ACOG Committee Opinion No. 357. American College of Obstetricians and Gynecologists. Obstet Gynecol 2006;108:1615–22.

Box 14

Periodic Assessment: Ages 40–64 Years

Screening

History

Reason for visit
Health status: medical, surgical, family
Dietary/nutrition assessment
Physical activity
Use of complementary and alternative medicine
Tobacco, alcohol, other drug use
Abuse/neglect
Sexual practices
Urinary and fecal incontinence

Physical Examination

Height
Weight
Body mass index (BMI)
Blood pressure
Oral cavity
Neck: adenopathy, thyroid
Breasts, axillae
Abdomen
Pelvic examination
Skin*

Laboratory Testing

Periodic

Cervical cytology (every 2–3 years after three consecutive negative test results if no history of cervical intraepithelial neoplasia 2 or 3, immunosuppression, human immunodeficiency virus [HIV] infection, or diethylstilbestrol exposure in utero)[†]

Mammography (every 1–2 years beginning at age 40 years; yearly beginning at age 50 years)

Lipid profile assessment (every 5 years beginning at age 45 years)

Colorectal cancer screening (beginning at age 50 years), using one of the following options:

1. Yearly patient-collected fecal occult blood testing[‡]
2. Flexible sigmoidoscopy every 5 years
3. Yearly patient-collected fecal occult blood testing[‡] plus flexible sigmoidoscopy very 5 years
4. Double contrast barium enema every 5 years
5. Colonoscopy every 10 years

Fasting glucose testing (every 3 years after age 45 years)

Thyroid-stimulating hormone screening (every 5 years beginning at age 50 years)

Human immunodeficiency virus (HIV) testing[§]

High-Risk Groups*

Hemoglobin level assessment
Bacteriuria testing
Fasting glucose testing
Sexually transmitted disease testing
Tuberculosis skin testing
Lipid profile assessment
Thyroid-stimulating hormone testing
Hepatitis C virus testing
Colorectal cancer screening

Evaluation and Counseling

Sexuality[||]

High-risk behaviors
Contraceptive options for prevention of unwanted pregnancy, including emergency contraception
Sexually transmitted diseases
–Partner selection
–Barrier protection
Sexual function

Fitness and Nutrition

Dietary/nutrition assessment
Exercise: discussion of program
Folic acid supplementation (0.4 mg/d before age 50 years)
Calcium intake

Psychosocial Evaluation

Family relationships
Intimate partner violence
Work satisfaction
Retirement planning
Lifestyle/stress
Sleep disorders

Cardiovascular Risk Factors

Family history
Hypertension
Dyslipidemia
Obesity
Diabetes mellitus
Lifestyle

Health/Risk Behaviors

Hygiene (including dental)
Hormone therapy
Injury prevention
–Safety belts and helmets
–Occupational hazards
–Recreational hazards
–Exercise and sports involvement
–Firearms
–Hearing
Breast self-examination[¶]

Chemoprophylaxis for breast cancer (for high-risk women)**
Skin exposure to ultraviolet rays
Suicide: depressive symptoms
Tobacco, alcohol, other drug use

Immunizations

Periodic

Influenza vaccine (annually beginning at age 50 years)
Tetanus–diphtheria–pertussis booster (every 10 years)

High-Risk Groups

Measles–mumps–rubella vaccine
Hepatitis A vaccine
Hepatitis B vaccine
Influenza vaccine
Meningococcal vaccine
Pneumococcal vaccine
Varicella vaccine

Leading Causes of Death

1. Malignant neoplasms
2. Diseases of the heart
3. Cerebrovascular diseases
4. Chronic lower respiratory diseases
5. Accidents
6. Diabetes mellitus
7. Chronic liver disease and cirrhosis
8. Septicemia
9. Suicide
10. Human immunodeficiency virus (HIV) disease

Leading Causes of Morbidity

Arthritis/osteoarthritis	Mental disorders, including affective and neurotic disorders
Asthma	
Cancer	Musculoskeletal symptoms
Cardiovascular disease	Nose, throat, ear, and upper respiratory infections
Depression	
Diabetes mellitus	Obesity
Disorders of the urinary tract	Pneumonia
Headache/migraine	Sexually transmitted diseases
Hypertension	Ulcers
Menopause	Vision impairment

*See Table 2.

[†]For a more detailed discussion of cervical cytology screening, including the use of human papillomavirus DNA testing and screening after hysterectomy, see Cervical cytology screening. ACOG Practice Bulletin No. 45. American College of Obstetricians and Gynecologists. Obstet Gynecol 2003;102:417–27.

[‡]Fecal occult blood testing (FOBT) requires two or three samples of stool collected by the patient at home and returned for analysis. A single stool sample for FOBT obtained by digital rectal examination is not adequate for the detection of colorectal cancer.

[§] Physicians should be aware of and follow their states' HIV screening requirements. For a more detailed discussion of HIV screening, see Branson BM, Handsfield HH, Lampe MA, Janssen RS, Taylor AW, Lyss SB, et al. Revised recommendations for HIV testing of adults, adolescents, and pregnant women in health care settings. Centers for Disease Control and Prevention. MMWR Recomm Rep 2006;55(RR-14):1–17; quiz CE1–4.

[||]Preconception and genetic counseling is appropriate for certain women in this age group.

[¶]Despite a lack of definitive data for or against breast self-examination, breast self-examination has the potential to detect palpable breast cancer and can be recommended.

**For a more detailed discussion of risk assessment and chemoprevention therapy, see Selective estrogen receptor modulators. ACOG Practice Bulletin No. 39. American College of Obstetricians and Gynecologists. Obstet Gynecol 2002;100:835–43.

Primary and preventive care: periodic assessments. ACOG Committee Opinion No. 357. American College of Obstetricians and Gynecologists. Obstet Gynecol 2006;108:1615–22.

Box 15

Periodic Assessment: Ages 65 Years and Older

Screening

History

Reason for visit

Health status: medical, surgical, family

Dietary/nutrition assessment

Physical activity

Use of complementary and alternative medicine

Tobacco, alcohol, other drug use, and concurrent medication use

Abuse/neglect

Sexual practices

Urinary and fecal incontinence

Physical Examination

Height

Weight

Body mass index (BMI)

Blood pressure

Oral cavity

Neck: adenopathy, thyroid

Breasts, axillae

Abdomen

Pelvic examination

Skin*

Laboratory Testing

Periodic

Cervical cytology (every 2–3 years after three consecutive negative test results if no history of cervical intraepithelial neoplasia 2 or 3, immunosuppression, human immunodeficiency virus [HIV] infection, or diethylstilbestrol exposure in utero)[†]

Urinalysis

Mammography

Lipid profile assessment (every 5 years)

Colorectal cancer screening using one of the following methods:

1. Yearly patient-collected fecal occult blood testing[‡]

2. Flexible sigmoidoscopy every 5 years

3. Yearly patient-collected fecal occult blood testing[‡] plus flexible sigmoidoscopy every 5 years

4. Double contrast barium enema every 5 years

5. Colonoscopy every 10 years

Fasting glucose testing (every 3 years)

Bone density screening[§]

Thyroid-stimulating hormone screening (every 5 years)

High-Risk Groups*

Hemoglobin level assessment

Sexually transmitted disease testing

Human immunodeficiency virus (HIV) testing

Tuberculosis skin testing

Thyroid-stimulating hormone screening

Hepatitis C virus testing

Colorectal cancer screening

Evaluation and Counseling

Sexuality

Sexual function

Sexual behaviors

Sexually transmitted diseases

—Partner selection

—Barrier protection

Fitness and Nutrition

Dietary/nutrition assessment

Exercise: discussion of program

Calcium intake

Psychosocial Evaluation

Neglect/abuse

Lifestyle/stress

Depression/sleep disorders

Family relationships

Work/retirement satisfaction

Cardiovascular Risk Factors

Hypertension

Dyslipidemia

Obesity

Diabetes mellitus

Sedentary lifestyle

Health/Risk Behaviors

Hygiene (including dental)

Hormone therapy

Injury prevention

—Safety belts and helmets

—Prevention of falls

—Occupational hazards

—Recreational hazards

—Exercise and sports involvement

—Firearms

Visual acuity/glaucoma

Hearing

Breast self-examination[‖]

Chemoprophylaxis for breast cancer (for high-risk women)[¶]

Skin exposure to ultraviolet rays

Suicide: depressive symptoms

Tobacco, alcohol, other drug use

Immunizations

Periodic

Tetanus–diphtheria booster (every 10 years)

Influenza vaccine (annually)

Pneumococcal vaccine (once)

*High-Risk Groups***

Hepatitis A vaccine

Hepatitis B vaccine

Meningococcal vaccine

Varicella vaccine

Leading Causes of Death

1. Diseases of the heart
2. Malignant neoplasms
3. Cerebrovascular diseases
4. Chronic lower respiratory diseases
5. Alzheimer disease
6. Influenza and pneumonia
7. Diabetes mellitus
8. Nephritis, nephrotic syndrome, and nephrosis
9. Accidents
10. Septicemia

Leading Causes of Morbidity

Arthritis/osteoarthritis	Mental disorders
Asthma	Musculoskeletal symptoms
Cancer	Nose, throat, ear, and upper respiratory infections
Cardiovascular disease	
Chronic obstructive pulmonary diseases	Obesity
	Osteoporosis
Diabetes mellitus	Pneumonia
Diseases of the nervous system and sense organs	Ulcers
	Urinary incontinence
Hearing and vision impairment	Urinary tract infections
Hypertension	Vertigo

*See Table 2.

[†]For a more detailed discussion of cervical cytology screening, including the use of human papillomavirus DNA testing and screening after hysterectomy, see Cervical cytology screening. ACOG Practice Bulletin No. 45. American College of Obstetricians and Gynecologists. Obstet Gynecol 2003;102:417–27.

[‡]Fecal occult blood testing (FOBT) requires two or three samples of stool collected by the patient at home and returned for analysis. A single stool sample for FOBT obtained by digital rectal examination is not adequate for detection of colorectal cancer.

[§]In the absence of new risk factors, subsequent bone density screening should not be performed more frequently than every 2 years.

[‖]Despite a lack of definitive data for or against breast self-examination, breast self-examination has the potential to detect palpable breast cancer and can be recommended.

[¶]For a more detailed discussion of risk assessment and chemoprevention therapy, see Selective estrogen receptor modulators. ACOG Practice Bulletin No. 39. American College of Obstetricians and Gynecologists. Obstet Gynecol 2002;100:835–43.

Primary and preventive care: periodic assessments. ACOG Committee Opinion No. 357. American College of Obstetricians and Gynecologists. Obstet Gynecol 2006;108:1615–22.

Table 2. High-Risk Factors

Intervention	High-Risk Factor
Bacteriuria testing	Diabetes mellitus
Bone density screening*	Postmenopausal women younger than 65 years: history of prior fracture as an adult; family history of osteoporosis; Caucasian; dementia; poor nutrition; smoking; low weight and BMI; estrogen deficiency caused by early (age younger than 45 years) menopause, bilateral oophorectomy or prolonged (longer than 1 year) premenopausal amenorrhea; low lifelong calcium intake; alcoholism; impaired eyesight despite adequate correction; history of falls; inadequate physical activity
	All women: certain diseases or medical conditions and those who take certain drugs associated with an increased risk of osteoporosis
Colorectal cancer screening†	Colorectal cancer or adenomatous polyps in first-degree relative younger than 60 years or in two or more first-degree relatives of any ages; family history of familial adenomatous polyposis or hereditary nonpolyposis colon cancer; history of colorectal cancer, adenomatous polyps, inflammatory bowel disease, chronic ulcerative colitis, or Crohn disease
Fasting glucose testing	Overweight (BMI greater than or equal to 25); family history of diabetes mellitus; habitual physical inactivity; high-risk race/ethnicity (eg, African American, Hispanic, Native American, Asian, Pacific Islander); have given birth to a newborn weighing more than 9 lb or have a history of gestational diabetes mellitus; hypertension; high-density lipoprotein cholesterol level less than or equal to 35 mg/dL; triglyceride level greater than or equal to 250 mg/dL; history of impaired glucose tolerance or impaired fasting glucose; polycystic ovary syndrome; history of vascular disease
Fluoride supplementation	Live in area with inadequate water fluoridation (less than 0.7 ppm)
Genetic testing/counseling	Considering pregnancy and: patient, partner, or family member with history of genetic disorder or birth defect; exposure to teratogens; or African, Cajun, Caucasian, European, Eastern European (Ashkenazi) Jewish, French Canadian, Mediterranean, or Southeast Asian ancestry
Hemoglobin level assessment	Caribbean, Latin American, Asian, Mediterranean, or African ancestry; history of excessive menstrual flow
HAV vaccination	Chronic liver disease, clotting factor disorders, illegal drug users, individuals who work with HAV-infected nonhuman primates or with HAV in a research laboratory setting, individuals traveling to or working in countries that have high or intermediate endemicity of hepatitis A
HBV vaccination	Hemodialysis patients; patients who receive clotting factor concentrates; health care workers and public safety workers who have exposure to blood in the workplace; individuals in training in schools of medicine, dentistry, nursing, laboratory technology, and other allied health professions; injecting drug users; individuals with more than one sexual partner in the previous 6 months; individuals with a recently acquired STD; all clients in STD clinics; household contacts and sexual partners of individuals with chronic HBV infection; clients and staff of institutions for the developmentally disabled; international travelers who will be in countries with high or intermediate prevalence of chronic HBV infection for more than 6 months; inmates of correctional facilities
HCV testing	History of injecting illegal drugs; recipients of clotting factor concentrates before 1987; chronic (long-term) hemodialysis; persistently abnormal alanine aminotransferase levels; recipients of blood from donors who later tested positive for HCV infection; recipients of blood or blood-component transfusion or organ transplant before July 1992; occupational percutaneous or mucosal exposure to HCV-positive blood
HIV testing	More than one sexual partner since most recent HIV test or a sex partner with more than one sexual partner since most recent HIV test, seeking treatment for STDs, drug use by injection, history of prostitution, past or present sexual partner who is HIV positive or bisexual or injects drugs, long-term residence or birth in an area with high prevalence of HIV infection, history of transfusion from 1978 to 1985, invasive cervical cancer, adolescents who are or ever have been sexually active, adolescents entering detention facilities. Offer to women seeking preconception evaluation.
Influenza vaccination	Anyone who wishes to reduce the chance of becoming ill with influenza; chronic cardiovascular or pulmonary disorders, including asthma; chronic metabolic diseases, including diabetes mellitus, renal dysfunction, hemoglobinopathies, and immunosuppression (including immunosuppression caused by medications or by HIV); residents and employees of nursing homes and other long-term care facilities; individuals likely to transmit influenza to high-risk individuals (eg, household members and caregivers of the elderly, children aged from birth to 59 months, and adults with high-risk conditions); those with any condition (eg, cognitive

(continued)

Table 2. High-Risk Factors (continued)

Intervention	High-Risk Factor
Influenza vaccination (continued)	dysfunction, spinal cord injury, seizure or other neuromuscular disorder) that compromises respiratory function or the handling of respiratory secretions, or that increases the risk of aspiration; health care workers
Lipid profile assessment	Family history suggestive of familial hyperlipidemia; family history of premature (age younger than 50 years for men, age younger than 60 years for women) cardiovascular disease; diabetes mellitus; multiple coronary heart disease risk factors (eg, tobacco use, hypertension)
Mammography	Women who have had breast cancer or who have a first-degree relative (ie, mother, sister, or daughter) or multiple other relatives who have a history of premenopausal breast or breast and ovarian cancer
Meningococcal vaccination	Adults with anatomic or functional asplenia or terminal complement component deficiencies, first-year college students living in dormitories, microbiologists routinely exposed to Neisseria meningitidis isolates, military recruits, travel to hyperendemic or epidemic areas
MMR vaccination	Adults born in 1957 or later should be offered vaccination (one dose of MMR) if there is no proof of immunity or documentation of a dose given after first birthday; individuals vaccinated in 1963–1967 should be offered revaccination (two doses); health care workers, students entering college, international travelers, and rubella-negative postpartum patients should be offered a second dose.
Pneumococcal vaccination	Chronic illness, such as cardiovascular disease, pulmonary disease, diabetes mellitus, alcoholism, chronic liver disease, cerebrospinal fluid leaks, functional asplenia (eg, sickle cell disease) or splenectomy; exposure to an environment where pneumococcal outbreaks have occurred; immunocompromised patients (eg, HIV infection, hematologic or solid malignancies, chemotherapy, steroid therapy). Revaccination after 5 years may be appropriate for certain high-risk groups.
Rubella titer assessment	Childbearing age and no evidence of immunity
STD testing	History of multiple sexual partners or a sexual partner with multiple contacts, sexual contact with individuals with culture-proven STD, history of repeated episodes of STDs, attendance at clinics for STDs, women with developmental disabilities; routine screening for chlamydial infection for all sexually active women aged 25 years or younger and other asymptomatic women at high risk for infection; routine screening for gonorrheal infection for all sexually active adolescents and other asymptomatic women at high risk for infection; sexually active adolescents who exchange sex for drugs or money, use intravenous drugs, are entering a detention facility, or live in a high prevalence area should also be tested for syphilis.
Skin examination	Increased recreational or occupational exposure to sunlight; family or personal history of skin cancer; clinical evidence of precursor lesions
Thyroid-stimulating hormone testing	Strong family history of thyroid disease; autoimmune disease (evidence of subclinical hypothyroidism may be related to unfavorable lipid profiles)
Tuberculosis skin testing	HIV infection; close contact with individuals known or suspected to have tuberculosis; medical risk factors known to increase risk of disease if infected; born in country with high tuberculosis prevalence; medically underserved; low income; alcoholism; intravenous drug use; resident of long-term care facility (eg, correctional institutions, mental institutions, nursing homes and facilities); health professional working in high-risk health care facilities
Varicella vaccination	All susceptible adults and adolescents, including health care workers; household contacts of immunocompromised individuals; teachers; daycare workers; residents and staff of institutional settings, colleges, prisons, or military installations; adolescents and adults living in households with children; international travelers; nonpregnant women of childbearing age

Abbreviations: BMI indicates body mass index; HAV, hepatitis A virus; HBV, hepatitis B virus; HCV, hepatitis C virus; HIV, human immunodeficiency virus; MMR, measles–mumps–rubella; STD, sexually transmitted disease.

*For a more detailed discussion of bone density screening, see Osteoporosis. ACOG Practice Bulletin 50. American College of Obstetricians and Gynecologists. Obstet Gynecol 2004;103:203–16.

†For a more detailed discussion of colorectal cancer screening, see Smith RA, von Eschenbach AC, Wender R, Levin B, Byers T, Rothenberger D, et al. American Cancer Society guidelines for the early detection of cancer: update of early detection guidelines for prostate, colorectal, and endometrial cancers. Also: update 2001—testing for early lung cancer detection. Prostate Cancer Advisory Committee, ACS Colorectal Cancer Advisory Committee, ACS Endometrial Cancer Advisory Committee [published erratum appears in CA Cancer J Clin 2001;51:150]. CA Cancer J Clin 2001;51:38–75; quiz 77–80.

Primary and preventive care: periodic assessments. ACOG Committee Opinion No. 357. American College of Obstetricians and Gynecologists. Obstet Gynecol 2006;108:1615–22.

Screening Tests

How can the obstetrician–gynecologist decide when a screening test is warranted? Guidelines for obtaining and interpreting evidence regarding screening recommendations have been published (1). A number of characteristics must be considered in determining whether the benefits of screening exceed the risks and whether net benefits are cost-effective (2). Following are characteristics of ideal screening tests:

- *Characteristics of the disease:* Ordering batteries of diagnostic tests is an inefficient approach to identifying illness. Ordering screening tests to detect a specific disease or risk factor is a more cost-effective approach. Furthermore, the disease should be a serious threat to life or well-being, and the prevalence of the disease and its natural history should be understood. Additionally, early diagnosis of the disease should lead to an improved outcome.

- *Characteristics of the management of the disease:* For screening to be warranted, there must be an effective and acceptable intervention for patients with positive test results. Diagnostic tests and treatments for such persons should be readily available and affordable, and the treatments themselves should do more good than harm.

- *Characteristics of the screening test:* The screening test should be safe, simple, affordable, and acceptable to individuals being screened. Furthermore, a screening test must be valid and reliable. Test reliability is the extent to which a test yields reproducible results.

The validity of a screening test typically is described by four characteristics: *sensitivity, specificity, positive predictive value,* and *negative predictive value* (see "Principles of Evidence-Based Medicine"). Of these characteristics, positive predictive value is the characteristic of greatest value to the clinician. *Accuracy* is a distinct term that refers to the proportion of test results that are correct (2).

- *Sensitivity:* The ability of a test to detect those patients with the disease (ie, the number of individuals correctly identified as diseased, divided by the total number of diseased individuals). Thus, sensitivity also can be considered as the true positives ÷ (true positives + false negatives).

- *Specificity:* The ability of a test to detect those patients without the disease (ie, the number of individuals correctly identified as disease-free, divided by the total number without disease). Thus, specificity also can be considered as true negatives ÷ (true negatives + false positives).

- *Positive predictive value:* The proportion of individuals who test positive who actually have the disease (ie, the number of individuals with a positive test who are diseased, divided by the total number who test positive). Thus, positive predictive value also can be considered as true positives ÷ (true positives + false positives).

- *Negative predictive value:* The proportion of those who test negative who actually are disease-free (ie, the number of individuals with a negative test who are disease-free, divided by the total number who test negative). Thus, negative predictive value also can be considered as true negatives ÷ (true negatives + false negatives).

- *Accuracy:* The proportion of individuals who are correctly identified as being diseased or free of disease, divided by the total number of individuals tested. Thus, accuracy also can be considered as (true positives + true negatives) ÷ (true positives + false positives + true negatives + false negatives).

Because there usually is an overlap in test values between individuals with and without a disease, there is a need to predetermine cut points in test values that define whether the person is likely to have the disease or to be disease-free. These predetermined cut points often result in a trade-off between sensitivity and specificity, such that highly sensitive tests often will have low specificity and vice versa. The higher the sensitivity, the lower the number of false-negative test results; the higher the specificity, the lower the number of false-positive test results. The sensitivity and specificity of a screening test usually are based on public health considerations.

Obstetrician–gynecologists must make important decisions regarding the implications of positive and negative screening test results. It is particularly important to understand the role of disease prevalence in interpreting positive predictive value. In settings where disease prevalence is low, even a very sensitive test may have a low positive predictive value. Thus, the obstetrician–gynecologist can interpret a positive screening test result only in light of the prevalence of the disease being screened.

The U.S. Preventive Services Task Force

The benefits of a screening test rest largely on the clinical effectiveness of the test. In 1984, the U.S. Public Health Service commissioned the U.S. Preventive Services Task Force to evaluate the use of preventive services, including screening tests, by systematically reviewing available evidence of clinical effectiveness. The first Task Force determined that a screening test had to meet two requirements to be considered effective:

1. The test must be able to detect a target condition a) earlier than the condition would be detected without screening and b) with sufficient accuracy

to avoid producing large numbers of false-positive and false-negative test results.

2. Screening for and treating persons with early disease should improve health outcomes (ie, reduce disease-specific morbidity or mortality) compared with treating patients with signs or symptoms of the disease.

Even when screening tests accurately diagnose early disease, they are not considered useful unless the condition is treatable or preventable. Thus, treatment efficacy becomes a key consideration in evaluating screening effectiveness.

Initially very limited in topics for screening, the Guide to Clinical Preventive Services has evolved to cover more topics. The third Task Force is currently making recommendations regarding screening tests, counseling interventions, immunizations, and chemoprevention for people without symptoms or signs of the relevant condition (3). Current topics are available from the U.S. Preventive Services Task Force web site (see Resources).

The U.S. Preventive Services Task Force continues to conduct systematic reviews of evidence for the effectiveness of prevention services, including screening tests. The quality of the evidence is assessed on the basis of research design hierarchy, in which a proper randomized controlled trial has the highest score. In addition, the Task Force has added ratings of "good," "fair," and "poor" to assess the internal validity of each study, as well as the body of evidence for each key question regarding the preventive service and the overall body of evidence for the entire preventive service.

The Task Force translated the review of the evidence into recommendations for practice by assigning one of five possible letter codes, ranging from "A" (the Task Force strongly recommends that clinicians routinely provide the preventive service) to "I" (the Task Force concludes that the evidence is insufficient to make a recommendation) (see Table 1). As systematic reviews and recommendations from the Task Force are completed, the Agency for Health Care Research and Quality makes them available on its web site.

Screening Controversies

A number of health care organizations publish guidelines for the use of screening services based on age and population. These guidelines vary in part because of differences in interpretation of data on effectiveness and costs of screening. For example, although the use of annual screening mammography is recommended consistently for women aged 50 years and older, recommendations for younger women have been inconsistent. The American College of Obstetricians and Gynecologists (ACOG) recommends that mammography be performed every 1–2 years for women aged 40–49 years and annually thereafter (4), but the American Cancer Society (ACS) recommends annual mammography for all women aged 40 years and older (5).

Cervical cytology screening programs have reduced cervical cancer incidence and mortality rates dramatically in the United States. The Pap test is one of the most successful screening strategies and is the most cost-effective cancer screening program in history; however, controversies remain regarding the optimal use of this important tool. The American College of Obstetricians and Gynecologists and ACS recommend that all women begin to receive screening for cervical cancer approximately 3 years after initiation of vaginal intercourse but not later than age 21 years. However, ACS recommends screening at that point with either a Pap test every year or liquid-based cytologic testing every 2 years, whereas ACOG recommends annual screening (4, 5). The American College of Obstetricians and Gynecologists and ACS recommend that most women aged 30 years and older with three normal test results in a row may be screened every 2–3 years. However, ACS recommends that screening may stop at age 70 years for most women who have had three or more normal test results in a row and no abnormal test results in the preceding 10 years (5). In contrast, ACOG has no such upper age limit (6).

As policy-making bodies increasingly adopt the evidence-based approach to decision making, guidelines for screening become increasingly consistent. Because guidelines change often, becoming outdated as new technologies and research affect practice, physicians should refer to the most recent recommendations.

The few major discrepancies in screening recommendations from various authorities should not cause obstetrician–gynecologists to lose sight of agreements in recommendations for the vast majority of screening practices. Implementation of recommended screening practices, along with other clinical preventive services (including counseling and immunizations), will improve the health of women.

References

1. Barratt A, Irwig L, Glasziou P, Cumming RG, Raffle A, Hicks N, et al. Users' guides to the medical literature: XVII. How to use guidelines and recommendations about screening. Evidence-Based Medicine Working Group. JAMA 1999;281:2029–34.

2. Grimes DA, Schulz KF. Uses and abuses of screening tests [published erratum appears in Lancet 2008;371:1998]. Lancet 2002;359:881–4.

3. Harris RP, Helfand M, Woolf SH, Lohr KN, Mulrow CD, Teutsch SM, et al. Current methods of the US Preventive Services Task Force: a review of the process. Am J Prev Med 2001;20(suppl):21–35.

4. Primary and preventive care: periodic assessments. ACOG Committee Opinion No. 357 American College of Obstetricians and Gynecologists. Obstet Gynecol 2006; 108:1615–22.

5. Smith RA, Cokkinides V, Eyre HJ. American Cancer Society guidelines for the early detection of cancer, 2006. CA Cancer J Clin 2006;56:11–25; quiz 49–50.

6. Cervical cytology screening. ACOG Practice Bulletin No. 45. American College of Obstetricians and Gynecologists. Obstet Gynecol 2003;102:417–27.

Risk Assessment

Sharon T. Phelan

Risk factors for common health problems have been identified among selected age groups, such as teenagers and postmenopausal women. Screening programs to identify those common risk factors enable health care providers to provide care and patient education to prevent or delay the adverse consequences of disease (Box 16).

Adolescents

Puberty is the hallmark of early adolescence, when dramatic changes in the appearance and function of the body are accompanied by major changes in intellectual and social functioning. This section reviews the physical and emotional growth that occurs in early adolescence (approximately age 9–15 years) and risk behavior trends for adolescent girls. Understanding normative patterns of physical and psychosocial development enables health care providers to address the concerns of maturing adolescents and their parents.

Physical Development

Physical development, as signaled by breast development (thelarche), growth of pubic hair (pubarche), or both at a mean age 10 years, is sequential and proceeds over a 2-year period (range, 1–6 years). Menstrual function, or menarche, occurs on average at 12.8 years, within 2.3 years after breast budding and a little more than 1 year after girls have completed their largest growth spurt (mean age of peak height velocity, 11.5 years). Menstrual irregularity generally is considered normal during this time; achieving regular ovulatory cycle can take 1–2 years (1). Puberty is considered delayed if thelarche has not occurred by age 13 years or menarche has not occurred by age 16 years (2). Puberty is considered precocious when girls younger than 8 years experience physical changes.

The onset of puberty can be stressful for all girls, but it is especially disruptive to the emotional well-being of those who mature at younger ages. Early-maturing girls

---

Resources

Risk Assessment

American Cancer Society
http://www.cancer.org

American College of Preventive Medicine
http://acpm.org

U.S. Preventive Services Task Force
http://www.ahrq.gov/clinic/uspstfix.htm

---

tend to exhibit higher rates of depressive symptomatology, to associate with older peer groups, and to experience more conflict with their parents than girls who mature on time or late. Related to these factors is the increased likelihood that young adolescents who appear older will engage in substance use and early sexual activity. Despite their physically mature appearance, many early-maturing adolescents lack the emotional and cognitive maturity to resist negative influences from older individuals who befriend them. Because girls who mature early are more likely to be overweight and to have a negative body image than later-maturing adolescents (3), they are at increased risk of developing eating disorders.

Risk Behaviors

Despite recently declining rates, substance use among young adolescents is still common. According to the Monitoring the Future Study, an ongoing survey of the behaviors of secondary-school students, in 2006 approximately 39% of approximately 15,000 eighth-grade students reported having tried alcohol, and approximately 18% reported having been drunk (4), which is a decrease of approximately one third over the past decade. Two national studies (4, 5) demonstrate that 23% of high school students have smoked in the past month, and approximately 9% smoked 20 or more cigarettes in a single day in the past month. Beyond immediate health risks, the use of cigarettes, alcohol, or marijuana potentially serves as a gateway to harder drug use and increases the likelihood of substance dependence in adulthood (6).

Cigarette smoking and alcohol use are associated with adolescent development of depressive symptoms and early sexual risk-taking behaviors (7, 8). Because of the negative health consequences associated with early onset of substance use, screening for substance use has been recommended for preadolescents as young as 9 years (9).

Early sexual activity is a cause for concern, given that young adolescents tend to use condoms infrequently, to have sexual intercourse while under the influence of alcohol or drugs, and to choose partners who have engaged in high-risk behaviors (5). Currently, there is an increase in birthrates for teenagers after a number of years of decreasing rates. It is unclear if this change represents a minor variation or the beginning of a new trend. Adolescent birthrates had declined in the past decade, with the steepest rate of decline (23%) among African-American girls; the lowest rate of decline

---

Box 16

Routine Tests and Immunizations by Age

13–18 Years
- Pap test
- Chlamydia and gonorrhea testing
- Tetanus–diphtheria–pertussis booster
- Hepatitis B vaccine
- Human papillomavirus vaccine
- Meningococcal vaccine

19–39 Years
- Pap test
- Chlamydia test
- Human immunodeficiency virus test
- Human papillomavirus vaccine
- Tetanus–diphtheria–pertussis booster

40–64 Years
- Pap test
- Human immunodeficiency virus test
- Tetanus–diphtheria–pertussis booster
- Mammography
- Lipid profile assessment
- Colorectal cancer screening
- Fasting glucose screening
- Thyroid-stimulating hormone screening
- Flu vaccine
- Herpes zoster vaccine

65 Years and Older
- Pap test
- Mammography
- Colorectal cancer screening
- Herpes zoster vaccine
- Pneumococcal vaccine
- Flu vaccine
- Urinalysis
- Bone density screening
- Fasting glucose screening
- Lipid profile assessment
- Thyroid-stimulating hormone screening
- Tetanus–diphtheria booster

(9%) was among Hispanic girls (10). Slowly declining birthrates among Hispanic adolescents have been attributed to low use of contraceptives, low levels of knowledge about self-protection, and a lower incidence of abortions.

Early sexual debut and associated risk-taking behaviors increase adolescents' exposure to sexually transmitted diseases (STDs) (11). Chlamydia and gonorrhea pose immediate and long-term health consequences, including pelvic inflammatory disease, ectopic pregnancy, and infertility. Infection with human papillomavirus, another prevalent STD threatening U.S. adolescent girls, increases the risk of cervical cancer.

Adolescent girls are at increased risk of STDs not only because of their health-compromising behavior but also because of physiological reasons. Biologic risk factors that increase adolescent vulnerability include cervical ectopy (the presence of large areas of columnar, rather than stratified, squamous epithelium on the ectocervix), inadequate cervical mucous production, and underdeveloped immune responses (12). Given the potentially devastating consequences of STDs, physicians should discuss risks and self-protective behaviors relevant to sexual activity with young adolescent patients and should encourage parents to communicate with their daughters about these health issues (see Box 17) (13).

Emotional Development

For most Americans, the transition from childhood to adolescence brings a desire for increased independence and autonomy. This transition has been portrayed as an inevitably stressful time of intense familial conflict, but this depiction is exaggerated. Conflicts usually stem from differing viewpoints on how much freedom should be granted to adolescents, but such conflicts usually do not threaten the bond of healthy parent–child relationships. Early adolescents experience more episodes of negative emotion and more frequent mood changes than do preadolescents and adults (14). This characteristic is due in part to hormonal changes in puberty. However, the causes of mood swings are not entirely biologic. The degree to which adolescents experience mood disruptions depends on many nonbiologic factors, including peer acceptance, school performance, and family problems (15–17). Changes in schools and in family demands and responsibilities are likely to be stressful for adolescents, especially for those with less well-developed coping strategies (18).

Although episodes of depressed mood are typical in early adolescence, mood disorders are not considered normal. Compared with boys, girls in early adolescence are highly vulnerable to developing depressive disorders, which places them at higher risk of suicidal ideation. The 2006 Youth Risk Behavior Surveillance System survey showed that the prevalence rate of adolescents who are considering suicide is as high as 24% among ninth-grade girls, which is almost double the rate reported by boys who are the same age (5).

Confidentiality

When physicians screen their patients for high-risk behaviors, the provision of confidentiality is much more likely to result in honest responses and, thus, facilitate

---

Box 17

American College of Obstetricians and Gynecologists Recommendations for Screening for Sexually Transmitted Diseases

Routine Screening

- Sexually active women 25 years and younger should be routinely screened for chlamydial infection.
- All sexually active adolescents should be routinely screened for gonorrhea.
- Women with developmental disabilities should be screened for sexually transmitted diseases (STDs).
- HIV screening is recommended for women aged 19–64 years and adolescents who are or ever have been sexually active.*

Screening Based on Risk Factors

- Women with history of multiple sexual partners or a sexual partner with multiple contacts, sexual contact within individuals with culture-proven STDs, a history of repeated episodes of STDs, or attendance at clinics for STDs should be regularly screened for STDs.
- HIV screening is indicated for women with more than one sexual partner since most recent HIV test or a sexual partner with more than one sexual partner since most HIV test, current treatment for STDs, a history of drug use by injection, a history of prostitution, a past or present sexual partner who is HIV positive or bisexual or who injects drugs, long-term residence or birth in an area with a high-prevalence of HIV infection, a history of transfusion between 1978 and 1985, or invasive cervical cancer; adolescents who are or ever have been sexually active; and adolescents entering detention facilities. Testing should be offered to women seeking preconception care.
- Asymptomatic women aged 26 years and older who are at high risk of infection should be routinely screened for chlamydial infection and gonorrhea.

Abbreviations: HIV indicates human immunodeficiency virus; STDs, sexually transmitted diseases.

*Physicians should be aware of and follow their states' HIV screening requirements.

Modified from American College of Obstetricians and Gynecologists. Primary and preventive care: periodic assessments. ACOG Committee Opinion No. 357. Obstet Gynecol 2006;108:1615–22 and American College of Obstetricians and Gynecologists. Sexually transmitted diseases in adolescents. ACOG Committee Opinion No. 301. Obstet Gynecol 2004;104:891–8.

---

ning programs, drug and alcohol programs, and Title V maternal and child health programs. In addition, all states have statutes that address the rights of minors to consent to health care services. Because a minor's ability to consent differs among states, physicians should be aware of the laws of their individual states. Also, some states require reporting of sexual activity or pregnancy in very young teenagers to children, youth, and family divisions. Such cases should be reported especially if the partner is older, because of concerns of sexual or child abuse. Because most parents will ask questions about their child's visit, it is best to address confidentiality at the initial meeting. It is helpful to explain to parents that confidential services facilitate the development of responsible decision-making skills relevant to their children's health. Because confidentiality also should extend to test results, it may be necessary to work out alternative arrangements for payment of services with dependent adolescents at the initial visit (19).

Reproductive-Aged Women

Reproductive awareness should be a part of the routine health care of all women of childbearing age, from menarche to menopause. Reproductive health screening can help promote patient awareness of risks, health-enhancing behaviors, and family planning options.

Family Planning

Women should be assessed for the need for family planning and contraception, including emergency contraception. A woman's contraceptive needs change according to her age, other aspects of her health, lifestyle, and interest in future childbearing. In addition to contraceptive needs, women should consider the other health benefits and risks of specific methods. After an initial assessment, a woman's contraceptive needs should be reevaluated periodically to ensure that her health profile and preferences have not changed. New options and choices are available, allowing women much more flexibility (see "Family Planning").

Preconception Care

Women should be encouraged to plan their pregnancies for optimal outcome by identifying risks and minimizing exposure to them. A woman's plans for childbearing should be reviewed during routine reproductive heath screening (20). Women who are planning a pregnancy should undergo preconception counseling to identify if pregnancy might pose a risk, if a woman is at risk of having a baby with a birth defect, and if a woman needs to make a change in her health status or lifestyle to promote a healthy pregnancy (21). The components of such a program include extensive history gathering (including medical information; information on medication and

treatment and referral for other services. Federal law affords some protection for adolescents' confidentiality in obtaining care in settings, such as Title X family plan-

substance use or abuse, reproductive history, nutritional status—especially extremes of nutrition—and environmental or work exposures) and physical assessment (including body mass index and dental status). The patient then should be counseled regarding risk factors and appropriate lifestyle changes to promote a successful pregnancy.

More in-depth genetic counseling may be appropriate for couples with genetic concerns or identifiable risks of having a child with heritable abnormalities. Recognizing positive carrier status before conception enables couples to understand the risks outside the emotional context of pregnancy and allows time for more thorough evaluation. Women should be advised of the effect of advancing maternal age on their ability to have children and the risk of birth defects and complications of pregnancy.

Hereditary Risk Assessment and Screening

Because of the human genome project, more and more illnesses are being found to have an identifiable genetic component. This number will continue to grow and will require practitioners to review their standard questions and screens to be sure they are current. There tend to be two prime times when a more detailed family history is gathered and affects care: the new patient intake history and the preconception or prenatal history. Some hereditary disorders are more pertinent to screening before or early in a pregnancy. They include cystic fibrosis, neural tube defect, fragile X syndrome, polycystic kidney disease, neurofibromatosis, Marfan syndrome, various dystrophies, and others as indicated by age and ethnicity.

Other hereditary concerns affect the woman and her ongoing health. A patient with menorrhagia might require testing for a clotting disorder. A patient with the history of a deep vein thrombosis or pulmonary embolism without a good reason may benefit from a thrombophilia testing to see if she requires long-term anticoagulation. Many hemoglobinopathies affect women and their pregnancies and should be considered in women with anemia and in women in high-risk ethnic groups. A strong family history of cardiovascular (CV) disease, diabetes mellitus (type 1 and 2), bleeding disorders, high lipid levels, thyroid disorders, or glaucoma should prompt early screening and possibly more frequent screening. The patient should be informed of her increased long-term risks and be encouraged to make lifestyle changes or seek intervention to minimize the genetic expression (22).

One area that has become more specific in screening and potentially genetic testing is hereditary cancer syndromes. These syndromes predispose women at younger age to hereditary ovarian and breast cancer. Often the patients with a given gene mutation are at greater risk of other specific cancers, hence the classification of hereditary cancer syndromes.

BRCA

BRCA1 and *BRCA2* increase the lifetime risk of breast cancer to 65–85%, compared with the background risk of 12%. Approximately 1–3% of women have this high risk of developing breast cancer due to an inherited predisposition. Lifetime risk is higher than background risk at any age group but accounts only for approximately 5% of all cases of breast cancer. One third of patients with *BRCA* mutations will have a diagnosis of breast cancer before age 50 years. Therefore, screening should start at age 30 years, if not earlier (22). However, screening is challenging in the young patient because mammography is not reliable even with the adjunct use of breast ultrasonography. The American Cancer Society's guideline recommends magnetic resonance imaging screening for women with *BRCA* mutations, untested first-degree relatives of women with *BRCA* mutations, and any patient with a family history predictive of a lifetime cancer risk of at least 25% (23).

A *BRCA* mutation increases the risks of ovarian cancer (8–13% of newly diagnosed ovarian cancers) and fallopian tube cancer, which are more difficult to screen. Women with *BRCA1* have a 35–56% risk of developing ovarian cancer by age 70 years; *BRCA2* carriers have a 10–27% risk. For this reason, the National Comprehensive Cancer Network recommends that women with *BRCA1* or *BRCA2* mutations who do not receive a risk-reducing bilateral salpingo-oophorectomy be screened for ovarian cancer twice yearly with transvaginal ultrasonography and CA 125. The use of oral contraceptive pills until a bilateral salpingo-oophorectomy or menopause also appears to decrease the risk of ovarian cancer in this population (22, 24). Recent studies show a relationship between *BRCA1* and *BRCA2* and an increased risk of prostate cancer in male relatives (25).

Hereditary Nonpolyposis Colorectal Cancer

Hereditary nonpolyposis colorectal cancer (HNPCC), or Lynch syndrome, is an autosomal-dominant syndrome that is more genetically heterogeneous than recognized before; at least four genes are associated with HNPCC, which accounts for 3–6% of colon cancer cases. Not only is the risk of colon cancer (60–80% lifetime risk) increased; so are the risks of gastric, endometrial (40–60% lifetime risk), ovarian (12% lifetime risk), hepatobiliary, and urinary tract cancers (26). This syndrome accounts for 2–3% of all cases of endometrial and colon cancer. In fact, the endometrial cancer may be the first or sentinel cancer. Diagnosis often is established by family history. The diagnostic criteria include the following:

- Three or more relatives have an HNPCC-associated cancer, including cancer of the colon, endometrium, ovary, small bowel, ureter, or renal pelvis.

- Two or more successive generations are affected.
- Cancer is diagnosed in at least one individual who is younger than 50 years.
- Familial adenomatosis polyposis (FAP) should be excluded in any colorectal cancers (27).

FAMILIAL ADENOMATOUS POLYPOSIS

Familial adenomatous polyposis also is genetically heterogeneous. At least two genes are associated with FAP. The affected patient will be found to have hundreds of colonic polyps at an early age. The patient also may have osteomas, dental abnormalities, and hepatoblastomas (28).

Before patients undergo genetic testing, they need to have counseling regarding the risks and benefits of such testing and of the impact the results may have on the patients and their families. Medical, psychologic, and financial risks may be associated with finding out that one is a carrier of a hereditary cancer gene mutation. Although most clinicians can provide basic counseling, many patients may benefit from more extensive counseling provided by a genetic counselor or medical geneticist. It is important to discuss issues of confidentiality relative to employment, insurance, and other family members, especially issues relating to state or federal requirements regarding genetic screening, reporting, disclosure, breach of confidentiality, and discrimination based on genetic information (29).

Perimenopause

As most women approach menopause, they experience irregular menstrual function, as well as the menopausal symptoms of hot flushes and vaginal dryness. They should be counseled about prevention of osteoporosis and modifications in lifestyle with regard to diet, exercise, and routine health assessments. Perimenopause is a time of risk of excessive weight gain and the associated health risks.

Prevention of unintended pregnancy assumes increasing importance during the perimenopausal years. Pregnancy rates have increased over the past decade. Although some pregnancies are planned, up to 75% of pregnancies in women older than 40 years are unintended. It is difficult to determine exactly when there is no longer a need for contraception; approximately 85% of women are postmenopausal by 55 years. Therefore, fertility control should be encouraged (see "Family Planning").

Postmenopausal Women

A century ago, the average life expectancy for women was slightly more than 50 years. Today it is 80 years, and with continuing medical advances it will probably be higher in the future. Because the number of U.S. women older than 60 years during the next decade will be increasing thanks to the baby boomer generation, the goal for physicians who care for these women should be to prevent morbidity and postpone death. These goals must be achieved within a framework of maintaining quality of life. Many of the conditions affecting older women are covered in more detail elsewhere in this volume. This section focuses on screening for conditions and problems for which the older woman is at risk.

Aging

As women age, their physical abilities slowly decline. Also they undergo a progressive decrease in bone mineralization, muscle mass, cardiopulmonary reserve, microsomal enzyme activity, sensory acuity, and connective tissue integrity (30). Whereas knowledge acquired with socialization tends to remain stable in older women, the speed of acquisition and retrieval of new information, creativity, fluidity of thought, and the ability to solve problems decrease. Assessing these mental and physical losses is an important part of examinations.

Difficulties in adjusting to changes in self-image may be stressful. Loss of family and friends increases with age. By reaching age 65 years or older, 36% of women and 16% of men are living alone. Also, 12% of the women older than 65 years and 7% of the men are living in poverty (31) and often have associated financial and social problems. Loss of independence also may occur.

Cardiovascular Disease and Stroke

Heart disease is the leading cause of death in women older than 65 years: 1,553 in 100,000 women died of heart disease in 2004, compared with 1,082 in 100,000 for all cancer mortalities (32). Risk factors for coronary artery disease include cigarette smoking, hypertension, diabetes mellitus, age older than 55 years or premature menopause, a family history of premature coronary artery disease, and high-density lipoprotein cholesterol (HDL-C) concentration less than 40 mg/dL (HDL-C level greater than 60 mg/dL is protective). In addition, obese and physically inactive women may be at increased risk of coronary artery disease (33). All women should undergo lipid profile assessment every 5 years beginning at age 45 years (21).

Cerebrovascular disease is the third leading cause of death in the United States, after heart disease and cancer. Risk factors include hypertension, smoking, and diabetes mellitus. Counseling should include encouraging the patient to stop smoking.

Cancer Risks

Cancer is the second most common cause of death in women, so it is desirable to detect it in the precancerous or early invasive stage. This detection is possible for cervical cancer with the Pap test and for breast cancer with mammography. Current guidelines for using these modalities should be applied. Individuals in high-risk groups should be screened with colonoscopy approximately every 1–2 years or more often (34). For patients who are not at high risk, the preferred screening method is a colonoscopy every 10 years. If that screening is not possible, other appropriate methods include annual studies for fecal occult blood testing, sigmoidoscopy, or both every 5 years starting at age 50 years. If bleeding or polyps are noted, colonoscopy should be used (35).

The incidence of lung cancer increased dramatically in the second half of the 20th century, probably because of the increased number of women who initiated smoking starting in the 1940s and continuing through today. Deaths from lung cancer are more common than deaths from breast cancer, even though the incidence of breast cancer is much greater. The reason is the lack of an adequate screening method for early detection of lung cancer. This fact is yet another reason to counsel women to stop smoking.

Ovarian cancer and pancreatic cancer are common causes of female mortality. However, they are difficult to diagnose in the early, treatable stage because in many cases they do not produce symptoms. At present, no screening tests are available for these diseases.

The risk of skin cancer also increases with age. Risk factors for melanoma include having fair skin and hair color, a family history of melanoma, large congenital nevi, and pigmented lesions that meet the criteria for dysplastic nevi (macular and papular components, irregular borders, variegated pigmentation within the same lesion, and a diameter of 5–12 mm) (36). An annual full skin examination is recommended for women older than 50 years to detect evidence of squamous cell cancer, basal cell cancer, and melanoma.

Metabolic Diseases

Hypothyroidism is much more common in old women than in young women. Symptoms and signs include lethargy, constipation, dry skin, alopecia, memory impairment, and depression. Unfortunately, these symptoms and signs often are ascribed to menopause, depression, or aging. Many patients with hypothyroidism are obese and may have markedly elevated cholesterol and triglyceride levels. The prevalence of hypothyroidism in otherwise healthy individuals is approximately 5%. Determination of thyroid stimulating hormone levels is a good screening test for hypothyroidism. It is reasonable to screen older women every 1–2 years, but there is no consensus on this practice. Women with elevated cholesterol levels or with the symptoms described should be tested for hypothyroidism (21, 37).

Hyperthyroidism is less common in elderly individuals, but it does occur. Symptoms include decreased energy, weight loss, muscle weakness, rapid pulse rate, and elevated systolic blood pressure. Elderly women with hyperthyroidism also may present with atrial fibrillation or congestive heart failure. Women who present with these symptoms should be tested for hyperthyroidism (21, 37).

Type 1 diabetes mellitus is caused by the destruction of pancreatic islet cells. Although it usually occurs in childhood, it may occur at any age. Type 2 diabetes mellitus usually is seen in older patients than type 1 diabetes mellitus because of relative insulin and glucose insensitivity and impairment of insulin release. Diabetes affects an increasing number of women in the U.S. population, and obesity is a definite risk factor. African-American women receive the diagnosis of diabetes mellitus at twice the rate of white women, with the overall rate increasing with age. Other risk factors include a family history of diabetes mellitus and gestational diabetes mellitus. Women with these risk factors should probably be screened for glucose intolerance (38, 39).

Urinary and Fecal Incontinence

Urinary incontinence is a common problem in older women; it affects as many as 15% of older women living in their own homes and as many as 40% of women living in nursing homes (40, 41). Continence is a complicated issue that involves the interaction among the patient's neurologic state, mental status, anatomic condition, and hormonal balance. In some cases, medications may complicate or even be the cause of the problem. Embarrassment may prevent the patient from bringing this problem to the attention of her physician. The physician should ask the patient whether she is ever incontinent of urine and, if the answer is affirmative, then should question the patient as to the type and extent of the incontinence.

Likewise, with fecal incontinence, it is important to ask the patient whether she is incontinent of gas or stool. If she does experience incontinence, the physician should perform a physical examination and appropriate testing as the first steps in correcting the problem.

Osteoporosis

Approximately 13–18% of U.S. women aged 50 years and older have osteoporosis; another 37–50% have low bone mass (osteopenia) (42). Osteoporosis is caused by increased bone absorption and reduced bone formation. These changes lead to decreased bone density and resulting fractures. Evidence has indicated that osteoporosis of the maxillary and mandibular bones also may be responsible for tooth loss and resulting nutritional concerns. Thus, a woman's dentist may be the first to identify her osteoporosis (43).

Osteoporosis is generally a slow process that begins in the fourth decade of life and is accelerated by several risk factors, particularly genetics (see "Osteoporosis") (42). Bone mineral density testing to diagnose osteoporosis should be recommended for postmenopausal women who 1) are 65 years or older, 2) are younger than 65 years but have one or more risk factors for osteoporosis, or 3) have had fractures. These women should be counseled about such preventive measures as calcium consumption, weight-bearing exercises, smoking cessation, moderation of alcohol intake, and fall prevention strategies.

Exercise

It is important to encourage aging women to maintain or develop an active exercise program. Even if they have chronic illness, exercise may improve symptoms and even arrest the condition. Women should be encouraged to participate in three types of exercise: 1) endurance, 2) resistance, and 3) balance training. Endurance training improves CV status. Resistance training improves muscle mass and strength and slows the rate of bone loss. Balance training improves balance, which may help prevent falls (44). However, strenuous or excessive exercise can cause injuries, so older women should gradually build up to an exercise program that promotes these three components.

Safety Factors

Most safety issues would seem to be a matter of common sense for physicians and patients, yet often they are not considered as carefully as they should be. The annual health maintenance visit is a good time to discuss safety issues with patients, particularly as they may affect an aging person. Active older women who ride bicycles, horses, motorcycles, or scooters, or those who roller skate or ice skate, should be asked whether they wear a helmet as protective gear during these activities. Because balance often is a problem for older individuals, the use of very high heels should be discouraged. The use of good footwear for athletic activities should be encouraged. Aging women should be cautioned not to move as rapidly as they used to because of the potential for balance problems.

Another issue is safety in the home. Screening should include domestic violence inquiries and questions about the presence, safe storage, and the use of firearms in the home. (35).

Finally, physicians should evaluate the patient's vision and hearing and recommend corrective measures, if needed. Corrective glasses or hearing aids can be obtained where necessary, and referral for cataract surgery or other corrective eye therapy can be made. If there are concerns regarding vision or cognition, it may be wise to encourage family members to seek evaluation of the patient's driving and independent living arrangements.

Drug Interactions

It is difficult to reach old age without having some illnesses or at least unpleasant symptoms. Therefore, most elderly individuals use some form of medication, and many use multiple medications. These medications may consist of prescription drugs, over-the-counter medications, and alternative therapies. The patient should be encouraged to bring all the medications she is taking to the annual health maintenance visit, where their use, adverse effects, and drug interactions should be discussed.

The dosages for many medications that are appropriate for women during the reproductive years may be inappropriate in older patients for a number of reasons, including decreased lean body mass, changes in renal and hepatic function, and increased sensitivity to side effects. Drugs always should be prescribed in the lowest dosage possible in an older individual and be increased as necessary. When a drug is prescribed, it is important for the patient to understand the reasons for taking the prescribed drug, the potential benefits and side effects that may be expected, and the dosage schedule that has been ordered. The physician should be satisfied that the patient understands the directions, can read the label, can remove the cap from the bottle, and has some system for remembering whether she has taken the medication. If necessary, a family member should be included in the explanation of the directions for medication use.

Dental Problems

Although tooth loss may be attributed to osteoporosis, most tooth loss experienced by older individuals is related to periodontal disease. Of women older than 55 years, 44% have periodontal disease. The mouth should be examined for the presence of this condition, and regular dental examinations should be encouraged.

Mental Health Problems

Of patient visits to primary care physicians, 50–60% are for signs and symptoms that have a behavioral or emotional component and 25% of patient visits are for psychiatric disorders. Women have a 2–3 times greater risk of depression than do men in their lifetime (45). Depression is common and may be associated with bereavement, disappointment, or other types of loss. Social isolation may intensify the problem. Depression may be transient and in many cases requires no therapy. Mild antidepressant agents may be helpful over the short period.

Major depression is a greater problem. The average woman has approximately a 20% chance of having a major depressive disorder at some time during her life. Depressed women appear tired, sad, and disinterested. Often they speak slowly, have difficulty concentrating, and answer questions after a delay of several seconds. Women should be screened for depression using the American Psychiatric Association's diagnostic criteria (46, 47). The presence of five or more of these criteria is considered indicative of depression; depressed mood and loss of interest or pleasure in most activities are considered the most serious symptoms of depression (see "Mental Health Issues").

A decline in cognitive functioning (eg, problems remembering names or appointments or difficulty solving complex problems) is a normal part of the aging process. If the decline is not within normal limits given the person's age, evaluation should determine whether the impairment is attributable to a specific mental disorder (eg, depression) or a medical or neurologic condition (eg, stroke or hypothyroidism) that can be treated (47).

Sexuality

Sexuality is a behavioral phenomenon influenced by many factors, including the health and physiological state of both members of a couple and the importance that each individual places on sexual activity as a source of comfort and gratification. It is strongly influenced by other associations in a person's life, including psychologic, biologic, and relationship factors. With advancing age, sexual function and satisfaction may decrease. Failing health and many medications may contribute to a decrease in function. However, sexual activity can and should be enjoyed into old age. The physician should ascertain if there are problems with sexual behavior and present options when possible.

References

1. Strasburger VC, Brown RT. Growth and development. In: Adolescent medicine: a practical guide. 2nd ed. Philadelphia (PA): Lippincott–Raven; 1998. p. 1–22.

2. Adams Hillard PJ. Menstruation in young girls: a clinical perspective. Obstet Gynecol 2002;99:655–62.

3. Striegel-Moore RH, McMahon RP, Biro FM, Schreiber G, Crawford PB, Voorhees C. Exploring the relationship between timing of menarche and eating disorder symptoms in Black and White adolescent girls. Int J Eat Disord 2001;30:421–33.

4. Johnston LD, O'Malley PM, Bachman JG, Schulenberg JE. Montoring the future national results on adolescent drug use: overview of key findings, 2007. Bethesda (MD): National Institute on Drug Abuse; 2008. Available at: http://www.monitoringthefuture.org/pubs/monographs/overview2007.pdf. Retrieved November 12, 2008.

5. Eaton DK, Kann L, Kinchen S, Ross J, Hawkins J, Harris WA, et al. Youth risk behavior surveillance—United States, 2005. Centers for Disease Control and Prevention. MMWR Surveill Summ 2006;55:1–108.

6. Lynskey MT, Heath AC, Bucholz KK, Slutske WS, Madden PA, Nelson EC, et al. Escalation of drug use in early-onset cannabis users vs co-twin controls. JAMA 2003;289: 427–33.

7. Paxton RJ, Valois RF, Watkins KW, Huebner ES, Drane JW. Associations between depressed mood and clusters of health risk behaviors. Am J Health Behav 2007;31:272–83.

8. Brooks TL, Harris SK, Thrall JS, Woods ER. Association of adolescent risk behaviors with mental health symptoms in high school students. J Adolesc Health 2002;31:240–6.

9. DuRant RH, Smith JA, Kreiter SR, Krowchuk DP. The relationship between early age of onset of initial substance use and engaging in multiple health risk behaviors among young adolescents. Arch Pediatr Adolesc Med 1999;153: 286–91.

10. Hamilton BE, Martin JA, Ventura SJ. Births; preliminary data for 2006. Natl Vital Stat Rep 2007;56(7):1–18. Available at: http://www.cdc.gov/nchs/data/nvsr/nvsr56/nvsr56_07.pdf. Retrieved November 14, 2008.

11. Kahn JA, Rosenthal SL, Succop PA, Ho GY, Burk RD. Mediators of the association between age of first sexual intercourse and subsequent human papillomavirus infection. Pediatrics 2002;109:E5.

12. Collins SI, Mazloomzadeh S, Winter H, Rollason TP, Blomfield P, Young LS, et al. Proximity of first intercourse to menarche and the risk of human papillomavirus infection: a longitudinal study. Int J Cancer 2005;114:498–500.

13. Sexually transmitted diseases in adolescents. ACOG Committee Opinion No. 301. American College of Obstetricians and Gynecologists. Obstet Gynecol 2004; 104:891–8.

14. Arnett JJ. Adolescent storm and stress, reconsidered. Am Psychol 1999;54:317–26.

15. Simantov E, Schoen C, Klein JD. Health-compromising behaviors: why do adolescents smoke or drink?: identifying underlying risk and protective factors. Arch Pediatr Adolesc Med 2000;154:1025–33.

16. Galaif ER, Sussman S, Newcomb MD, Locke TF. Suicidality, depression, and alcohol use among adolescents: a review of empirical findings. Int J Adolesc Med Health 2007;19:27–35.

17. DuBois DL, Silverthorn N. Natural mentoring relationships and adolescent health: evidence from a national study. Am J Public Health 2005;95:518–24.

18. Burgess Dowdell E. Alcohol use, smoking, and feeling unsafe: health risk behaviors of two urban seventh grade classes. Issues Compr Pediatr Nurs 2006;29:157–71.

19. The initial reproductive health visit. ACOG Committee Opinion No. 335. American College of Obstetricians and Gynecologists. Obstet Gynecol 2006;107:1215–9.

20. American College of Obstetricians and Gynecologists. Guidelines for women's health care. 3rd ed. Washington, DC: ACOG; 2007.

21. Primary and preventive care: periodic assessments. ACOG Committee Opinion No. 357. American College of Obstetricians and Gynecologists. Obstet Gynecol 2006; 108:1615–22.

22. Dent R, Warner E. Screening for hereditary breast cancer. Semin Oncol 2007;34:392–400.

23. Saslow D, Boetes C, Burke W, Harms S, Leach MO, Lehman CD, et al. American Cancer Society guidelines for breast screening with MRI as an adjunct to mammography.

American Cancer Society Breast Cancer Advisory Group [published erratum appears in CA Cancer J Clin 2007;57:185]. CA Cancer J Clin 2007;57:75–89.

24. Kehoe SM, Kauff ND. Screening and prevention of hereditary gynecologic cancers. Semin Oncol 2007;34:406–10.

25. Rosen EM, Fan S, Goldberg ID. BRCA1 and prostate cancer. Cancer Invest 2001;19:396–412.

26. Soravia C, van der Klift H, Brundler MA, Blouin JL, Wijnen J, Hutter P, et al. Prostate cancer is part of the hereditary non-polyposis colorectal cancer (HNPCC) tumor spectrum. Am J Med Genet 2003;121A:159–62.

27. Elective and risk-reducing salpingo-oophorectomy. ACOG Practice Bulletin No. 89. American College of Obstetricians and Gynecologists. Obstet Gynecol 2008;111:231–41.

28. Matloff ET, Brierley KL, Chimera CM. A clinician's guide to hereditary colon cancer. Cancer J 2004;10:280–7.

29. Offit K, Thom P. Ethical and legal aspects of cancer genetic testing. Semin Oncol 2007;34:435–43.

30. Stenchever MA. Care of aging women. Clin Update Womens Health Care 2004;III(1):1–79.

31. Spraggins RE. We the people: women and men in the United States: Census 2000 special report: CENSR-20. Washington, DC: U.S. Census Bureau; 2005. Available at: http://www.census.gov/prod/2005pubs/censr-20.pdf. Retrieved November 12, 2008.

32. National Center for Health Statistics. Health data for all ages (HDAA). Hyattsville (MD): NCHS; 2008. Available at: http://www.cdc.gov/nchs/health_data_for_all_ages.htm. Retrieved November 12, 2008.

33. Executive Summary of The Third Report of The National Cholesterol Education Program (NCEP) Expert Panel on Detection, Evaluation, And Treatment of High Blood Cholesterol In Adults (Adult Treatment Panel III). Expert Panel on Detection, Evaluation, and Treatment of High Blood Cholesterol in Adults. JAMA 2001;285:2486–97.

34. Smith RA, von Eschenbach AC, Wender R, Levin B, Byers T, Rothenberger D, et al. American Cancer Society guidelines for the early detection of cancer: update of early detection guidelines for prostate, colorectal, and endometrial cancers. Also: update 2001--testing for early lung cancer detection. ACS Prostate Cancer Advisory Committee. ACS Colorectal Cancer Advisory Committee. ACS Endometrial Cancer Advisory Committee [published erratum appears in CA Cancer J Clin 2001;51:150]. CA Cancer J Clin 2001;51:38–75; quiz 77–80.

35. Colonoscopy and colorectal cancer screening and prevention. ACOG Committee Opinion No. 384. American College of Obstetricians and Gynecologists. Obstet Gynecol 2007; 110:1199–202.

36. Greene MH, Clark WH Jr, Tucker MA, Kraemer KH, Elder DE, Fraser MC. High risk of malignant melanoma in melanoma-prone families with dysplastic nevi. Ann Intern Med 1985;102:458–65.

37. Eskelinen SI, Vahlberg TJ, Isoaho RE, Lopponen MK, Kivela SL, Irjala KM. Associations of thyroid-stimulating hormone and free thyroxine concentrations with health and life satisfaction in elderly adults. Endocr Pract 2007; 13:451–7.

38. National Center for Health Statistics. Age specific prevalence of diagnosed diabetes by race/ethnicity and sex in the United States, 2005. Hyattsville (MD): NCHS; 2005. Available at: http://www.cdc.gov/diabetes/statistics/prev/national/fig2004.htm. Retrieved November 12, 2008.

39. Harris MI, Flegal KM, Cowie CC, Eberhardt MS, Goldstein DE, Little RR, et al. Prevalence of diabetes, impaired fasting glucose, and impaired glucose tolerance in U.S. adults. The Third National Health and Nutrition Examination Survey, 1988–1994. Diabetes Care 1998;21:518–24.

40. Cigolle CT, Langa KM, Kabeto MU, Tian Z, Blaum CS. Geriatric conditions and disability: the Health and Retirement Study. Ann Intern Med 2007;147:156–64.

41. Morley JE. Urinary incontinence and the community-dwelling elder: a practical approach to diagnosis and management for the primary care geriatrician. Clin Geriatr Med 2004;20:427–35, v–vi.

42. Osteoporosis. ACOG Practice Bulletin No. 50. American College of Obstetricians and Gynecologists. Obstet Gynecol 2004;103:203–16.

43. Civitelli R, Pilgram TK, Dotson M, Muckerman J, Lewandowski N, Armamento-Villareal R, et al. Alveolar and postcranial bone density in postmenopausal women receiving hormone/estrogen replacement therapy: a randomized, double-blind, placebo-controlled trial [published erratum appears in Arch Intern Med 2004;164:96]. Arch Intern Med 2002;162:1409–15.

44. Hale RW. Women and exercise. Clin Update Womens Health Care 2004;III(3):1–68.

45. Dell D. Mood and anxiety disorders. Clin Update Womens Health Care 2008;VII(2):1–98.

46. Lapid MI, Rummans TA. Evaluation and management of geriatric depression in primary care. Mayo Clin Proc 2003;78:1423–9.

47. American Psychiatric Association. Diagnostic and statistical manual of mental disorders: DSM-IV-TR. 4th ed., text revision. Washington, DC: American Psychiatric Association; 2000.

Role of Exercise, Diet, and Medical Intervention in Weight Management

Raul Artal, George A. Bray, Catherine M. Champagne, and Gerald S. Zavorsky

Overweight and Obesity

Epidemiology

The epidemic of obesity that began in the 1980s continues unabated (1). This worldwide epidemic increases health concerns for women. Reports from the World Health Organization (2) and the National Heart, Lung, and Blood Institute recommend the use of the body mass index (BMI), which is defined as weight in kilograms divided by height in meters squared (Table 3). Use of the waist circumference to gauge the degree of central adiposity also is recommended (1, 2).

More than 30% of adult Americans are obese, and the prevalence of obesity is higher in women than in men (33.4% compared with 27.5%), based on direct measurement. The prevalence of obesity in children and adults has increased more than 50% in the past decade (3). The progression of this epidemic in the United States is shown in Figure 8. This epidemic also has led to concerns regarding the widespread development of diabetes mellitus, heart disease, and complications associated with these disorders. A recent report shows that more than 100,000 deaths in the United States each year are caused by obesity (4). Although obesity represents excessive caloric intake, obese individuals often are malnourished in regard to nutrients. Thus, the ability to assess nutritional status is important to clinical care.

A major consequence of obesity is an increase in mortality rates. It has been estimated that obesity is responsible for approximately 100,000–300,000 deaths each year. As body weight (usually expressed in BMI) increases, there is a curvilinear increase in the risk of mortality, mostly increased deaths from heart disease, diabetes mellitus, hypertension, and cancer. This relationship exists for men, women, and all ethnic groups that have been studied, but the steepness of the increase in mortality rates varies among groups. Obesity is associated with the following morbidities: metabolic syndrome, diabetes mellitus, gallbladder disease, sleep apnea, musculoskeletal disease, psychosocial distress, and cancer (breast, endometrial, colon and gallbladder). There also is an increased risk of CV disease, which can be attributed to a number of factors, including 1) a decrease in high-density lipoprotein cholesterol levels that is associated with insulin resistance and obesity and 2) an increase in plasminogen activator inhibitor-1. Studies of weight loss have shown that these levels return to normal with weight loss (2, 5). Obesity also is associated with hypertension. At least two events may account for the increase in the severity of hypertension: 1) an increase in insulin, which increases sodium reabsorption by the renal tubule, and 2) the change in vascular resistance and cardiac function needed to compensate for the higher blood flow in obese individuals.

Causes

LIFESTYLE FACTORS

Several lifestyle factors play a role in the development of obesity, many as early as in childhood. These factors include diet, an active compared with a sedentary lifestyle, and cessation of smoking. The consumption of sugar or high-fructose beverages by children may enhance the risk of rapid weight gain. Given that the standard serving of a cola drink has gone from 6 ounces to 24 ounces or more, the caloric intake has increased dramatically from this source.

A second relationship between obesity and carbohydrate intake involves the rate at which glucose is absorbed, expressed as the glycemic index. A food with a high glycemic index is readily digested and produces a large and rapid increase in plasma glucose levels. A food with a low glycemic index, however, is digested more slowly and is associated with a slower and lower increase in glucose levels. Foods with a high glycemic index do not suppress food intake as much as foods with a low glycemic index. Foods with a low glycemic index include fruits and vegetables that tend to have fiber, plus legumes and whole wheat. Potatoes, white rice, and white bread have a high glycemic index (6).

Resources

Diet, Exercise, and Weight Management

American College of Sports Medicine
http://www.acsm.org

American Council on Exercise
http://www.acefitness.org

American Dietetic Association
http://www.eatright.org

Office of the Surgeon General
http://www.surgeongeneral.gov

U.S. Food and Drug Administration
http://www.fda.gov

Table 3. Body Mass Index Chart

	Normal						Overweight					Obese										Extreme Obesity															
BMI	19	20	21	22	23	24	25	26	27	28	29	30	31	32	33	34	35	36	37	38	39	40	41	42	43	44	45	46	47	48	49	50	51	52	53	54
Height (inches)															Body Weight (pounds)																					
58	91	96	100	105	110	115	119	124	129	134	138	143	148	153	158	162	167	172	177	181	186	191	196	201	205	210	215	220	224	229	234	239	244	248	253	258
59	94	99	104	109	114	119	124	128	133	138	143	148	153	158	163	168	173	178	183	188	193	198	203	208	212	217	222	227	232	237	242	247	252	257	262	267
60	97	102	107	112	118	123	128	133	138	143	148	153	158	163	168	174	179	184	189	194	199	204	209	215	220	225	230	235	240	245	250	255	261	266	271	276
61	100	106	111	116	122	127	132	137	143	148	153	158	164	169	174	180	185	190	195	201	206	211	217	222	227	232	238	243	248	254	259	264	269	275	280	285
62	104	109	115	120	126	131	136	142	147	153	158	164	169	175	180	186	191	196	202	207	213	218	224	229	235	240	246	251	256	262	267	273	278	284	289	295
63	107	113	118	124	130	135	141	146	152	158	163	169	175	180	186	191	197	203	208	214	220	225	231	237	242	248	254	259	265	270	278	282	287	293	299	304
64	110	116	122	128	134	140	145	151	157	163	169	174	180	186	192	197	204	209	215	221	227	232	238	244	250	256	262	267	273	279	285	291	296	302	308	314
65	114	120	126	132	138	144	150	156	162	168	174	180	186	192	198	204	210	216	222	228	234	240	246	252	258	264	270	276	282	288	294	300	306	312	318	324
66	118	124	130	136	142	148	155	161	167	173	179	186	192	198	204	210	216	223	229	235	241	247	253	260	266	272	278	284	291	297	303	309	315	322	328	334
67	121	127	134	140	146	153	159	166	172	178	185	191	198	204	211	217	223	230	236	242	249	255	261	268	274	280	287	293	299	306	312	319	325	331	338	344
68	125	131	138	144	151	158	164	171	177	184	190	197	203	210	216	223	230	236	243	249	256	262	269	276	282	289	295	302	308	315	322	328	335	341	348	354
69	128	135	142	149	155	162	169	176	182	189	196	203	209	216	223	230	236	243	250	257	263	270	277	284	291	297	304	311	318	324	331	338	345	351	358	365
70	132	139	146	153	160	167	174	181	188	195	202	209	216	222	229	236	243	250	257	264	271	278	285	292	299	306	313	320	327	334	341	348	355	362	369	376
71	136	143	150	157	165	172	179	186	193	200	208	215	222	229	236	243	250	257	265	272	279	286	293	301	308	315	322	329	338	343	351	358	365	372	379	386
72	140	147	154	162	169	177	184	191	199	206	213	221	228	235	242	250	258	265	272	279	287	294	302	309	316	324	331	338	346	353	361	368	375	383	390	397
73	144	151	159	166	174	182	189	197	204	212	219	227	235	242	250	257	265	272	280	288	295	302	310	318	325	333	340	348	355	363	371	378	386	393	401	408
74	148	155	163	171	179	186	194	202	210	218	225	233	241	249	256	264	272	280	287	295	303	311	319	326	334	342	350	358	365	373	381	389	396	404	412	420
75	152	160	168	176	184	192	200	208	216	224	232	240	248	256	264	272	279	287	295	303	311	319	327	335	343	351	359	367	375	383	391	399	407	415	423	431
76	156	164	172	180	189	197	205	213	221	230	238	246	254	263	271	279	287	295	304	312	320	328	336	344	353	361	369	377	385	394	402	410	418	426	435	443

The practical guide: identification, evaluation, and treatment of overweight and obesity in adults. National Heart, Lung, and Blood Institute and North American Association for the Study of Obesity. Bethesda (MD): National Institutes of Health; 2000.

An inverse relationship was found between calcium intake and the risk of having a BMI in the highest quartile. Although the studies are conflicting, one study found that increasing supplemental calcium from 0 mg/d to nearly 2,000 mg/d led to a reduction in BMI of approximately 5 units (7). These data may suggest that low calcium intake has a role in the current epidemic of obesity.

The relationship between the frequency of meals and the development of obesity has not been determined. The frequency of eating does affect lipid and glucose metabolism. When normal-weight women eat several small meals per day, their serum cholesterol concentrations are lower than when they eat a few large meals per day. Similarly, mean blood glucose concentrations are lower when meals are eaten frequently.

A pattern of conscious limitation of food intake is called "restrained" eating, commonly termed "dieting." Higher restraint scores in women are associated with lower body weights. Weight loss is associated with an increase in restraint, indicating that higher levels of conscious control can maintain lower weight. Greater increases in restraint were correlated with greater weight loss, but also with a higher risk of lapses, loss of control, and overeating.

Weight gain also is common when women stop smoking and is at least partly mediated by nicotine withdrawal (8). The average weight gain is 4–5 kg, but it can be much greater. Because of the predictability of weight gain after smoking cessation, all patients who plan to stop smoking should consider an exercise program, a decreased caloric intake, and the use of bupropion.

Finally, a sedentary lifestyle also decreases energy expenditure and promotes weight gain in women. Energy-sparing devices in the workplace and at home may enhance the tendency to gain weight. In fact, reduced energy expenditure may be a greater contributor to obesity than increased food intake. According to *Physical Activity and Health: A Report of the Surgeon General*, the percentage of adult Americans participating in physical activity decreases steadily with age, and reduced energy expenditure in adults and children predicts weight gain (9). In the United States, the amount of time spent watching television is related to BMI and obesity in children; the number of automobiles is related to the degree of obesity in adults.

MEDICAL AND PHARMACOLOGIC FACTORS

Several clinical entities can lead to obesity, and clinicians must diagnose them correctly and initiate the proper treatment when they exist. Some of these entities are genetic and relatively rare, such as proopiomelanocortin deficiency, Prader–Willi syndrome, and Bardet–Biedl syndrome. Hypothalamic obesity, which is

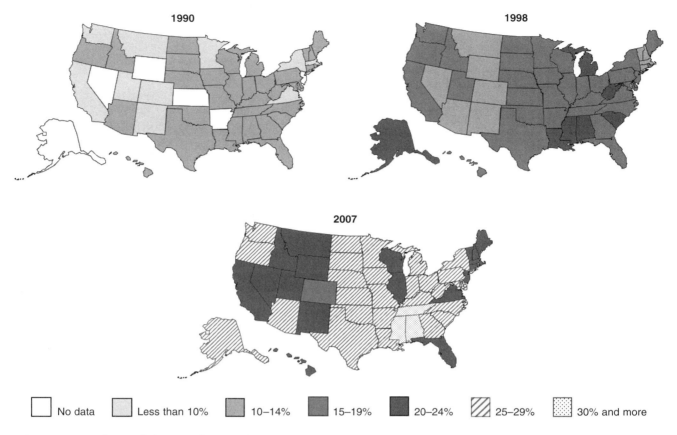

Figure 8. Prevalence of obesity in the United States in 1990, 1998, and 2007. Obesity is defined as a body mass index equal to or greater than 30 or 30 lb overweight for a person who is 5'4" tall. (Centers for Disease Control and Prevention. U.S. obesity trends 1985–2007. Atlanta [GA]: CDC; 2008. Available at: http://www.cdc.gov/nccdphp/dnpa/obesity/trend/maps. Retrieved November 12, 2008.)

rare in humans (10, 11), may be caused by trauma, tumor, inflammatory disease, surgery in the posterior fossa, or increased intracranial pressure; its associated signs and symptoms include neurologic abnormalities or generalized endocrine disorder. Cushing syndrome (or pseudo Cushing) has the cardinal feature of obesity. Hypothyroidism can cause a modest weight gain because of a generalized slowing of the metabolism.

More than 50% of women with polycystic ovary syndrome (PCOS) are obese. The cardinal features of this syndrome are oligomenorrhea, hirsutism, and polycystic ovaries. Insulin resistance is present in normal and overweight women with PCOS (12). The factors responsible for the association of PCOS and obesity are not understood. Treatment with metformin will improve many of these symptoms and signs, including insulin resistance.

Several drugs, including a variety of psychoactive agents and hormones, can cause weight gain (13). The weight gain generally is not sufficient to cause obesity, except occasionally in patients treated with high-dose corticosteroid psychoactive drugs or with valproate. Weight gain occurs in patients with diabetes mellitus who receive insulin; sulfonylurea, which enhances endogenous insulin release; and glitazones, which act on the peroxisome proliferator-activated receptor-γ receptor to increase insulin sensitivity (14).

Weight gain also may be a result of a psychiatric disorder, such as binge-eating disorder or night-eating syndrome. Binge-eating disorder is a psychiatric illness that primarily affects women. It is characterized by uncontrolled episodes of eating, usually in the evening. Women with this disorder may respond to treatment with drugs that modulate levels of serotonin.

Night-eating syndrome is the consumption of at least 25% (and usually more than 50%) of the total energy consumed per day between the evening meal and the following morning. It is one of the patterns of disturbed eating in obese women. Night-eating syndrome is related to sleep disturbances and may be a component of sleep apnea, in which daytime somnolence and nocturnal wakefulness often are found.

Special Concerns by Age

Individuals can become overweight at any age, but obesity is more common at certain ages (10, 11). Specific risks apply to specific age groups in women: adolescents and young adults, adults (pregnant women), and older women.

ADOLESCENTS AND YOUNG ADULTS

Weight in adolescence becomes a progressively better predictor of weight in adulthood. Adolescents who are above the 95th percentile for weight have a 5–20-fold greater risk of being overweight in adulthood than adolescents whose weight is below the 95th percentile. During adolescence, parental overweight is a less important predictor than it is for younger children, or it has already had its effect. However, adolescence is a unique period of intensive physical, psychosocial, and cognitive development. Nutritional needs are greatest during this period, when adolescents gain up to 50% of their adult weight, more than 20% of their adult height, and 50% of their adult skeletal mass (15). Many individuals establish lifelong eating habits during this period. Young women from low socioeconomic backgrounds are at greatest risk for poor dietary patterns (16). Many adolescents rely on high-fat, high-fructose foods (containing sugar or high-fructose corn syrup) for much of their intake or skip meals as a method of weight control. The diets of adolescents often lack adequate amounts of fruit and vegetables and sufficient amounts of vitamins A and C, folic acid, calcium, iron, and fiber.

Because most bone deposition occurs during adolescence, adequate calcium and vitamin D intake is important at that time. Many teenagers do not consume the daily requirement of 1,300 mg of calcium (17). It is important to recognize that adolescents who drink more soft drinks consume less milk and, thus, less calcium. Dairy products, calcium-enriched orange juice, and calcium supplements can help to overcome this problem. Iron deficiency as a result of growth, menses, and poor diet also is common in adolescent females.

Obesity is becoming an appreciable health problem among adolescents. In 2004, 17% of U.S. adolescents aged 12–19 years were overweight (18)—triple the prevalence two decades earlier. In some cultures, one of the consequences of overweight, as perceived by the young women themselves, is social discrimination, which is associated with poor self-esteem and depression. The prevalence of type 2 diabetes mellitus, previously considered an adult disease, has increased substantially in children and adolescents (19).

PREGNANT WOMEN

Weight gain during pregnancy and the effect of pregnancy on subsequent weight gain are important causes of overweight in women. Pregnancy may be associated with a permanent increase in weight (20).

During pregnancy women have increased requirements for iron and require adequate intake of calcium and the B vitamins. Folic acid intake ideally should be increased before conception and be continued through the pregnancy. Inadequate weight gain during pregnancy, especially in underweight women, increases the risk of infants who are born small for gestational age, as well as subsequent obesity in the child. Excessive weight gain or prepregnancy obesity increases the risk of infant macrosomia and adult obesity, as well as many obstetric issues for the mother. Obesity has been demonstrated to be an independent risk factor for spontaneous abortion (21, 22), neural tube defects, and having twins. Obesity has been associated with an increased risk of gestational hypertension, gestational diabetes mellitus, fetal macrosomia, and stillbirth.

Pregnancy is an opportune time for lifestyle modification for an individual who has been sedentary. Pregnancy should not be a state of confinement; in the absence of complications, women can continue to engage in physical activities. Women with uncomplicated pregnancies, with or without a previously sedentary lifestyle, should be encouraged to participate in aerobic and strength-conditioning exercises (23–25). Physicians should adopt the absolute and relative contraindications to exercise as per the American College of Obstetricians and Gynecologists guidelines (23).

Sedentary women tend to gain additional weight and retain it after pregnancy (26). Health care providers are still reluctant to prescribe lifestyle modification in pregnancy that includes judicious diet and exercise (27). For details on exercise during pregnancy and the postpartum period, see the current edition of *Precis: Obstetrics*.

USERS OF ORAL CONTRACEPTIVES

Oral contraceptive use has been reported to cause weight gain in some women, although this effect is diminished with low-dose estrogen pills. One study evaluated 49 healthy women taking low-dose oral contraceptives (30 mg ethinyl estradiol) (28). Weight gain was similar in the women taking oral contraceptives and in the control group, with 33% gaining weight with an average gain of 1 lb. Just as important, approximately 20% of the women in both groups lost weight.

OLDER WOMEN

In the Study of Women's Health Across the Nation, BMI was significantly higher in menopausal women than in premenopausal women (29). Because fat distribution becomes more centrally located, these increases in weight were associated with an increase in CV risk factors and insulin levels (30). A slower metabolic rate and decreased physical activity may be involved in weight gain during the menopausal years.

Elderly individuals often have poor dietary intake because of inadequate finances, ill-fitting dental appliances, or the inability or lack of desire to prepare healthful foods and a loss of smell, which makes food seem less delicious. Older people often find that their tastes have changed, and they favor sweet, easy-to-eat foods rich in refined carbohydrates (eg, bread, cereal, and sweet rolls) over more healthful items.

Older women often lack vitamins A and C, folate, and potassium because of an inadequate intake of fruit and vegetables (31). Vitamin B_{12} status may be poor because of inadequate consumption of protein-rich foods and an age-related decline in vitamin B_{12} absorption. Calcium status may be inadequate because of lactose intolerance or a low intake of dairy foods. Many old people spend a considerable amount of time indoors, and vitamin D synthesis and activation decrease with age. Although clinical zinc deficiencies are uncommon, old women often have marginal zinc levels because of low intake of protein-rich foods (31).

Reduced physical activity and a decrease in metabolic rate with aging require that old women choose foods with high nutrient density and low energy density. An aging patient with a caloric intake of less than 1,600 kcal per day is at risk for inadequate intake of vitamins and minerals. A multiple vitamin and mineral supplement can provide nutritional insurance to older women.

Principles of Nutritional Assessment

Assessment of a patient's nutritional status through the use of a number of instruments can help to identify a potential lack of essential nutrients for health. Among these instruments are the food frequency questionnaire, the diet and lifestyle history (Box 18), and 24-hour recall. These techniques can take time and may be performed most effectively by a clinic staff person.

As part of the physical examination, the patient's height, weight, and waist circumference should be measured to determine weight and BMI. Actual measurement is important because most patients will overestimate their height and underestimate their weight. The current approach to the assessment of overweight and obese women is summarized in Figure 9. For more details, clinicians should refer to the guidelines of the National Heart, Lung, and Blood Institute (5) and the North American Association for the Study of Obesity (32). A BMI between 18.5 and 25 is considered normal for most American women. The BMI is divided into five-unit intervals that are used to define overweight and various levels of obesity (Table 3) (2, 5).

The BMI must be interpreted in an ethnically sensitive context, because the amount of body fat for a given BMI differs among ethnic groups. For Japanese Americans and other Asians, a BMI greater than 23 has the same association with disease as does a BMI greater than 25 for whites. For African Americans, probably for Hispanics, and possibly for descendants of Polynesians, a BMI of 27 is probably equivalent to a BMI of 25 in whites. Once the BMI has been determined, assessment should include central fat distribution measured as of waist circumference. The rate of weight gain (greater than 1 kg per year is high) and level of physical activity are additional criteria for determining the risk from a given BMI.

Box 18

Sample Questions for Basic Nutrition and Lifestyle History

- I would like to know everything you ate and drank yesterday.
- When did you first have something to eat or drink, and what did you have? _____
- When was the next time you ate or drank something? _____ (continue)
- Do you avoid any foods for any reason (religious, cultural, likes or dislikes, or food sensitivity or allergy)?
- Yes ____ No ____ Which ones? _____
- How often do you eat away from home? _____
- Do you drink alcoholic beverages? Yes ____ No ____ How often? _____ How much? _____
- Do you take any vitamin, mineral, or other supplements? Yes ____ No ____ What kind? _____ How much? _____
- Do you exercise? Yes ____ No ____ What kind? _____ How often? _____
- Do you smoke cigarettes? Yes _____ No ____
- Has your weight changed in the past 5 years? Yes ____ No ____ How? _____
- Are you trying to lose (or gain) weight? Yes ____ No ____ How? _____ Why? _____
- Are you on a special diet? Yes ____ No ____ What kind? _____ Why? _____
- Do you have problems with planning and preparing meals for yourself or your family? Yes ____ No ____ If so, for what reasons? _____

Fat located in the abdominal and visceral fat depots carries a higher risk of diseases associated with obesity than does extra fat on the hips and thighs (33). A waist circumference greater than 88 cm in women carries a higher risk of CV disease outcomes than does a high BMI (34).

General Strategies for Prevention and Treatment of Obesity

The first goal of weight control should be to prevent obesity or its progression, because obesity is difficult to manage effectively once it has developed. Because of the greater risk of obesity in women, identifying women

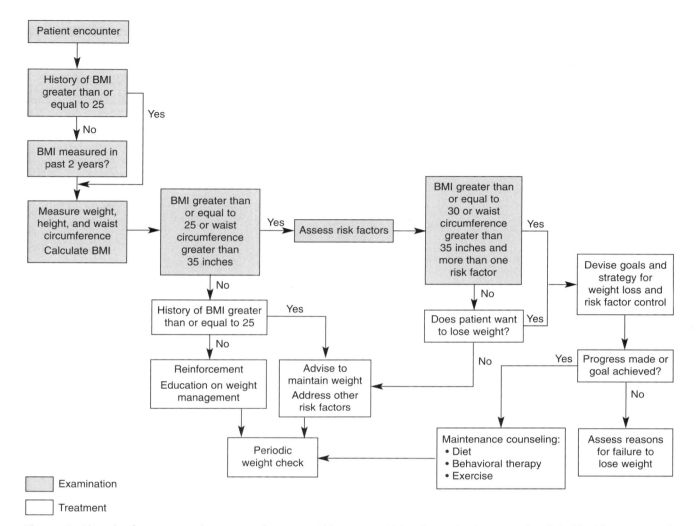

Figure 9. Algorithm for assessing the overweight patient. Abbreviation: BMI indicates body mass index. (Modified from National Heart, Lung, and Blood Institute [NHLBI], National Institute for Diabetes and Digestive and Kidney Diseases [NIDDK]. Clinical guidelines on the identification, evaluation, and treatment of overweight and obesity in adults. The evidence report. NIH Publication No. 98–4083. Bethesda [MD]: NIH; 1998. Available at: http://www.nhlbi.nih.gov/guidelines/obesity/ ob_gdlns.pdf. Retrieved November 12, 2008.)

at high risk is an important challenge for physicians. Women with one or more overweight parents are at substantially greater risk of becoming overweight. Socioeconomic and cultural norms also may affect a woman's risk of obesity.

Establishing a Dialogue

A patient's perception of her weight often is not what the physician might expect. The patient's peer group and community often have a major effect on the patient's idea of what is an acceptable weight and what is obese. Many patients who are clearly obese, with a BMI greater than 35, will see themselves as overweight—not obese. Furthermore, many women fear hormone therapy and its risk of breast cancer more than they care about obesity, a condition that actually increases that risk more than does hormone therapy and also increases CV risks. Therefore, a frank dialogue is

necessary to ascertain the patient's knowledge and feelings about her weight (Box 19).

Behavioral and Lifestyle Strategies

The initial step in helping a patient manage her weight is to determine whether she is ready to make lifestyle changes. The "stages of change" is a useful concept for this purpose (35).

One important aspect of the behavioral strategy for weight loss is having realistic expectations. A plateau in body weight will occur after all forms of management have been used. For most treatments, including behavioral therapy, dietary change, and exercise, the average weight loss plateau is less than 10% below the baseline weight. Although this amount of weight loss has real health benefits, it is nonetheless seen as frustratingly low for many women and physicians. Thus, despite what total weight a patient wishes to lose, the initial

Nutrition Facts	Amount/serving	%DV*	Amount/serving	%DV*
Serv. Size 4 crackers (15g)	**Total Fat** 1g	**2%**	**Total Carb.** 12g	**4%**
Servings 10	Sat. Fat 0g	**0%**	Fiber 0g	**0%**
Calories 60	*Trans* Fat 0g		Sugars 0g	
Fat Cal. 10	**Cholest.** 0mg	**0%**	**Protein** 2g	
Percent Daily Values (DV) are based on a 2,000 calorie diet.	**Sodium** 75mg	**3%**		
	Vitamin A 0% • Vitamin C 0% • Calcium 0% • Iron 4%			

Figure 10. Nutrition facts label.

goal should be set at 10% of body weight. Only after this goal is accomplished should the patient and physician reassess the patient's readiness to attempt another 10% loss. An initial loss of 5–10% of body weight should be considered a success by both parties, or the patient may stop treatment altogether.

The patient also can be encouraged to use a defined eating plan and to adopt an exercise or activity plan. Women who are successful in losing weight and maintaining weight loss tend to monitor their behavior, eat low-fat diets, increase their physical activity, and practice positive self-thinking and techniques for stress reduction.

DIETARY CHANGES

Achieving a healthy diet should be one of the main objectives, in addition to the reduction of energy intake. MyPyramid is a tool available from the U.S. Department of Agriculture. It is based on the concept that one size does not fit all, and it offers personalized eating plans and interactive tools to help plan and assess food choices so the patient can make better choices from food groups. The food plans are not for specific health conditions; they focus on healthy choices for healthy individuals who want to achieve the best dietary plan. Physical activity is covered as well. MyPyramid makes recommendations for all the life stages beginning from age 2 years.

One tool that can help women understand calorie and nutrient intake is the nutrition facts label (Fig. 10). It is important to look at the portion size. Often it is much smaller than the patient might expect.

A number of popular diets—eg, the low-fat diet, low-carbohydrate diet, and Mediterranean diet—have been studied (36). The major differences between these diets involve fat and carbohydrate levels. Popular diets can be grouped into three categories: 1) very low fat, 2) moderate fat, and 3) high fat. When advising patients, it is important to stress the need for moderation and variety in all diets. It is preferable to recommend a moderate reduction in fat and carbohydrates, which will keep protein at the high level, rather than extreme reductions of either fat or carbohydrates. The use of meal replacements, either frozen entrées or various commercial products, also can be recommended. It is advisable for patients to take a multivitamin pill, because it is sometimes difficult to get all the necessary micronutrients while dieting.

A clinical trial compared four popular diets: the Atkins diet, the Zone diet, the Weight Watchers diet, and the Ornish diet (37). After 1 year, there was no significant difference in the weight loss of patients using any of the four diets. The principal determinant of weight loss was the degree of adherence to the diet, not the diet itself. The more patients adhered to the diet, the more weight they lost.

EXERCISE

Exercise is another strategy for balancing energy intake and expenditure; it may be a primary treatment of weight loss or serve as a preventive strategy against weight regain. Walking briskly for 1 hour burns approximately 100 kcal per mile. To lose 1 lb of body weight a week from exercise alone, an individual should walk 5 miles per day, 7 days per week. For this reason, exercise alone has not been effective as a primary weight loss technique. However, it still has appreciable health benefits.

Initiating an exercise program is the first step in beginning a healthy lifestyle. Most individualized exercise programs include initial conditioning, improvement, and maintenance stages. The initial conditioning stage lasts typically 4 weeks and serves as a primer to familiarize the participant with exercise training. Treadmill running and walking, aerobics, and stationary cycling are appropriate activities, because they all engage large muscle groups. During this stage, a warm-up of 10–15 minutes should be initiated, followed by moderate-intensity aerobic activities at approximately 45% of heart rate. An extended (10- to 15-minute) cool-down then would include stretching (38). The duration at this stage may be only approximately 20 minutes of CV exercise, with 10 minutes of warm-up and 10 minutes of cool down.

Exercise adherence may decrease if the program is initiated too aggressively.

The goal of the improvement stage of the exercise program is to provide a gradual increase in the overall exercise stimulus to allow for appreciable improvements and adaptations in aerobic fitness. This stage is more rapid and typically lasts 4–8 months. The intensity is progressively raised to 50–85% of heart rate. Duration is increased consistently, with increments of no more than 20% each week until the patient is able to exercise at a moderate to vigorous intensity continuously for approximately 30 minutes (38). Interval training (high-intensity exercise with short periods of rest) can be used to gradually increase exercise intensity. An example of interval training would be 1 minute at 85% of heart rate, followed by a 1-minute rest at 30% of heart rate, repeated 6 times in a 20-minute session.

The goal of the maintenance stage is to maintain the aerobic fitness gained during the improvement stage. This stage is long term. A further improvement in aerobic fitness is minimal, but continuing the same workouts allows individuals to maintain current fitness.

In previously sedentary old women and men, aerobic capacity can improve by 20–30% in response to 6–12 months' training (39, 40). However, the training response will differ, and not every participant will improve to the same extent. A vigorous exercise program enhances the level of fitness regardless of genetic background, with the limits for aerobic capacity linked closely to natural endowment (41). Of two individuals in the same exercise program, one might show a 10-fold greater improvement compared with the other. Cardiovascular capacity declines with detraining (stopping of training), age, and a decline in aerobic capacity. Interestingly, three weeks of bed rest results in a more profound deterioration of aerobic capacity and CV fitness than does 30 years of aging (42).

MEDICATIONS

Only two medications, sibutramine and orlistat, are approved by the U.S. Food and Drug Administration for long-term use in weight loss therapy (43). When used as monotherapy, either agent can produce a weight loss of 5–10%. Obesity is a chronic disease that has many causes. When the medications for a chronic disease are discontinued, the disease is expected to recur. Thus, the medications work only when they are used. This argument applies to medications used to treat patients with obesity.

SURGERY

Several surgical procedures currently are available for the treatment of patients with obesity: 1) vertical banded gastroplasty, 2) gastric bypass, 3) gastric band (Lap-Band), and 4) duodenal–intestinal bypass (Scopinaro procedure). Liposuction is not a treatment for obesity. A surgical intervention may be considered for a patient with a BMI greater than 40 or for a patient with a BMI greater than 35 with comorbid conditions, such as diabetes mellitus, treated hypertension, sleep apnea, or appreciable dyslipidemia.

Women who undergo bariatric surgery may develop deficiencies in iron, vitamin B_{12}, folate, and calcium. Thus, they should be monitored for such deficiencies and receive appropriate treatment. Weight loss may result in an unexpected return of fertility, so contraceptive use should be discussed with these patients. Pregnancy has occurred successfully after all of these bariatric procedures. In general, the infants tend to be smaller than infants born to the same mother before the bariatric operation, and no associated adverse perinatal outcomes seem to occur.

Management Strategies by Age

Table 4 outlines the treatment strategies for overweight and obese females by age groupings (11). Preventive strategies should be directed toward individuals with risk factors for weight gain. Recommendations should include lifestyle changes, such as increased physical activity (which would benefit most adults), and good dietary practices, including a diet lower in saturated fat.

Behavioral strategies should be added to the lifestyle strategies for women in the overweight category. Behavioral change is particularly important for adolescents who are overweight, because intervening in this group can reduce the degree of overweight in adult life. Behavioral programs carried out in controlled settings can result in weight losses averaging nearly 10%.

By age 60 years, most women who will become overweight have already done so. Thus, the focus is on treatment of those women who are overweight or obese. In this age group, there may be an argument for treating the comorbid conditions directly and paying less attention to treating the clinical obesity through weight loss. The issue of treating body weight in women who are older than 75 years is controversial.

Table 4. Treatment Strategies for Obesity by Age Categories

Predictors of Overweight	Treatment Strategies		
	At Risk of Preoverweight	Preclinical Overweight	Clinical Overweight
Age Less Than 10 Years			
Positive family history, genetic defects (dysmorphic-Prader–Willi, Bardet–Biedel, and Cohen syndromes)	Family counseling and reducing inactivity	Family behavioral therapy, exercise, and low-fat and low-energy diet	Treatment of comorbid conditions, exercise, and low-energy dense diet
Age 11 Years to 50 Years			
Family history of diabetes or obesity, endocrine disorders (polycystic ovary syndrome), multiple pregnancies, marriage, smoking cessation, and use of medications	Reducing sedentary lifestyle, low-fat and low-energy dense diet, and portion control	Behavioral therapy, low-fat and low-energy dense diet, and reducing sedentary lifestyle	Treatment of comorbid conditions, drug treatment for overweight, reducing sedentary lifestyle, low-fat and low-energy dense diet, behavioral therapy, and surgery
Age 51 Years to 75 Years			
Menopause, decreasing growth hormone levels, decreasing testosterone levels, smoking cessation, and use of medications	Few individuals remain here	Behavioral therapy, low-fat and low-energy dense diet, and reducing sedentary lifestyle	Treatment of comorbid conditions, drug treatment for overweight, reducing sedentary lifestyle, low-fat and low-energy dense diet, behavioral therapy, and surgery

Bray GA. Contemporary diagnosis and management of obesity and the metabolic syndrome. 3rd ed. Newtown (PA): Handbooks in Health Care Co.; 2003.

References

1. Gregg EW, Cheng YJ, Cadwell BL, Imperatore G, Williams DE, Flegal KM, et al. Secular trends in cardiovascular disease risk factors according to body mass index in US adults [published erratum appears in JAMA 2005;294:182]. JAMA 2005;293:1868–74.

2. Obesity: preventing and managing the global epidemic. Report of a WHO consultation. World Health Organ Tech Rep Ser 2000;894:i–xii, 1–253.

3. Mokdad AH, Bowman BA, Ford ES, Vinicor F, Marks JS, Koplan JP. The continuing epidemics of obesity and diabetes in the United States. JAMA 2001;286:1195–200.

4. Flegal KM, Graubard BI, Williamson DF, Gail MH. Excess deaths associated with underweight, overweight, and obesity. JAMA 2005;293:1861–7.

5. Clinical Guidelines on the Identification, Evaluation, and Treatment of Overweight and Obesity in Adults--The Evidence Report. National Institutes of Health [published erratum appears in Obes Res 1998;6:464]. Obes Res 1998;6(suppl 2):51S209S.

6. Roberts SB, Pi-Sunyer FX, Dreher M, Hahn R, Hill JO, Kleinman RE, et al. Physiology of fat replacement and fat reduction: effects of dietary fat and fat substitutes on energy regulation. Nutr Rev 1998;56:S29–41; discussion S41–9.

7. Davies KM, Heaney RP, Recker RR, Lappe JM, Barger-Lux MJ, Rafferty K, et al. Calcium intake and body weight. J Clin Endocrinol Metab 2000;85:4635–8.

8. O'Hara P, Connett JE, Lee WW, Nides M, Murray R, Wise R. Early and late weight gain following smoking cessation in the Lung Health Study. Am J Epidemiol 1998;148:821–30.

9. U.S. Department of Health and Human Services. Physical activity and health: a report of the Surgeon General. Atlanta (GA): U.S. Department of Health and Human Services, Centers for Disease Control and Prevention, National Center for Chronic Disease Prevention and Health Promotion; 1996. Available at: http://www.cdc.gov/nccdphp/sgr/pdf/sgrfull.pdf. Retrieved November 12, 2008.

10. Bray GA. Risks of obesity. Prim Care 2003;30:281–99, v–vi.

11. Bray GA. Contemporary diagnosis and management of obesity and the metabolic syndrome. 3rd ed. Newtown (PA): Handbooks in Health Care Co.; 2003.

12. Ehrmann DA. Polycystic ovary syndrome. N Engl J Med 2005;352:1223–36.

13. Allison DB, Mentore JL, Heo M, Chandler LP, Cappelleri JC, Infante MC, et al. Antipsychotic-induced weight gain: a comprehensive research synthesis. Am J Psychiatry 1999;156:1686–96.

14. Smith SR, De Jonge L, Volaufova J, Li Y, Xie H, Bray GA. Effect of pioglitazone on body composition and energy

expenditure: a randomized controlled trial. Metabolism 2005;54:24–32.

15. World Health Organization. Nutrition for health and development: a global agenda for combating malnutrition. Geneva: WHO; 2000. Available at: http://www.who.int/mip2001/files/2231/NHDprogressreport2000.pdf. Retrieved November 12, 2008.

16. U.S. Department of Agriculture, Agricultural Research Service. Food and nutrirent intakes by individuals in the United States, by sex and age, 1994–1996. Washington, DC: USDA; 1998.

17. Optimal calcium intake. NIH Consens Statement 1994;12:1–31. Available at http://consensus.nih.gov/1994/1994 OptimalCalcium097html.htm. Retrieved November 12, 2008.

18. Ogden CL, Carroll MD, Curtin LR, McDowell MA, Tabak CJ, Flegal KM. Prevalence of overweight and obesity in the United States, 1999-2004. JAMA 2006;295:1549–55.

19. Libman I, Arslanian S. Type 2 diabetes in childhood: the American perspective. Horm Res 2003;59(suppl 1):69–76.

20. Smith DE, Lewis CE, Caveny JL, Perkins LL, Burke GL, Bild DE. Longitudinal changes in adiposity associated with pregnancy. The CARDIA Study. Coronary Artery Risk Development in Young Adults Study. JAMA 1994;271:1747–51.

21. Wang JX, Davies MJ, Norman RJ. Obesity increases the risk of spontaneous abortion during infertility treatment. Obes Res 2002;10:551–4.

22. Lashen H, Fear K, Sturdee DW. Obesity is associated with increased risk of first trimester and recurrent miscarriage: matched case-control study. Hum Reprod 2004;19:1644–6.

23. Exercise during pregnancy and the postpartum period. ACOG Committee Opinion No. 267. American College of Obstetricians and Gynecologists. Obstet Gynecol 2002;99:171–3.

24. Davies GA, Wolfe LA, Mottola MF, MacKinnon C. Joint SOGC/CSEP clinical practice guideline: exercise in pregnancy and the postpartum period. Society of Obstetricians and Gynaecologists of Canada. SOGC Clinical Practice Obstetrics Committee. Can J Appl Physiol 2003;28:330–41.

25. Artal R, O'Toole M. Guidelines of the American College of Obstetricians and Gynecologists for exercise during pregnancy and the postpartum period. Br J Sports Med 2003;37:6–12; discussion 12.

26. Gunderson EP, Abrams B, Selvin S. The relative importance of gestational gain and maternal characteristics associated with the risk of becoming overweight after pregnancy. Int J Obes Relat Metab Disord 2000;24:1660–8.

27. Artal R. Weight gain recommendations in pregnancy [editorial]. Expert Rev Obstet Gynecol 2008;3:November 14, 2008,143–5. Available at: http://www.expert–revies.com/doi/pdf/10.1586/17474108.3.2.143. Retrieved November 14, 2008.

28. Reubinoff BE, Grubstein A, Meirow D, Berry E, Schenker JG, Brzezinski A. Effects of low-dose estrogen oral contraceptives on weight, body composition, and fat distribution in young women. Fertil Steril 1995;63:516–21.

29. Matthews KA, Abrams B, Crawford S, Miles T, Neer R, Powell LH, et al. Body mass index in mid-life women: relative influence of menopause, hormone use, and ethnicity [published erratum appears in Int J Obes Relat Metab Disord 2002;26:1150]. Int J Obes Relat Metab Disord 2001;25:863–73.

30. Wing RR, Matthews KA, Kuller LH, Meilahn EN, Plantinga P. Waist to hip ratio in middle-aged women. Associations with behavioral and psychosocial factors and with changes in cardiovascular risk factors. Arterioscler Thromb 1991;11:1250–7.

31. Russell RM. New views on the RDAs for older adults. J Am Diet Assoc 1997;97:515–8.

32. Aronne LJ, editor. A practical guide to drug–induced weight gain. Minneapolis (MN): Healthcare Information Programs; 2002.

33. Wajchenberg BL, Bosco A, Marone MM, Levin S, Rocha M, Lerario AC, et al. Estimation of body fat and lean tissue distribution by dual energy X-ray absorptiometry and abdominal body fat evaluation by computed tomography in Cushing's disease. J Clin Endocrinol Metab 1995;80:2791–4.

34. Balkau B, Deanfield JE, Despres JP, Bassand JP, Fox KA, Smith SC Jr, et al. International Day for the Evaluation of Abdominal Obesity (IDEA): a study of waist circumference, cardiovascular disease, and diabetes mellitus in 168,000 primary care patients in 63 countries. Circulation 2007;116:1942–51.

35. Prochaska JO, DiClemente CC, Norcross JC. In search of how people change. Applications to addictive behaviors. Am Psychol 1992;47:1102–14.

36. Shai I, Schwarzfuchs D, Henkin Y, Shahar DR, Witkow S, Greenberg I, et al. Weight loss with a low-carbohydrate, Mediterranean, or low-fat diet. Dietary Intervention Randomized Controlled Trial (DIRECT) Group. N Engl J Med 2008;359:229–41.

37. Dansinger ML, Gleason JA, Griffith JL, Selker HP, Schaefer EJ. Comparison of the Atkins, Ornish, Weight Watchers, and Zone diets for weight loss and heart disease risk reduction: a randomized trial. JAMA 2005;293:43–53.

38. American College of Sports Medicine. ACSM's guidelines for exercise testing and prescription. 8th ed. Baltimore (MD): LWW; 2009.

39. Topp R, Ditmyer M, King K, Doherty K, Hornyak J 3rd. The effect of bed rest and potential of prehabilitation on patients in the intensive care unit. AACN Clin Issues 2002;13:263–76.

40. Shephard RJ, Rankinen T, Bouchard C. Test-retest errors and the apparent heterogeneity of training response. Eur J Appl Physiol 2004;91:199–203.

41. McArdle WD, Katch FI, Katch VL. Exercise physiology: energy, nutrition and human performance. 5th ed. Philadelphia (PA): Lippincott Williams and Wilkins; 2001.

42. McGuire DK, Levine BD, Williamson JW, Snell PG, Blomqvist CG, Saltin B, et al. A 30-year follow-up of the Dallas Bedrest and Training Study: I. Effect of age on the cardiovascular response to exercise. Circulation 2001;104:1350–7.

43. Li Z, Maglione M, Tu W, Mojica W, Arterburn D, Shugarman LR, et al. Meta-analysis: pharmacologic treatment of obesity. Ann Intern Med 2005;142:532–46.

Complementary and Alternative Medicine

Tracy Gaudet

The use of complementary and alternative approaches for health and disease management is steadily increasing in this country, and women are the primary users (1). The number of visits to alternative health care providers exceeds the number of visits to primary health care providers (2). Although there is evidence supporting many of these approaches, many others are potentially dangerous or fraudulent (1). Women frequently make decisions regarding treatment options without the advice of medically trained individuals, and most patients do not inform their physicians of their use of alternative approaches (3). Obstetrician–gynecologists are in an excellent position to help guide patients in their treatment choices, including guiding them away from potentially dangerous alternative treatments and supporting the use of potentially beneficial treatments.

Types of Complementary and Alternative Medicine

Complementary and alternative medicine (CAM) is defined by the National Center for Complementary and Alternative Medicine as a group of diverse medical and health care systems, practices, and products that are not currently considered to be part of conventional medicine (4). The spectrum of therapies, practitioners, and products within this grouping is extremely broad but can be categorized into five major groupings (Box 20).

Potential Benefits and Adverse Reactions

Biologically Based Therapies

Biologically based medicine is the most conceptually accessible area of CAM. Botanicals are the source of the active components in approximately 25% of prescription medications and 60% of over-the-counter drugs. Some botanicals may have clinical effectiveness. In the United States, however, these products are not regulated by the U.S. Food and Drug Administration (FDA) because they qualify as dietary supplements. The fact that the FDA does not regulate these products creates the potential for issues regarding standardization of products, as well as the potential for adulteration or mislabeling. There also is a lack of pharmacokinetic evaluation. Known or potential drug–botanical interactions exist, and patients should be screened for their use. See Table 5 for some potential drug–botanical interactions.

Manipulative-Based Therapies

There is some evidence documenting the value of massage therapy. It is an effective stress-reduction technique and can result in physical relaxation, reduced anxiety, increased circulation, improved immune function, and pain relief. Specific indications for massage include acute low back pain and lymphedema (lymphatic massage).

Resources

Complementary and Alternative Medicine

National Center for Complementary and Alternative Medicine
http://www.nccam.nih.gov

Box 20

Complementary and Alternative Medicine Categories

The National Institutes of Health has categorized complementary and alternative medicine into five domains:

- *Biologically based therapies:* substances found in nature, such as herbs, special diets, or vitamins (in doses outside those used in conventional medicine). Examples include botanicals, dietary supplements, vitamins, minerals, and orthomolecular medicine.

- *Manipulative-based therapies:* manipulation or movement of one or more body parts. Examples include chiropractic, osteopathy, and massage.

- *Mind-body-based therapies:* techniques designed to enhance the mind's ability to affect bodily function and symptoms. Examples include meditation, hypnosis, music, and prayer.

- *Energy-based therapies:* use of energy fields, such as magnetic fields or biofields (energy fields that some individuals believe surround and penetrate the human body). Examples include therapeutic touch, Quigong treatment, Reiki, and magnets.

- *Whole medical* systems: complete systems of theory and practice, which often have evolved apart from the conventional medical approaches. Examples include traditional Chinese medicine, acupuncture, and homeopathy.

Table 5. Potential Interactions With Drugs

Drug Class	Herb	Potential Interactions
Anticoagulants	Bilberry	Increased risk of bleeding (high dose)
	Chamomile	Increased risk of bleeding
	Co-enzyme Q10	Decreased effectiveness of anticoagulants
	Danshen	Increased risk of bleeding
	Dong quai	Increased risk of bleeding
	Feverfew	Increased risk of bleeding
	Garlic	Increased risk of bleeding
	Ginger	Increased risk of bleeding
	Ginkgo	Increased risk of bleeding
	Ginseng	Increased risk of bleeding
Anticonvulsants	Borage	Decreased seizure threshold
	Evening primrose oil	Decreased seizure threshold
	Valerian	Increased effects of barbiturates
Antidepressants	Ephedra	Increased effect of monoamine oxidase inhibitors
	Ginseng	Increased effect of monoamine oxidase inhibitors
	St. John's wort	Monoamine oxidase inhibitors—increased blood pressure
	Yohimbine	Tricyclics—hypertension; selective serotonin reuptake inhibitors—increased serotonin levels
Diuretics	Aloe	Increased risk of hypokalemia
	Cascara sagrada	Increased risk of hypokalemia
	Licorice	Increased risk of hypokalemia
Hypoglycemic agents	Aloe	Risk of hypoglycemia
	Ginseng	Risk of hypoglycemia
	Stinging nettle	Potential elevation of blood glucose level
Sedatives	Chamomile	Increased drowsiness
	Valerian	Increased risk of sedation

Data from O'Mathuna DP. Herb–drug interactions. Altern Med Alert 2003;6:37–43.
Gaudet T. Complementary and alternative medicine. Clin Update Womens Health Care 2004;III:1–82.

Massage should not be used in patients with bleeding disorders, phlebitis or thrombophlebitis, edema caused by heart or kidney failure, fever or infections that can be spread by blood or lymph circulation, and leukemia or lymphoma. Massage also should not be performed on or near malignant tumors and bone metastases; over bruises, unhealed scars, or open wounds; on or near recent fracture sites; or over joints or other tissues that are acutely inflamed.

Perhaps the most appreciable risk associated with manipulative-based therapies is stroke caused by chiropractic manipulation. Vertebrobasilar accidents occur mostly after a cervical manipulation with a rotatory component. Estimates of vertebrobasilar accidents range from 1 per 20,000 patients to 1 per 1 million cervical manipulations. The average age of patients with a vertebrobasilar accident is 38 years. The second most common complication of spinal manipulation is cauda equina syndrome related to progression of disk herniation. The incidence of cauda equina syndrome is estimated to be less than one per 1 million treatments.

Mind-Body–Based Therapies

Hypnosis is a mind-body–based therapy that has documented value in the treatment of a variety of psychologic conditions, pain control, and recovery from surgery. The effectiveness of mind–body approaches in stress reduction, which can secondarily affect many medical conditions, is well documented. In addition, the data on the use of mind–body approaches to reach desired physical and emotional states are growing. The potential effectiveness of hypnosis is perhaps best demonstrated by documented cases of invasive surgeries, such as cesarean deliveries, with no anesthesia other than hypnosis.

Hypnotized individuals occasionally report unanticipated negative effects during or after hypnosis. The spectrum of reported effects has encompassed minor transient symptoms such as headaches, dizziness, and nausea and less frequent symptoms of anxiety or panic, unexpected reactions to an inadvertently given suggestion, and difficulties in awakening from hypnosis. More serious reactions after hypnosis generally have been attributed to the misapplication of hypnotic techniques, failure to prepare the patient, or preexisting psychopathologic conditions or personality factors.

Energy-Based Therapies

Energy-based therapies are the least well researched and the most diverse of all CAM modalities. It is, therefore, not possible to address the potential benefits and risks of these therapies.

Whole Medical Systems

The whole medical system with the most research supporting its effectiveness is the Asian system of care, including acupuncture. A 1997 National Institutes of Health (NIH) Consensus Panel established that there was convincing evidence for the use of acupuncture in the treatment of postoperative dental pain, as well as nausea and vomiting. A number of other indications were considered promising and worthy of more research; they included headache, low back pain, stroke, addiction, asthma, premenstrual syndrome, osteoarthritis, carpal tunnel syndrome, and tennis elbow. Since that time, the evidence for the effectiveness of acupuncture in the treatment of a variety of clinical conditions has continued to grow. The NIH panel also stated that "data for acupuncture are as strong as those for many accepted Western medical therapies, and the incidence of adverse effects substantially lower than that of many accepted medical procedures used for the same conditions." There also is an extensive body of animal research supporting the neurophysiologic effects of acupuncture on the endorphin system.

The most common complications of acupuncture are minor bleeding and bruising. These complications rarely require treatment other than local pressure to the needle site for minor bleeding, and they occur in approximately 2% of all needles placed. The most appreciable risk of acupuncture in the past has been hepatitis. The risk of transmissible infection is eliminated by the one-time use of disposable needles. Pneumothorax is the second most appreciable risk of acupuncture.

Specific Conditions

Many patients seek alternative treatments for their conditions (Table 6). National survey data do not support the view that use of CAM therapy in the United States primarily reflects dissatisfaction with conventional care. Adults who use both kinds of care appear to value both and tend to be less concerned about their medical physician's disapproval than about their physician's inability to understand or incorporate CAM therapy use within the context of their medical management (3).

Many surgical patients use botanicals, do not tell their physicians or anesthesiologists about their use, and do not discontinue their use before surgery (1). Many of the most commonly used substances have effects that, when combined with anesthesia, can lead to the following complications: prolongation of anesthetic agents, coagulation disorders, cardiovascular effects, electrolyte disturbances, hepatotoxicity, and endocrine effects. It is prudent to ask patients to discontinue use of botanicals 1–2 weeks before surgery.

Quality Control

Licensing bodies for the myriad CAM providers are as varied as the approaches. Each state has approached the regulation of these professions in a different way. Quality control regarding products is equally challenging. Botanicals are regulated as dietary supplements in the United States. In 1994, the Dietary Supplement Health and Education Act was enacted. This act makes it legal to make "structure/function" claims, or to refer to the supplement's effect on the body's structure or function or to an individual's well-being without approval by the FDA. Products falling under the purview of the Dietary Supplement Health and Education Act are easy to recognize because their labels read as follows: "This product is not intended to diagnose, treat, cure, or prevent any disease."

Screening

One of the greatest barriers to the best practice of medicine regarding issues of CAM is a lack of communication. Most patients do not tell their physicians of their use of complementary or alternative therapies, even when the physicians are receptive to the topic. Given the prevalence of use and the potential for interactions with conventional approaches, it is imperative that questions regarding CAM be integrated into the patient history. Many patients simply do not think of sharing this information with their physicians, so direct and specific inquiry is necessary (3).

Although it is useful to know all the CAM that patients have used in the past or are currently using, it is particularly important to elicit a history of anything ingestible. If patients are seeing CAM practitioners, it is best to ask specifically if they have recommended any supplements or botanicals. For example, Asian medicine practitioners or acupuncturists often treat with botanical products or herbal teas. Naturopaths and chiropractors often recommend vitamins and supplements.

Table 6. Potentially Beneficial Complementary and Alternative Therapies Listed By Condition

Therapies by Condition	Putative Effects	Dose	Evidence-Based Support
Menstrual Disorders			
Biologically Based Therapies			
Calcium	Effects the symptoms of PMS and PMDD, including negative mood, water retention, and food cravings	900–1,200 mg per day in divided doses	Randomized controlled trial with 248 subjects in calcium arm reported reduced luteal phase symptoms (1).
			Randomized controlled trial with 33 subjects who completed crossover study showed reduction in PMS symptoms (2).
Magnesium	Decrease in PMS and dysmenorrheal symptoms and possible relief from the bowel effects of calcium supplementation	200–400 mg per day (divided), can be taken either cyclically during the luteal phase or continuously	Randomized controlled trial with 14 subjects in magnesium group reported reduced symptoms related to mood (3).
			Randomized controlled trial with 37 volunteers who completed the crossover showed reduced fluid retentions symptoms (4).
			Systematic review of three small randomized controlled trials showed a reduction in dysmenorrhea (5).
Vitamin B$_6$ (pyridoxine)	Less mastalgia, breast, pain, and mood changes in PMS and relieves dysmenorrhea symptoms	50–100 mg per day with meals; pyridoxine is benign in doses less than 100 mg per day, but neuropathies can be seen in doses of 200 mg per day or higher; doses greater than 200 mg per day may cause dependence and withdrawal; beware of interactions with other drugs; eg, anti-Parkinson medications	Weak evidence for reduction of PMS from a 1990 review of 12 randomized controlled trials (6) and some benefit in reduction of PMS and dysmenorrhea in a 2003 systematic review of randomized controlled trials (2).
Rose tea *Rosa gallica* (contains vitamin C and to a lesser extent vitamins B, E, K, and P)	Less dysmenorrhea, distress, and anxiety among adolescents	During the mid luteal phase: two cups per day for 12 days per cycle	Randomized controlled trial with 70 subjects in *Rosa gallica* group reported less symptoms in a 6-month follow-up study (7).
Manipulative Based Therapies			
Spinal manipulation	No evidence effective in the treatment of primary or secondary dysmenorrhea, PMS, or PMDD		Cochrane systematic review of randomized clinical trials (8)

(continued)

Table 6. Potentially Beneficial Complementary and Alternative Therapies Listed By Condition *(continued)*

Therapies by Condition	Putative Effects	Dose	Evidence-Based Support
	**Menstrual Disorders** *(continued)*		
	*Mind-Body–Based Therapies*		
Relaxation techniques	Treatment of PMS or PMDD	Relaxation response twice a day for 3 months	Randomized controlled trial with 16 subjects treated with relaxation monitored for 5 months reported less symptoms; most effective in nine subjects with most severe symptoms (9).
	*Whole Medical Systems*		
Acupuncture	Treatment of primary dysmenorrhea	30–40 minute therapy each week for 1 year with 12 needles	Randomized controlled trial with 11 subjects in real acupuncture group showed benefit in dysmenorrhea (10).
	Improvement in PMS symptoms	De qi effect obtained every second day (7 days) for a period of 30 minutes a day during luteal phase	Randomized controlled trial with 18 subjects in acupuncture arm showed reduced PMS symptoms. Four subjects continued their previous medication during acupuncture trial (11).
	**Menopause**		
	*Biologically Based Therapies*		
Black cohosh (*Cimicifuga racemosa*)	Central mediation of vasomotor and other menopause symptoms	40–160 mg daily	Randomized controlled trial with 20 subjects in *Cimicifuga racemosa* arm showed benefit in menopausal symptoms and bone degradation (12).
			Randomized controlled trial with 80 subjects in black cohosh arm showed no benefit in menopausal symptoms (13).
Black cohosh (*Cimicifuga racemosa*) St. John's wort (*Hypericum perforatum*) combination	Menopause symptoms and depression	3.75 mg *Cimicfugae rhizoma* extract siccus (corresponds to 22.5–41 mg of rootstock) and 70 mg *Hyperici* herb extract siccus (corresponds to 245–350 mg of herb)	Randomized controlled trial with 150 subjects in treatment arm showed combination superior to placebo in alleviating climacteric complaints, including psychological component (14).
	*Mind-Body–Based Therapies*		
Relaxation techniques	Paced respiration may decrease central sympathetic activity and, therefore, may decrease frequency and severity of hot flashes.	Eight 1-hour biweekly treatments; relief may be short-lived; therefore, women should be disciplined about using relaxation techniques frequently (15)	Randomized controlled trial with 11 subjects in paced respiration group reported fewer symptoms (16).
			Randomized controlled trial with 11 subjects in relaxation group who reported less hot flash intensity and psychologic symptoms (17).

(continued)

Table 6. Potentially Beneficial Complementary and Alternative Therapies Listed By Condition (continued)

Therapies by Condition	Putative Effects	Dose	Evidence-Based Support
Menopause (continued)			
Whole Medical Systems			
Acupuncture	Improve or eliminate menopausal symptoms	Weekly for 3 weeks, then once every other week for a total of six 20–30 minute treatments	Eight women from a convenience sample were randomized to the experimental acupuncture group and showed fewer hot flushes and sleep disturbances (18).
		Weekly for 3 months, then monthly for 3 months	Pilot study with 15 subjects showed improvement in menopausal symptoms, but not libido (19).
Preconception, Infertility, and Pregnancy			
Biologically Based Therapies			
Concentrated bioflavonoids	Avoid secondary to increased risk of infant and early childhood lymphomas	N/A	Dietary bioflavonoids were shown to induce site-specific cleavage in the mixed lineage leukemia breakpoint cluster region in cell cultures (20).
Vitamin B_6 (pyridoxine)	Decreased nausea and vomiting	30 mg daily	Randomized controlled trial with 169 subjects taking pyridoxine for more than 17 weeks reported decreased severity of nausea (21).
		25 mg every 8 hours for 72 hours	Randomized controlled trial with 31 subjects in the pyridoxine group reported reduced nausea scores (22).
Ginger	Decreased nausea and vomiting	1 g per day	Randomized controlled trial with 32 subjects in the ginger group reported less severe nausea and vomiting in pregnancy (23).
Omega-3 fatty acids DHA	Maternal diet rich in DHA associated with increased offspring stereopsis at 3.5 years	32-week gestation food questionnaire of white fish and oily fish	Prospectively collected diet data from 4,733 women showed increased stereoacuity among 435 full term infant at 3.5 years (24).
Mind-Body–Based Therapies			
Stress reduction techniques	Treatment of infertility	Ten sessions of stress reduction, breathing, and cognitive behavioral exercises	Fifty-four subjects in uncontrolled pilot study had less anxiety, depression, and fatigue. Thirty-four percent of patients got pregnant within 6 months (25).
Continuous support during labor	Shorter labor, less analgesia, oxytocin, forceps, and cesarean delivery	Continuous one-on-one doula-like support versus intermittent support	Meta-analysis of 11 randomized controlled trials found greater beneficial impact on the five listed outcomes with continuous support (26).
Hypnosis	Pain relief in labor	Four prenatal education sessions beginning at 20 weeks of gestation	Systematic review of five randomized clinical trials, in which subjects rated their labor pain less severe and required less analgesia (27, 28).

(continued)

Table 6. Potentially Beneficial Complementary and Alternative Therapies Listed By Condition *(continued)*

Therapies by Condition	Putative Effects	Dose	Evidence-Based Support
Preconception, Infertility, and Pregnancy (continued)			
Whole Medical Systems			
Acupuncture	Supportive in the treatment of infertility	Twice a week for 4 weeks	Pilot study with 8 subjects found curative effect of acupuncture in pulsatility index of uterine arteries (29).
		Acupuncture lasting 25 minutes was performed 25 minutes before and after embryo transfer.	Eighty subjects who received acupuncture in randomized controlled trial had higher clinical pregnancy rates (30).
	Nausea and vomiting of pregnancy	Acupuncture or acupressure applied to the P6 point on the volar aspect of the wrist; durations 1 day to 4 weeks	Systematic review of randomized controlled trials reported 10 of 14 studies proved efficacy (2); results promising, but equivocal in NIH Consensus Statement (31); Cochrane review found P6 acupuncture equivocal (32).
	Version of breech	Stimulation of acupoint BL 67 by moxa (Japanese term for *Artemisia vulgaris*) rolls for 7 days, with treatment for additional 7 days if the fetus persisted in the breech presentation	One hundred and thirty subjects randomized to the intervention group showed increased fetal activity during the treatment period and cephalic presentation after the treatment period and at delivery (33).
	Management of labor	20 minute-session each week for 4 weeks starting at 36 weeks of gestation	Fifty seven subjects in case control study had shorter first stage of labor (34).
		20-minute session each week for 4 weeks starting at 35 weeks of gestation	Forty matched pairs in the treatment arm had a shorter first stage of labor pairs (35)
	Pain associated with cesarean birth	De qi elicited; needles left for a few minutes or through delivery	Systematic review of three randomized controlled trials showed less pain and reported less analgesia use (36).
	Nausea and vomiting associated with cesarean birth	Acupressure bands placed at P6 5 minutes before spinal anesthesia	Forty seven patients in randomized controlled trials who received acupressure reported reduced nausea and vomiting during and after cesarean delivery (37).
Surgical Patients			
Mind-Body–Based Therapies			
Hypnosis, imagery, music, and relaxation techniques	Reduced blood loss, decreased pain and medication use, increased return of bowel function, decreased psychologic stress, and decreased length of hospital stays	Music and therapeutic suggestion during surgery	Randomized controlled trial with 31 subjects in the intervention group reported less analgesic requirements (38).
		Therapeutic suggestion during neurolept-anesthesia	Randomized controlled trial with 36 subjects in the intervention arm reported less postoperative nausea and vomiting (39).

(continued)

Table 6. Potentially Beneficial Complementary and Alternative Therapies Listed By Condition *(continued)*

Therapies by Condition	Putative Effects	Dose	Evidence-Based Support
Surgical Patients (continued)			
Whole Medical Systems			
Acupuncture	No anesthetic agents needed for cesarean delivery, with blood pressure levels, heart rates, and respiratory rates remaining stable	Frequencies of electrical pulsatile stimulation were 2 Hz on both legs and 800 Hz for abdominal paraincisional needles	Population-based study of 25,271 cases and 16,649 cases in two time intervals showed success rates of 92.1% and 98.9%, respectively (40)
	Acupuncture preoperatively decreased pain, nausea and vomiting, analgesic requirement, and sympathoadrenal responses.	Preoperative insertion of intra-dermal needles at acupoints 2.5 cm from spinal vertebrae and maintained in position for 4 days	Controlled, double-blind study reported on 50 patients for upper abdominal surgery and 39 patients for lower abdominal surgery with reduced post-operative pain and analgesia use (41).

Abbreviations: DHA indicates docosahexaenoic acid; NIH, National Institutes of Health; PMDD, premenstrual dysphoric disorder; PMS, premenstrual syndrome.

1. Thys-Jacobs S, Starkey P, Bernstein D, Tian J. Calcium carbonate and the premenstrual syndrome: effects on premenstrual and menstrual symptoms. Premenstrual Syndrome Study Group. Am J Obstet Gynecol 1998;179:444–52.

2. Fugh-Berman A, Kronenberg F. Complementary and alternative medicine (CAM) in reproductive-age women: a review of randomized controlled trials. Reprod Toxicol 2003;17:137–52.

3. Facchinetti F, Borella P, Sances G, Fioroni L, Nappi RE, Genazzani AR. Oral magnesium successfully relieves premenstrual mood changes. Obstet Gynecol 1991;78:177–81.

4. Walker AF, De Souza MC, Vickers MF, Abeyasekera S, Collins ML, Trinca LA. Magnesium supplementation alleviates premenstrual symptoms of fluid retention. J Womens Health 1998;7:1157–65.

5. Proctor ML, Murphy PA. Herbal and dietary therapies for primary and secondary dysmenorrhoea. Cochrane Database of Systemic Reviews 2001, Issue 2. Art. No.: CD002124. DOI: 10.1002/14651858.CD002124.

6. Kleijnen J, Ter Riet G, Knipschild P. Vitamin B6 in the treatment of the premenstrual syndrome—a review [published erratum appears in Br J Obstet Gynaecol 1991;98:329–30]. Br J Obstet Gynaecol 1990;97:847–52.

7. Tseng YF, Chen CH, Yang YH. Rose tea for relief of primary dysmenorrhea in adolescents: a randomized controlled trial in Taiwan. J Midwifery Womens Health 2005;50:e51–7.

8. Proctor ML, Hing W, Johnson TC, Murphy PA. Spinal manipulation for primary and secondary dysmenorrhoea. Cochrane Database of Systemic Reviews 2006, Issue 3. Art. No.: CD002119. DOI: 10.1002/14651858.CD002119.pub3.

9. Goodale IL, Domar AD, Benson H. Alleviation of premenstrual syndrome symptoms with the relaxation response. Obstet Gynecol 1990;75:649–55.

10. Proctor ML, Smith CA, Farquhar CM, Stones RW. Transcutaneous electrical nerve stimulation and acupuncture for primary dysmenorrhoea. Cochrane Database of Systematic Reviews 2002, Issue 1. Art. No.: CD002123. DOI: 10.1002/14651858.CD002123.

11. Habek D, Habek JC, Barbir A. Using acupuncture to treat premenstrual syndrome. Arch Gynecol Obstet 2002;267:23–6.

12. Wuttke W, Seidlova-Wuttke D, Gorkow C. The Cimicifuga preparation BNO 1055 vs. conjugated estrogens in a double-blind placebo-controlled study: effects on menopause symptoms and bone markers. Maturitas 2003;44 Suppl 1:S67–77.

13. Newton KM, Reed SD, LaCroix AZ, Grothaus LC, Ehrlich K, Guiltinan J. Treatment of vasomotor symptoms of menopause with black cohosh, multibotanicals, soy, hormone therapy, or placebo: a randomized trial. Ann Intern Med 2006;145:869–79.

14. Uebelhack R, Blohmer JU, Graubaum HJ, Busch R, Gruenwald J, Wernecke KD. Black cohosh and St. John's wort for climacteric complaints: a randomized trial. Obstet Gynecol 2006;107:247–55.

15. Jones CR, Czajkowski L. Evaluation and management of insomnia in menopause. Clin Obstet Gynecol 2000;43:184–97.

16. Freedman RR, Woodward S. Behavioral treatment of menopausal hot flushes: evaluation by ambulatory monitoring. Am J Obstet Gynecol 1992;167:436–9.

17. Irvin JH, Domar AD, Clark C, Zuttermeister PC, Friedman R. The effects of relaxation response training on menopausal symptoms. J Psychosom Obstet Gynaecol 1996;17:202–7.

18. Cohen SM, Rousseau ME, Carey BL. Can acupuncture ease the symptoms of menopause? Holist Nurs Pract 2003;17:295–9.

19. Porzio G, Trapasso T, Martelli S, Sallusti E, Piccone C, Mattei A, et al. Acupuncture in the treatment of menopause-related symptoms in women taking tamoxifen. Tumori 2002;88:128–30.

20. Strick R, Strissel PL, Borgers S, Smith SL, Rowley JD. Dietary bioflavonoids induce cleavage in the MLL gene and may contribute to infant leukemia. Proc Natl Acad Sci U S A 2000;97:4790–5.

21. Vutyavanich T, Wongtra-ngan S, Ruangsri R. Pyridoxine for nausea and vomiting of pregnancy: a randomized, double-blind, placebo-controlled trial. Am J Obstet Gynecol 1995;173:881–4.

(continued)

Table 6. Potentially Beneficial Complementary and Alternative Therapies Listed By Condition *(continued)*

22. Sahakian V, Rouse D, Sipes S, Rose N, Niebyl J. Vitamin B6 is effective therapy for nausea and vomiting of pregnancy: a randomized, double-blind placebo-controlled study. Obstet Gynecol 1991;78:33-6.

23. Vutyavanich T, Kraisarin T, Ruangsri R. Ginger for nausea and vomiting in pregnancy: randomized, double-masked, placebo-controlled trial. Obstet Gynecol 2001;97:577-82.

24. Williams C, Birch EE, Emmett PM, Northstone K. Stereoacuity at age 3.5 y in children born full-term is associated with prenatal and postnatal dietary factors: a report from a population-based cohort study. Avon Longitudinal Study of Pregnancy and Childhood Study Team. Am J Clin Nutr 2001;73:316-22.

25. Domar AD, Seibel MM, Benson H. The mind/body program for infertility: a new behavioral treatment approach for women with infertility. Fertil Steril 1990;53:246-9.

26. Scott KD, Berkowitz G, Klaus M. A comparison of intermittent and continuous support during labor: a meta-analysis. Am J Obstet Gynecol 1999;180:1054-9.

27. Martin AA, Schauble PG, Rai SH, Curry RW Jr. The effects of hypnosis on the labor processes and birth outcomes of pregnant adolescents [published erratum appears in J Fam Pract 2001;50:749]. J Fam Pract 2001;50:441-3.

28. Cyna AM, McAuliffe GL, Andrew MI. Hypnosis for pain relief in labour and childbirth: a systematic review. Br J Anaesth 2004;93:505-11.

29. Stener-Victorin E, Waldenstrom U, Andersson SA, Wikland M. Reduction of blood flow impedance in the uterine arteries of infertile women with electro-acupuncture. Hum Reprod 1996;11:1314-7.

30. Paulus WE, Zhang M, Strehler E, El-Danasouri I, Sterzik K. Influence of acupuncture on the pregnancy rate in patients who undergo assisted reproduction therapy. Fertil Steril 2002;77:721-4.

31. Acupuncture. National Institutes of Health. 1997;15(5):1-34.

32. Jewell D, Young G. Interventions for nausea and vomiting in early pregnancy. Cochrane Database of Systematic Review 2003, Issue 4. Art. No.: CD000145. DOI: 10.1002/14651858.CD000145.

33. Neri I, Fazzio M, Menghini S, Volpe A, Facchinetti F. Non-stress test changes during acupuncture plus moxibustion on BL67 point in breech presentation. J Soc Gynecol Investig 2002;9:158-62.

34. Zeisler H, Tempfer C, Mayerhofer K, Barrada M, Husslein P. Influence of acupuncture on duration of labor. Gynecol Obstet Invest 1998;46:22-5.

35. Tempfer C, Zeisler H, Heinzl H, Hefler L, Husslein P, Kainz C. Influence of acupuncture on maternal serum levels of interleukin-8, prostaglandin F2alpha, and beta-endorphin: a matched pair study. Obstet Gynecol 1998;92:245-8.

36. Lee H, Ernst E. Acupuncture for labor pain management: a systematic review. Am J Obstet Gynecol 2004;191:1573-9.

37. Harmon D, Ryan M, Kelly A, Bowen M. Acupressure and prevention of nausea and vomiting during and after spinal anaesthesia for caesarean section. Br J Anaesth 2000;84:463-7.

38. Nilsson U, Rawal N, Unestahl LE, Zetterberg C, Unosson M. Improved recovery after music and therapeutic suggestions during general anaesthesia: a double-blind randomised controlled trial. Acta Anaesthesiol Scand 2001;45:812-7.

39. Eberhart LH, Doring HJ, Holzrichter P, Roscher R, Seeling W. Therapeutic suggestions given during neurolept-anaesthesia decrease postoperative nausea and vomiting. Eur J Anaesthesiol 1998;15:446-52.

40. Wang DW, Jin YH. Present status of cesarean section under acupuncture anesthesia in China. Fukushima J Med Sci 1989;35:45-52.

41. Kotani N, Hashimoto H, Sato Y, Sessler DI, Yoshioka H, Kitayama M, et al. Preoperative intradermal acupuncture reduces postoperative pain, nausea and vomiting, analgesic requirement, and sympathoadrenal responses. Anesthesiology 2001;95:349-56.

When patients are asked this history directly in an atmosphere of respect, they usually are very disclosing, and the most appreciable barrier has been broken. Screening is especially important in patients who have conditions that may place them at particular risk of botanical interactions or adverse reactions.

Integrating Complementary and Alternative Techniques in Clinical Practice

Complementary and alternative therapies and their integration into treatment plans for women is a developing area. More often than not, conclusive scientific data are lacking. A useful framework for making decisions in these circumstances is as follows:

1. *Evaluate the potential to do harm.*

    a. *Direct harm, eg, the potential of the therapy itself to cause harm.* Sometimes there are data; at other times, it is necessary to use conservative medical judgment. In the most basic terms, any product ingested or any procedure that is invasive should be considered as a potential source of toxicity or risk. For example, it is feasible to think that undergoing chelation therapy or ingesting megadoses of vitamins or botanicals has the potential to do direct harm.

    b. *Indirect harm that can occur in two ways.* First, effective treatments might be postponed in a belief that an unproven therapy offers a cure. Second, patients might be financially exploited by paying for useless therapies.

2. *Evaluate the potential to be of benefit.*

    a. *Direct evidence; ie, what is the research on the effectiveness of this treatment?* There are varying levels of research in many applicable areas, including the use of acupressure and acupuncture with *hyperemesis gravidarum* and the use of mind–body approaches in surgery. The Natural Standards database is a very good source for an overview of the data and also provides information sheets that can be given to the patient.

b. *Cultural experience*. The use of certain approaches with purported success across centuries is another form of data. If there is no evidence or rationale for potential harm, a therapy may be explored on the basis of cultural experience.

c. *Personal belief*. The beliefs of the patient are appreciable and can be a powerful therapeutic ally. In the face of no evidence of harm, a strong belief in a therapy is an important factor to consider.

3. *Evaluate the "delivery system."* If a provider delivers the therapy, knowing his or her training and skill is important, as in conventional medicine. If the approach involves a product, knowing the quality of the company or product is equally important.

4. *Evaluate the integration*. Some approaches and some practitioners will integrate well with conventional medicine; others will not. Well-integrated care is essential. If therapies or therapists are not amenable to integration, they should not be recommended.

References

1. Barnes PM, Powell-Griner E, McFann K, Nahin RL. Complementary and alternative medicine use among adults: United States, 2002. Adv Data 2004;(343):1–19.

2. Eisenberg DM, Davis RB, Ettner SL, Appel S, Wilkey S, Van Rompay M, et al. Trends in alternative medicine use in the United States, 1990–1997: results of a follow-up national survey. JAMA 1998;280:1569–75.

3. Eisenberg DM, Kessler RC, Van Rompay MI, Kaptchuk TJ, Wilkey SA, Appel S, et al. Perceptions about complementary therapies relative to conventional therapies among adults who use both: results from a national survey. Ann Intern Med 2001;135:344–51.

4. National Center for Complementary and Alternative Medicine. What is CAM? CAM basics. Bethesda (MD): NCCAM; 2007. Available at: http://nccam.nih.gov/health/whatiscam/pdf/D347.pdf. Retrieved November 12, 2008.

Cardiovascular Disease

J. V. (Ian) Nixon and Rachel A. Rabinowitz

Cardiovascular (CV) disease, which includes hypertension, coronary heart disease, cerebrovascular disease, heart failure, and peripheral artery disease, is the leading cause of death among men and women in the United States (1). It claims more lives each year than cancer, chronic lung disease, diabetes mellitus, and accidents combined (2). In 2004, 32% of deaths occurred prematurely (ie, before age 77 years). Death rates from CV disease are higher in females than in males. Because more women survive to advanced ages, the total number of women dying of CV disease every year is increasing (1).

Women often rely on their obstetrician–gynecologists for their routine medical care. Thus, obstetrician–gynecologists are in a unique position to diagnose and manage CV disease—in particular, hypertension, coronary artery disease, and associated risk factors. Screening for CV disease risk factors is an important intrinsic component of general medical management. Physicians responsible for the general medical care of their patients must screen for, assess, and manage or facilitate management of known and identified CV disease factors, including lifestyle, diet, exercise, tobacco use, hypertension, dyslipidemia, and diabetes mellitus. It is important to counsel patients on the benefits of cessation of smoking (3). The earlier the modifications to lifestyle are initiated, the greater the benefit incurred by the patient (4). Guidelines are available for the management of hypertension, dyslipidemia, or an established diagnosis of coronary artery disease (5, 6, 7); there also are guidelines for the prevention of CV disease in women (8).

Hypertension and dyslipidemia are appreciable risk factors for CV disease, and they commonly coexist. The presence of one risk factor should alert the treating physician to the possible existence of the other (1). Recent data have shown that the aggressive pursuit of blood pressure and cholesterol control is of marked benefit to patients who are at increased CV risk (9).

Resources

Cardiovascular Disease

American College of Cardiology
http://www.acc.org

American Heart Association
http://www.americanheart.org

National Heart, Lung, and Blood Institute
http://www.nhlbi.nih.gov

Hypertension

Hypertension has been reviewed in a monograph from the American College of Obstetricians and Gynecologists (10). Hypertension affects at least 65 million adults in the United States (1). More than two thirds of people older than 65 years have hypertension (5). In the United States, African-American women have a higher prevalence of hypertension (47%) than do Caucasian women (32%) or Hispanic women (31%) (5). African Americans also have a higher prevalence of hypertension at a young age and a higher prevalence of prehypertension, defined as a systolic blood pressure of 120–140 mm Hg (10).

A significant number of patients with hypertension do not receive that diagnosis or are treated inadequately (11). Only 70% of Americans with hypertension are aware that they have it, only 60% are being treated, and only 34% have blood pressure that is controlled to levels recommended by the guidelines (5). Lack of diagnosis and inadequate treatment are particularly evident in minority populations and the elderly (5, 12).

The relationship between blood pressure and CV risk is continuous, consistent, and independent of other CV risk factors (5). The higher the blood pressure, the greater the risk of CV disease, especially stroke (13). An aggressive approach to blood pressure control is effective in reducing CV disease risk, including the risk of stroke, coronary artery disease, and renal disease (1, 5, 14, 15). National guidelines recommend decreasing blood pressure to less than 140/90 mm Hg, with lower levels recommended in diabetic patients with hypertension (5). Blood pressure control can be achieved and maintained in most patients, but it may require combination therapy with two or more antihypertensive drugs. There is no upper age limit for the management of hypertension; studies of patients older than 65 years repeatedly show the benefits of antihypertensive therapies (14).

Diagnosis

Health care providers should be aware of the variables in measuring blood pressure and the need for precision. Obtaining an accurate blood pressure reading is essential to the diagnosis of hypertension (Box 21). The classification of hypertension is shown in Table 7. Hypertension is generally defined as a systolic pressure greater than 140 mm Hg or a diastolic pressure greater than 90 mm Hg, over three measurements performed at different times over several weeks (5). Repeated mea-

Box 21

Establishing the Blood Pressure Level

Establishing the correct blood pressure level should include the following steps:

1. Measure the blood pressure level of the patient in a sitting position, preferably in a chair, after 5 minutes of rest.

2. Confirm that the patient has not smoked or consumed caffeine for 30 minutes before the measurement.

3. Confirm that the cuff size is appropriate for the arm circumference. The bladder length should encircle approximately 80% of the arm circumference.

4. Inflate the bladder to 30 mm Hg above the level where the radial pulse is occluded to avoid the possibility of the auscultatory gap.

5. Note that the systolic blood pressure level is the appearance of the first sound (phase I Korotkoff) and the diastolic blood pressure level is the disappearance of sound (phase V Korotkoff).

6. Repeat the measurement after 2 minutes and average the readings.

7. Measure the blood pressure in both arms. Subsequently, all blood pressure measurements should be taken from the arm with the higher blood pressure level.

8. Do not base the diagnosis on a single encounter.

Peng TC. Hypertension. Clin Update Womens Health Care 2005;IV(5):1–76.

surements are important because for 20–30% of patients, elevated blood pressure readings are related to "white-coat hypertension," a well-characterized clinical syndrome that may be associated with target-organ damage.

Individuals with prehypertension (systolic pressure levels of 130–139 mm Hg and diastolic pressure levels less than 89 mm Hg) are at increased risk for progression to hypertension (see Table 7) (1). Lifestyle modifications should be directed at such patients to decrease their risk of progression to hypertension. In a recent prospective study of patients with prehypertension, progression to hypertension was appreciably decreased in the treatment group (16).

More than 95% of individuals with hypertension have essential hypertension, and less than 5% have secondary hypertension. Inquiries regarding the signs and symptoms of a secondary etiology should be made when assessing a patient's other risk factors for CV disease, including family history, lifestyle, dyslipidemia, diabetes mellitus, and medication use.

Management

The management of hypertension incorporates therapeutic and nontherapeutic options. The nontherapeutic options include a thorough assessment of risk factors, such as smoking, obesity, dyslipidemia, diabetes mellitus, older age, and the presence of CV disease. Nonpharmacologic interventions may be used for initial therapy. Persistently elevated blood pressure levels require pharmacologic treatment (5, 10).

Table 7. Classification and Management of Blood Pressure Levels for Adults

Class	Systolic/Diastolic Blood Pressure Levels (mm Hg)	Treatment	Follow-Up
Normal	Below 120/80	None	Check in 2 years
Prehypertension	130–139/80–89	Lifestyle modification	Check in 1 year
Stage 1 hypertension	140–159/90–99	Lifestyle modification and therapy	Check every 2 months after blood pressure controlled
Stage 2 hypertension	Greater than 160/100	Lifestyle modification and therapy (usually with multiple drugs)	Check every 2 months after blood pressure controlled (often requires referral to a specialist)

The scheduling of follow-up appointments for blood pressure level monitoring obviously depends on patient reliability and compliance. The frequency of follow-up also is modified by the presence or absence of other cardiovascular risk factors and any target organ disease.
Chobanian AV, Bakris GL, Black HR, Cushman WC, Green LA, Izzo JL Jr, et al. The Seventh Report of the Joint National Committee on Prevention, Detection, Evaluation, and Treatment of High Blood Pressure: the JNC 7 report. National Heart, Lung, and Blood Institute Joint National Committee on Prevention, Detection, Evaluation, and Treatment of High Blood Pressure; National High Blood Pressure Education Program Coordinating Committee [published erratum appears in JAMA 2003;290:197]. JAMA 2003;289:2560–72.

Nonpharmacologic Interventions

A number of lifestyle modifications have been proved effective for reducing blood pressure:

- *Reducing weight.* Obesity is the single most common covariable found with hypertension (1). Blood pressure elevations quantitatively increase in direct proportion to body fat. For women, obesity is associated with a higher risk of CV events than for men and may occur with a clustering of risk factors, termed *metabolic syndrome.* In obese patients, weight loss of as little as 10 lb through diet and exercise has been shown to appreciably decrease blood pressure levels (17). A diet high in fruit and vegetables and low in fat, such as the Dietary Approaches to Stop Hypertension (DASH) diet, is recommended by the American Heart Association (18).

- *Initiating an exercise program.* Regular aerobic physical activity also is important for weight reduction and CV fitness. Studies have shown that moderate physical activity, such as 30–45 minutes of brisk walking on most days of the week, can decrease blood pressure levels (19).

- *Limiting sodium intake.* Recent studies have demonstrated that reducing sodium intake to 2.4 g per day can reduce blood pressure effectively. Doing so requires limiting the amount of salt added to food and choosing foods that are very low in salt (17, 19).

- *Limiting alcohol.* Excessive alcohol intake is another important risk factor for high blood pressure; it also can cause resistance to antihypertensive therapy. The American Heart Association recommends that women not consume more than one drink per day on average, because greater amounts may be associated with adverse consequences, such as an increased risk of breast cancer (1).

- *Smoking cessation.* A number of smoking cessation aids are now available (1).

- *Reducing stress.* A stressful lifestyle is associated with CV disease (1).

Pharmacologic Interventions

The strategy for treating hypertension is to individualize therapy according to patient demographic profiles and comorbidities. A person's sex does not appear to affect response to antihypertensive medication. A low dose of a single, long-acting antihypertensive agent usually is the initial step in treating hypertension. Commencing therapy in this manner maximizes tolerance and compliance while avoiding abrupt changes in blood pressure. If hypertension has not been controlled after several weeks, the dose can be increased. Only approximately 50% of patients achieve a target blood pressure of less than 140/90 mm Hg with monotherapy; thus, a second drug may be added (5). Using low doses of two drugs not only can improve efficacy but also can minimize the risk of dose-dependent adverse effects (5, 20).

Many antihypertensive drugs and combinations of antihypertensive drugs are available in the United States (Table 8). Clinical trials have shown that diuretics reduce morbidity and mortality in patients with hypertension (5). Diuretics are an effective first step in antihypertensive therapy (21). Because diuretics and β-blockers can cause elevations of triglyceride levels, the recommended first-step treatment for hypertensive patients with multiple CV risk factors is a calcium channel blocker or an angiotensin-converting enzyme (ACE) inhibitor, both of which have virtually no effect on the lipid profile (21). β-Blockers are preferred for patients with migraine, angina pectoris, history of myocardial infarction, and in some cases, heart failure. The ACE inhibitors (eg, benazepril, captopril, enalapril, and perindopril) offer advantages in patients with diabetes mellitus, heart failure, or left ventricular dysfunction. For African-American patients, diuretics and calcium channel blockers are more effective than β-blockers, ACE inhibitors, or angiotensin II receptor blockers. In older patients with isolated systolic hypertension, the preferred choice is a dihydropyridine calcium channel blocker (22).

Diuretics. Thiazide diuretics can be a cornerstone of therapy in patients with essential hypertension. Hydrochlorothiazide and chlorthalidone are the most widely used thiazide diuretics. Loop diuretics (eg, furosemide and bumetanide) are reserved for patients with coexisting renal insufficiency. Patients taking thiazide diuretics for hypertension should have periodic electrolyte assessment. Potassium-sparing diuretics, such as amiloride, triamterene, and spironolactone, can be used with other diuretics to prevent or reverse electrolyte losses. Other adverse effects of thiazides include hyperuricemia, glucose intolerance, and hyperlipidemia (22).

Diuretics are more effective than other antihypertensive agents for treating African Americans, the elderly, and patients who have hypertension associated with volume overload (congestive heart failure or renal insufficiency). When diuretics are not fully effective, a second agent may be needed, depending on the physiologic presentation, comorbidities, lifestyle, and treatment compliance of the patient.

β-Blockers. The β-blockers, like diuretics, are effective in decreasing CV disease mortality. However, β-blockers are less effective than diuretics for treating hypertension in African-American and elderly patients (22). β-Blockers produce a mild increase in serum potassium and blood sugar levels. Many β-blockers also affect lipid profiles. However, the lipid changes are minimal and may be offset by the beneficial effects of the β-blockers. Labetalol and carvedilol are nonselective β-blockers

Table 8. Drugs for Hypertension

Drug Class	Examples	Comments*
Diuretics		
Thiazides	Hydrochlorothiazide and chlorthalidone	Decrease rates of mortality, cerebrovascular accident, cerebrovascular disease, and isolated systolic hypertension; useful as first line therapy; effective in African Americans, elderly, and patients with volume overload hypertension (CHF and renal insufficiency); diuretics associated with hyperuricemia, glucose intolerance, and hyperlipidemia.
Loop diuretics	Furosemide and bumetanide	
Potassium sparing	Amiloride, triameterene, spironolactone, and eplerenone	
β-Blockers		
β-Adrenergic blockers	Atenolol, betaxolol, bisoprolol, metoprolol, nadolol, propranolol, and timolol	May be less effective in African Americans; in low doses bisoprolol, atenolol, metoprolol, acebetulol, and betaxolol are β-1 (cardiac) selective; intrinsic sympathomimetic activity less effective in increasing triglyceride levels and decreasing HDL levels; labetalol, equally effective in African Americans and Caucasians, and no effect on lipids; carvedilol promoted more for heart failure than hypertension.
β-Blockers with instrinsic sympathomimetic activity	Acebutolol, penbutolol, and pindolol	
β-Blockers with alpha blocking activity	Carvedilol and labetalol	
Calcium Channel Blockers		
Dihydropyridines	Amlodipine, felodipine, isradipine, nicardipine, nifedipine, and nisoldipine	Cause vasodilatation; dizziness, headache, lower extremity edema, and constipation are common.
Nondihydropyridines	Diltiazem and verapamil	
Angiotensin-Associated Drugs		
ACE inhibitors	Benazepril, captopril, enalapril, fosinopril, lisinopril, moxeiril, perindopril, quinapril, ramipril, and trandolapril	Used alone, less effective in African Americans; decrease mortality caused by CHD, increase survival in CHF and left ventricular dysfunction with myocardial infarction; preserve renal function in diabetes mellitus; and are associated with cough, especially in women.
Angiotensin II antagonists	Cadesartan, eprosartan, irbesartan, losartan, lomesartan, telmisartan, and valsartan	Effective in lowering blood pressure without the side effect of cough associated with ACE inhibitors.
Central 2 Agonists and Other Central-Acting Drugs		
	Clonidine, methyldopa, reserpine, and guanfacine	Side effects include sedation, dry mouth, and depression.
Vasodilators		
	Hydralazine and minoxidil	Associated with reflex tachycardia; usually administered with a blocker or central acting drug to decrease reflex tachycardia; hydralazine may cause a lupuslike reaction.

Abbreviations: ACE indicates angiotensin-converting enzyme; CHD, coronary heart disease; CHF, congestive heart failure; HDL, high density lipoprotein.

*For detailed information on side effects and dosages refer to Drugs for hypertension. Med Lett Drugs Ther 2001;43:17–22 and Chobanian AV, Bakris GL, Black HR, Cushman WC, Green LA, Izzo JL Jr, et al. The Seventh Report of the Joint National Committee on Prevention, Detection, Evaluation, and Treatment of High Blood Pressure: the JNC 7 report. National Heart, Lung, and Blood Institute Joint National Committee on Prevention, Detection, Evaluation, and Treatment of High Blood Pressure; National High Blood Pressure Education Program Coordinating Committee [published erratum appears in JAMA 2003;290:197]. JAMA 2003;289:2560–72.

Modified from Drugs for hypertension. Treat Guidel Med Lett 2005;3:34–48.

with α-adrenergic blocking activity. They generally do not affect lipid levels. The β-blockers commonly cause fatigue, depression, impotence, and decreased exercise tolerance (22). Contraindications to β-blocker use include asthma, chronic obstructive pulmonary disease, and conduction abnormalities of the heart. In patients with angina, abrupt discontinuation of β-blockers may cause rebound ischemia with myocardial infarction.

Angiotensin-Converting Enzyme Inhibitors. Angiotensin-converting enzyme inhibitors are effective and generally well tolerated in young and old patients. Most formulations can be given in a single daily dose and remain effective for 24 hours. However, in African Americans, concomitant use of a diuretic often is necessary for effective blood pressure control. Angiotensin-converting enzyme inhibitors do not affect plasma lipids or glucose tolerance. Studies have shown that they may reduce mortality in patients with coronary artery disease, prolong survival in individuals with heart failure or left ventricular dysfunction after a myocardial infarction, and preserve renal function in patients with diabetes mellitus (22). For these reasons, ACE inhibitors may be used as first-line therapy for hypertension in patients with prior myocardial infarction, congestive heart failure, or diabetic nephropathy. They may be used with other antihypertensive agents such as β-blockers, calcium channel blockers, α-blockers, and diuretics. They are not contraindicated in patients with asthma, chronic obstructive airway disease, depression, diabetes mellitus, or peripheral vascular disease. Although ACE inhibitors cause relatively few adverse effects, 10–25% of patients (especially women) develop a chronic dry cough, which may necessitate the discontinuation of therapy.

Angiotensin II Receptor Blockers. Angiotensin II receptor blockers produce hemodynamic effects equal to those of ACE inhibitors but carry less risk of producing a dry cough and other side effects. Studies have demonstrated that angiotensin II receptor blockers are as effective as ACE inhibitors, β-blockers, calcium channel blockers, and diuretics in the treatment of patients with mild to moderate hypertension. Recent studies have shown that angiotensin II receptor blockers are as effective as ACE inhibitors in reducing mortality in patients at high risk for CV events after myocardial infarction and associated evidence of heart failure (23). Angiotensin II receptor blockers also have been shown to be effective in patients with heart failure who are intolerant to ACE inhibitor therapy.

Calcium Channel Blockers. Calcium channel blockers are one of the most widely used classes of agents for treating hypertension. They are especially effective in old patients and are equally effective in African-American and Caucasian patients (5, 22). Because they have virtually no effect on lipids, they also are recom-

mended for patients with multiple CV risk factors. Some calcium channel blockers have multiple indications, including angina pectoris. In the patients studied in the ALLHAT trial (Antihypertensive and Lipid-Lowering Treatment to Prevent Heart Attack Trial), amlodipine had no detrimental effects when compared with a diuretic in patients with diabetes mellitus or renal disease (21).

Selective α-1-Adrenergic Blockers. The α-blocking agents have CV benefits beyond decreasing blood pressure levels. They tend to increase insulin sensitivity, decrease total cholesterol and low-density lipoprotein cholesterol (LDL-C) levels, and increase high-density lipoprotein cholesterol (HDL-C) levels. They may be useful for patients with hypertension and concomitant diabetes mellitus, glucose intolerance, or dyslipidemia. The α-blockers generally are used in combination antihypertensive therapy. Although postural hypotension was formerly a concern during the initiation of a nonselective α-blocker, the use of a selective α-blocker, such as doxazosin, alleviates much of this concern. Nevertheless, it is still recommended that α-blockers be titrated up from their lowest available doses. Other side effects of α-blocker therapy are tachycardia, weakness, dizziness, and mild fluid retention. The α-blockers may cause stress urinary incontinence in women (22).

MONITORING THERAPY

The patient's hypertension should be reevaluated 2–4 weeks after the initiation of therapy to determine the adequacy of blood pressure control, the degree of patient adherence, and the presence of adverse effects. Because compliance often is an issue, long-term follow-up every 3–6 months is recommended after the blood pressure is adequately controlled (5). Side effects are common, and reports of them should be solicited. If they are minimal and do not interfere with compliance, discontinuation of an antihypertensive medication should not be necessary. Continued use over several months may diminish or eliminate side effects. However, if the medication causes appreciable lifestyle problems, trials of alternative agents should be considered.

Coronary Artery Disease

Awareness of CV disease as the leading cause of death in women is almost twice as high (55%) in Caucasian women as in African-American and Hispanic women (30% and 27%, respectively) (8). Since 1979, whereas mortality from CV disease in men has decreased gradually (between 30% and 50%), mortality from CV disease in women has continued to increase (24). For coronary artery disease in particular during the same time, mortality for men and women has gradually diminished, but much more rapidly for men than for women (Fig. 11) (1, 24).

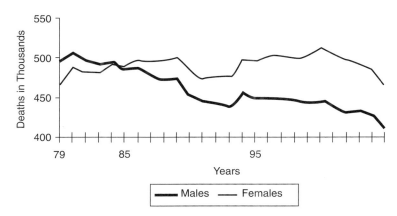

Figure 11. Cardiovascular disease mortality trends for males and females (United States 1979–2004). (From Rosamond W, Flegal K, Friday G, Furie K, Go A, Greenlund K, et al. Heart disease and stroke statistics—2007 update: a report from the American Heart Association Statistics Committee and Stroke Statistics Subcommittee. American Heart Association Statistics Committee and Stroke Statistics Subcommittee [published erratum appears in Circulation 2007;115:e172]. Circulation 2007;115[5]:e69–171.)

It is well accepted that for both sexes, the first presentation of coronary artery disease is an acute coronary syndrome. It also is well known that this first presentation occurs 10 years later in women (24). The worldwide INTERHEART study of 52,000 patients with acute coronary syndrome confirmed this delayed presentation in women, associated with a higher mortality and morbidity after the event (25). More premenopausal women are manifesting appreciably increased CV risk and an increased incidence of acute coronary syndrome equal to their male counterparts, with a significantly greater mortality rate (26). It is recognized that although the management of coronary artery disease in its acute and chronic presentations is the purview of a cardiologist, the condition often is noted first by a primary provider.

Diagnosis

The classic description of angina pectoris (dyspnea, palpitations, nausea, diaphoresis, lightheadedness, and dizziness) applies equally to men and to women. However, in women with myocardial infarction, more comorbidities, including hypertension, are present later in the course of symptoms; also, women have more high-risk complications, including heart failure and tachycardia (24). Because women who present with chest pain are more likely than men to have a noncardiac etiology, and because recent studies have shown a discordance between rates of coronary artery disease and the predicted probability of coronary disease, angina in women may be described as typical and atypical (24, 27). Nevertheless, women with multiple CV risk factors who present with chest pain, whether typical or atypical angina, warrant further work-up for possible coronary artery disease. Regardless of the result of the work-up, the completion emphasizes the importance of aggressive CV risk management (3). A consensus statement from the American Heart Association has recommended imaging (stress echocardiography and stress radionucleotide study) in symptomatic women undergoing stress testing (28, 29).

Management

The management of coronary artery disease incorporates therapeutic and preventive aspects (30, 31). Therapeutic management includes percutaneous intervention and coronary artery bypass surgery, in addition to medical management. The preventive aspects of effective CV risk management include effective counseling regarding diet, exercise, and cigarette smoking and the effective management of treatable CV risk factors, including hypertension, dyslipidemia, and diabetes mellitus.

PREVENTION

Dyslipidemia. The management of dyslipidemia as a CV risk factor is therapeutic and preventive; preventive management involves the use of therapeutic agents capable of significantly decreasing LDL-C levels and reducing CV risk (3). Because elevated serum total cholesterol, LDL-C, and triglyceride concentrations and decreased levels of HDL-C are recognized as risk factors for CV disease in men and women, various therapeutic agents have been advocated for modifying these parameters as a means of decreasing CV risk. Women are less likely then men to be aware of their abnormal cholesterol profiles (1). More than 50% of women in the United States have total cholesterol levels higher than 200 mg/dL, a level considered to be the upper limit of normal (1). The menopause adversely affects the lipid profile. Nearly 40% of women older than 55 years have elevated cholesterol levels (32).

In the past, postmenopausal women controlled their lipid levels by taking estrogen therapy, which reduces

LDL-C levels and increases HDL-C levels. However, the results of the Heart and Estrogen/Progestin Replacement Study Follow-up (33) and the Women's Health Initiative (34) indicate that therapy that combines estrogen and progestin does not reduce the risk of CV events in women with preexisting coronary heart disease and is not effective for the primary prevention of coronary heart disease in women who start hormone therapy more than 5 years after menopause. As a result, many postmenopausal women have discontinued hormone therapy, and their doing so has unmasked cholesterol disorders. This event has presented an opportunity for physicians to improve women's lipid profiles by using other effective therapies, such as statin agents.

Management directed at decreasing CV risk must address all risk factors and be supplemented by therapies that favorably modify the lipid profile and significantly reduce CV risk. The statin drugs fall into this category (3). Statins are used for primary prevention in patients without a diagnosis of coronary artery disease or a history of an acute coronary syndrome. Statins also are used in secondary prevention in patients with a documented diagnosis of coronary artery disease, acute coronary syndrome, or both. Until recently, primary prevention management was essentially the therapeutic management of an abnormal lipid profile (6). In a patient considered to be at increased CV risk for any apparent reason, a lipid profile was obtained; if it was abnormal, the patient was appropriately treated according to the therapeutic guidelines (3, 6).

The recent publication of the data from the ASCOT-LLA (Anglo-Scandinavian Cardiac Outcomes Trial—Lipid Lowering Arm), a primary prevention trial, has broadened the base of patients shown to benefit from primary preventive care (35) to include patients with hypertension and three other CV risk factors irrespective of the lipid profile of the individual. Patients at moderate or high CV risk with a relatively normal lipid profile and without a history of coronary artery disease, who are undergoing treatment of hypertension, will benefit from the use of a statin drug to decrease their overall CV risk (3). Significant reductions in coronary events by approximately 30% and reductions of CV events by 25% also have been documented with treatment with lovastatin in generally healthy men and women with average cholesterol levels and without coronary heart disease or hypertension (36).

Secondary prevention is an area of therapeutic management that continues to evolve. Consensus secondary preventive management was straightforward. All patients who had experienced an acute coronary syndrome or who had a history of coronary artery disease documented by a prior myocardial infarction, cardiac catheterization, or positive stress imaging study received statin therapy, irrespective of their cholesterol levels, for the rest of their lives. The selection and dose of the drug were nonissues. More recent studies have shown that the choice of drug, coupled with the aggressive titration of the dose of the statin drug, further improves the prognosis of the individual patient (3). The level of LDL-C in the monitoring of the titration of the dose of statin drug has become an indicator of the dosage of statin required by the individual patient (3). Until outcome data on the drugs become available, nonstatin therapies capable of efficiently reducing LDL-C levels are being used for preventive purposes only as supplementary therapy and not as replacement therapies (3).

Data on women in the completed preventive therapeutic trials are not adequate. Not all the trials included women and in the trials that did, females remained the minority of the patients (21.4%) (3). Nevertheless, in the primary and secondary prevention trials, there were no appreciable differences in reduction in outcomes in the treated or high-dose–treated groups in the female patients compared with the male patients (3).

The effective management of dyslipidemia incorporates effective risk factor management, including counseling on diet and exercise. Therapeutic management initially includes the maximal and effective use of statin therapies because of their pleiotropic properties, particularly their proven ability to decrease CV risk significantly; it also includes the complementary use of nonstatin therapies as supplementary therapies when and where necessary (3).

The currently available statin drugs (coenzyme A reductase inhibitors) are listed in Table 9. The table compares the doses of the different drugs. The selection of a particular statin drug is determined by the individual patient's LDL-C level and the LDL-C target (provided by the guidelines of the National Cholesterol Education Program III).

Statins are well tolerated, although some patients may develop myalgias, occasional instances of myopathy and elevated liver enzyme levels, and, rarely, rhabdomyolysis. As a precaution, regular liver function tests are advised. The incidence of adverse effects with statin use is remarkably low and does not appear to be dose

Table 9. Available Statin Drugs and Their Dose-for-Dose Comparative Efficacy

Agent	Doses (mg)				
Fluvastatin	40	80			
Pravastatin	20	40	80		
Lovastatin	20	40	80		
Simvastatin	10	20	40	0	
Atorvastatin	–	10	20	40	80
Rosuvastatin	–	5	10	20	40

Modified from Roberts WC. The rule of 5 and the rule of 7 in lipid-lowering by statin drugs [editorial]. Am J Cardiol 1997; 80:106–7.

related in all statins (3). Statins have not been tested in pregnant women and should not be used in this population. Lipid-regulating drugs are customarily discontinued before conception. Women of childbearing age who use statins must be counseled about the need for contraception to prevent pregnancy.

Obesity. Overweight and obesity management is clearly multifactorial. Weight loss relies appreciably on self-motivation. Thus, the counseling of overweight and obese patients is an integral part of the management of patients at increased risk for coronary artery disease. The risk of coronary artery disease associated with lack of physical activity is comparable with the increased risk observed for dyslipidemia, hypertension, and cigarette smoking (18). The American Heart Association issued recommendations about weight management to decrease the risk of coronary artery disease (see Resources). For more details on weight management, see "Role of Exercise, Diet, and Medical Intervention in Weight Management." Weight loss decreases blood pressure. Weight loss of 4.5 kg maintained for 36 months was found to reduce the progression from pre-hypertension to hypertension by 65% (37).

THERAPEUTIC MANAGEMENT

A number of drugs are used for the therapeutic, ancillary, and preventive management of coronary artery disease (30). Statin drugs have been discussed. Other drugs shown to be effective in CV risk reduction include aspirin, clopidogrel, β-blockers, and ACE inhibitors. Nitrates, β-blockers, and calcium channel blockers have been shown to be effective in therapeutic management (30). Several of these drugs—including β-blockers, ACE inhibitors, and calcium channel blockers—and their respective adverse effect profiles have been covered in the discussion of hypertension. Drugs not reviewed yet include aspirin, clopidogrel, and nitrates.

Aspirin. Multiple studies have shown the beneficial preventive capabilities of aspirin therapy in patients of both sexes with all forms of coronary artery disease. A meta-analysis of 140,000 patients in 300 studies confirmed these benefits, irrespective of the dose of aspirin used. Except where clear contraindications exist, aspirin is recommended for all patients with coronary artery disease (7, 38).

Clopidogrel. Clopidogrel is one of another group of agents capable of blocking platelet aggregation that is advocated for the prevention of CV disease in patients with acute and chronic forms of coronary artery disease (7). Clopidogrel may be used in patients who are unable to tolerate aspirin. Some data show a complementary benefit when aspirin and clopidogrel are given to patients with acute coronary syndromes or to patients undergoing percutaneous coronary intervention (7). The antiplatelet activity of clopidogrel, like that of aspirin,

lasts 4–8 days after drug discontinuation. The increased vulnerability to bleed of patients taking antiplatelet therapies continues for the same period.

Nitrates. Organic nitrates remain the most commonly used antianginal therapy. By relaxing smooth muscle, their vasodilatory effects occur in systemic arteries, including coronary arteries, and veins (30). Nitrates reduce the preload and the afterload to the heart, more particularly affecting preload. In patients with stable angina, nitrates improve exercise tolerance and time to electrocardiographic changes during treadmill exercise (38). There appears to be a synergistic effect with nitrates in patients with coronary disease when they are given in combination with calcium channel blockers and β-blockers (30). Nitrates may be administered in several different forms, which include topical, sublingual, oral, and intravenous routes. Adverse effects of nitrates include headaches, flushing, and hypotension. The use of nitrates in combination with phosphodiesterase-5 inhibitors, such as sildenophil, should be avoided because of possible prolonged life-threatening hypotension (30).

Mitral Valve Prolapse

Mitral valve prolapse (MVP), also known as systolic click murmur syndrome and Barlow syndrome, is a relatively common disorder (39). It affects approximately 2% of the general population and is twice as common in women as in men. Most patients with MVP are asymptomatic. Persons with more severe valve abnormalities and mitral regurgitation are at risk for the same complications as other patients with mitral valve disease, particularly infective endocarditis and arrhythmias. Patients with thickened or redundant mitral valves have an increased risk of endocarditis, mitral regurgitation, and mitral valve replacement. Sudden death associated with MVP is rare.

Mitral valve prolapse is defined as an abnormal systolic displacement of the mitral valve leaflets superiorly and posteriorly into the left atrium. It usually occurs as an isolated case in families and is considered to be an inherited connective tissue disease that is autosomal dominant with variable penetrance. It has been associated with a number of medical conditions, including hyperthyroidism, Marfan syndrome, Ehlers-Danlos syndrome, pseudoxanthoma elasticum, polyarteritis nodosa, osteogenesis imperfecta, myotonic dystrophy, and von Willebrand disease.

Symptoms of MVP rarely occur before adulthood. The most common symptom is palpitations. Atypical chest pain may occur; it may be recurrent and incapacitating but produces no evidence of ischemia on stress testing. Some patients also have reported fatigue and dyspnea associated with MVP.

Antibiotic prophylaxis to prevent endocarditis has been recommended for patients with MVP and auscultatory findings on echocardiography of valvular regurgitation, thickened leaflets, or both (40). Guidelines from the American Heart Association no longer recommend antibiotic prophylaxis in patients with mitral valve prolapse (41).

References

1. Rosamond W, Flegal K, Friday G, Furie K, Go A, Greenlund K, et al. Heart disease and stroke statistics--2007 update: a report from the American Heart Association Statistics Committee and Stroke Statistics Subcommittee. American Heart Association Statistics Committee and Stroke Statistics Subcommittee [published erratum appears in Circulation 2007;115:e172]. Circulation 2007;115:e69–171.

2. Minino AM, Heron MP, Smith BL. Deaths: preliminary data for 2004. 2006;54(19):1–49.

3. Nixon JV. Lower is better—the contemporary concept of low-density lipoprotein lowering in the preventive management of cardiovascular risk: does this apply to all patients? Prev Cardiol 2006;9:219–25; quiz 226–7.

4. Berenson GS, Srinivasan SR, Bao W, Newman WP 3rd, Tracy RE, Wattigney WA. Association between multiple cardiovascular risk factors and atherosclerosis in children and young adults. The Bogalusa Heart Study. N Engl J Med 1998;338:1650–6.

5. Chobanian AV, Bakris GL, Black HR, Cushman WC, Green LA, Izzo JL Jr, et al. The Seventh Report of the Joint National Committee on Prevention, Detection, Evaluation, and Treatment of High Blood Pressure: the JNC 7 report. National Heart, Lung, and Blood Institute Joint National Committee on Prevention, Detection, Evaluation, and Treatment of High Blood Pressure; National High Blood Pressure Education Program Coordinating Committee [published erratum appears in JAMA 2003;290:197]. JAMA 2003;289:2560–72.

6. Third Report of the National Cholesterol Education Program (NCEP) Expert Panel on Detection, Evaluation, and Treatment of High Blood Cholesterol in Adults (Adult Treatment Panel III) final report. National Cholesterol Education Program (NCEP) Expert Panel on Detection, Evaluation, and Treatment of High Blood Cholesterol in Adults (Adult Treatment Panel III). Circulation 2002; 106:3143–421.

7. Smith SC Jr, Allen J, Blair SN, Bonow RO, Brass LM, Fonarow GC, et al. AHA/ACC guidelines for secondary prevention for patients with coronary and other atherosclerotic vascular disease: 2006 update endorsed by the National Heart, Lung, and Blood Institute. American Heart Association. American College of Cardiology. National Heart, Lung, and Blood Institute. J Am Coll Cardiol 2006;47:2130–9.

8. Mosca L, Appel LJ, Benjamin EJ, Berra K, Chandra-Strobos N, Fabunmi RP, et al. Evidence-based guidelines for cardiovascular disease prevention in women. American Heart Association. Circulation 2004;109:672–93.

9. Kostis JB. The importance of managing hypertension and dyslipidemia to decrease cardiovascular disease. Cardiovasc Drugs Ther 2007;21:297–309.

10. Peng TC. Hypertension. Clin Update Womens Health Care 2005;IV(5):1–76.

11. Greenlund KJ, Croft JB, Mensah GA. Prevalence of heart disease and stroke risk factors in persons with prehypertension in the United States, 1999-2000. Arch Intern Med 2004;164:2113–8.

12. Hyman DJ, Pavlik VN. Characteristics of patients with uncontrolled hypertension in the United States [published erratum appears in N Engl J Med 2002;346:544]. N Engl J Med 2001;345:479–86.

13. Douglas JG, Bakris GL, Epstein M, Ferdinand KC, Ferrario C, Flack JM, et al. Management of high blood pressure in African Americans: consensus statement of the Hypertension in African Americans Working Group of the International Society on Hypertension in Blacks. Hypertension in African Americans Working Group of the International Society on Hypertension in Blacks. Arch Intern Med 2003;163:525–41.

14. Lewington S, Clarke R, Qizilbash N, Peto R, Collins R. Age-specific relevance of usual blood pressure to vascular mortality: a meta-analysis of individual data for one million adults in 61 prospective studies. Prospective Studies Collaboration [published erratum appears in Lancet 2003;361:1060]. Lancet 2002;360:1903–13.

15. Goldstein LB, Adams R, Alberts MJ, Appel LJ, Brass LM, Bushnell CD, et al. Primary prevention of ischemic stroke: a guideline from the American Heart Association/ American Stroke Association Stroke Council: cosponsored by the Atherosclerotic Peripheral Vascular Disease Interdisciplinary Working Group; Cardiovascular Nursing Council; Clinical Cardiology Council; Nutrition, Physical Activity, and Metabolism Council; and the Quality of Care and Outcomes Research Interdisciplinary Working Group: the American Academy of Neurology affirms the value of this guideline. American Heart Association/American Stroke Association Stroke Council; Atherosclerotic Peripheral Vascular Disease Interdisciplinary Working Group; Cardiovascular Nursing Council; Clinical Cardiology Council; Nutrition, Physical Activity, and Metabolism Council; Quality of Care and Outcomes Research Interdisciplinary Working Group; American Academy of Neurology [published erratum appears in Stroke 2007;38:207]. Stroke 2006;37:1583–633.

16. Julius S, Nesbitt SD, Egan BM, Weber MA, Michelson EL, Kaciroti N, et al. Feasibility of treating prehypertension with an angiotensin–receptor blocker. Trial of Preventing Hypertension (TROPHY) Study Investigators. N Engl J Med 2006;354:1685–97.

17. Effects of weight loss and sodium reduction intervention on blood pressure and hypertension incidence in overweight people with high-normal blood pressure. The Trials of Hypertension Prevention, phase II. The Trials of Hypertension Prevention Collaborative Research Group. Arch Intern Med 1997;157:657–67.

18. Krauss RM, Eckel RH, Howard B, Appel LJ, Daniels SR, Deckelbaum RJ, et al. AHA Dietary Guidelines: revision 2000: a statement for healthcare professionals from the Nutrition Committee of the American Heart Association. Circulation 2000;102:2284–99.

19. Pate RR, Pratt M, Blair SN, Haskell WL, Macera CA, Bouchard C, et al. Physical activity and public health. A recommendation from the Centers for Disease Control and Prevention and the American College of Sports Medicine. JAMA 1995;273:402–7.

20. Skolnik NS, Beck JD, Clark M. Combination antihypertensive drugs: recommendations for use. Am Fam Physician 2000;61:3049–56.

21. Major outcomes in high-risk hypertensive patients randomized to angiotensin-converting enzyme inhibitor or calcium channel blocker vs diuretic: The Antihypertensive and Lipid-Lowering Treatment to Prevent Heart Attack Trial (ALLHAT). ALLHAT Officers and Coordinators for the ALLHAT Collaborative Research Group. The Antihypertensive and Lipid-Lowering Treatment to Prevent Heart Attack Trial [published erratum appears in JAMA 2004; 291:2196]. JAMA 2002;288:2981–97.

22. Drugs for hypertension. Med Lett Drugs Ther 2001;43:17-22.

23. Pfeffer MA, McMurray JJ, Velazquez EJ, Rouleau JL, Kober L, Maggioni AP, et al. Valsartan, captopril, or both in myocardial infarction complicated by heart failure, left ventricular dysfunction, or both. Valsartan in Acute Myocardial Infarction Trial Investigators [published erratum appears in N Engl J Med 2004;350:203]. N Engl J Med 2003;349:1893–906.

24. Newby KL, Douglas PS. Cardiovascular disease in women. In: Libby P, Bonow RA, Zipes DP, editors. Braunwald's heart disease: a textbook of cardicovascular medicine. 8th ed. Philadelphia (PA): Saunders; 2008. p. 1955–66.

25. Yusuf S, Hawken S, Ounpuu S, Dans T, Avezum A, Lanas F, et al. Effect of potentially modifiable risk factors associated with myocardial infarction in 52 countries (the INTERHEART study): case-control study. INTERHEART Study Investigators. Lancet 2004;364:937–52.

26. Vaccarino V, Parsons L, Every NR, Barron HV, Krumholz HM. Sex-based differences in early mortality after myocardial infarction. National Registry of Myocardial Infarction 2 Participants. N Engl J Med 1999;341:217–25.

27. Shaw LJ, Merz CN, Pepine CJ, Reis SE, Bittner V, Kip KE, et al. The economic burden of angina in women with suspected ischemic heart disease: results from the National Institutes of Health—National Heart, Lung, and Blood Institute—sponsored Women's Ischemia Syndrome Evaluation. Women's Ischemia Syndrome Evaluation (WISE) Investigators. Circulation 2006;114:894–904.

28. Mieres JH, Shaw LJ, Arai A, Budoff MJ, Flamm SD, Hundley WG, et al. Role of noninvasive testing in the clinical evaluation of women with suspected coronary artery disease: Consensus statement from the Cardiac Imaging Committee, Council on Clinical Cardiology, and the Cardiovascular Imaging and Intervention Committee, Council on Cardiovascular Radiology and Intervention, American Heart Association. Cardiac Imaging Committee, Council on Clinical Cardiology, and the Cardiovascular Imaging and Intervention Committee, Council on Cardiovascular Radiology and Intervention, American Heart Association. Circulation 2005;111:682–96.

29. Shaw LJ, Vasey C, Sawada S, Rimmerman C, Marwick TH. Impact of gender on risk stratification by exercise and dobutamine stress echocardiography: long-term mortality in 4234 women and 6898 men. Eur Heart J 2005;26: 447–56.

30. Morrow DA, Gersh BJ. Chronic coronary artery disease. In: Libby P, Bonow RA, Zipes DP, editors. Braunwald's heart disease: a textbook of cardicovascular medicine. 8th ed. Philadelphia (PA): Saunders; 2008. p. 1353–418.

31. Sheikh AM, Crisco LV, Wenger NK. Angina, stable. Nixon JV, editor. AHA clinical cardiac consult. 2nd ed. Philadelphia (PA): Lippincott, Williams and Wilkins; 2007. 26–7.

32. Mosca L, Appel LJ, Benjamin EJ, Berra K, Chandra-Strobos N, Fabunmi RP, et al. Evidence-based guidelines for cardiovascular disease prevention in women. American Heart Association. Circulation 2004;109:672–93.

33. Grady D, Herrington D, Bittner V, Blumenthal R, Davidson M, Hlatky M, et al. Cardiovascular disease outcomes during 6.8 years of hormone therapy: Heart and Estrogen/progestin Replacement Study follow-up (HERS II). HERS Research Group [published erratum appears in JAMA 2002;288:1064]. JAMA 2002;288:49–57.

34. Rossouw JE, Anderson GL, Prentice RL, LaCroix AZ, Kooperberg C, Stefanick ML, et al. Risks and benefits of estrogen plus progestin in healthy postmenopausal women: principal results from the Women's Health Initiative randomized controlled trial. Writing Group for the Women's Health Initiative Investigators. JAMA 2002; 288:321–33.

35. Sever PS, Dahlof B, Poulter NR, Wedel H, Beevers G, Caulfield M, et al. Prevention of coronary and stroke events with atorvastatin in hypertensive patients who have average or lower-than-average cholesterol concentrations, in the Anglo-Scandinavian Cardiac Outcomes Trial—Lipid Lowering Arm (ASCOT-LLA): a multicentre randomised controlled trial. ASCOT investigators. Lancet 2003;361: 1149–58.

36. Downs JR, Clearfield M, Weis S, Whitney E, Shapiro DR, Beere PA, et al. Primary prevention of acute coronary events with lovastatin in men and women with average cholesterol levels: results of AFCAPS/TexCAPS. Air Force/Texas Coronary Atherosclerosis Prevention Study. JAMA 1998;279:1615–22.

37. Stevens VJ, Obarzanek E, Cook NR, Lee IM, Appel LJ, Smith West D, et al. Long-term weight loss and changes in blood pressure: results of the Trials of Hypertension Prevention, phase II. Ann Intern Med 2001;134:1–11.

38. Gibbons RJ, Abrams J, Chatterjee K, Daley J, Deedwania PC, Douglas JS, et al. ACC/AHA 2002 guideline update for the management of patients with chronic stable angina—summary article: a report of the American College of Cardiology/American Heart Association Task Force on Practice Guidelines (Committee on the Management of Patients With Chronic Stable Angina). American College of Cardiology; American Heart Association Task Force on Practice Guidelines. Committee on the Management of Patients With Chronic Stable Angina. Circulation 2003; 107:149–58.

39. Kuehn S, Herrman SC, Chaitman BR. Mitral valve prolapse, myxomatous degeneration of the heart. In: Nixon

JV, editor. AHA clinical cardiac consult. 2nd ed. Philadelphia (PA): Lippincott, Williams and Wilkins; 2007. p. 226–7.

40. Bonow RO, Carabello BA, Kanu C, de Leon AC Jr, Faxon DP, Freed MD, et al. ACC/AHA 2006 guidelines for the management of patients with valvular heart disease: a report of the American College of Cardiology/American Heart Association Task Force on Practice Guidelines (writing committee to revise the 1998 Guidelines for the Management of Patients With Valvular Heart Disease): developed in collaboration with the Society of Cardiovascular Anesthesiologists: endorsed by the Society for Cardiovascular Angiography and Interventions and the Society of Thoracic Surgeons. American College of Cardiology/ American Heart Association Task Force on Practice Guidelines. Society of Cardiovascular Anesthesiologists. Society for Cardiovascular Angiography and Interventions. Society of Thoracic Surgeons [published erratum appears in Circulation 2007;115:e409]. Circulation 2006;114: e84–231.

41. Wilson W, Taubert KA, Gewitz M, Lockhart PB, Baddour LM, Levison M, et al. Prevention of infective endocarditis: guidelines from the American Heart Association: a guideline from the American Heart Association Rheumatic Fever, Endocarditis, and Kawasaki Disease Committee, Council on Cardiovascular Disease in the Young, and the Council on Clinical Cardiology, Council on Cardiovascular Surgery and Anesthesia, and the Quality of Care and Outcomes Research Interdisciplinary Working Group. American Heart Association Rheumatic Fever, Endocarditis, and Kawasaki Disease Committee; American Heart Association Council on Cardiovascular Disease in the Young; American Heart Association Council on Clinical Cardiology; American Heart Association Council on Cardiovascular Surgery and Anesthesia; Quality of Care and Outcomes Research Interdisciplinary Working Group [published erratum appears in Circulation 2007;116: e376–7]. Circulation 2007;116:1736–54.

Substance Use

Cathy L. Melvin and William F. Rayburn

Physicians can play an important role by helping their patients to quit using tobacco, alcohol, and illicit drugs. It is especially important that obstetricians and gynecologists consider treatment options according to the pregnancy status of each patient, because the use of any of these substances poses significant risk to fetal, infant, and maternal health. Universal screening questions, brief intervention, and referral to treatment fall well within the purview of the obstetrician–gynecologist's role as a provider of primary care to women and may affect health outcomes.

Barriers to the use of screening tools for tobacco, alcohol, and illicit drug use exist for users and health care providers. Users may be reluctant to disclose their substance use to their physicians, may not believe that their physicians can help them quit, or may assume that they will get a lecture from their physicians instead of help with quitting (1). More than one third of current smokers report that they were never asked about their smoking status or urged to quit by their clinician (2, 3). Fewer than 15% of smokers who saw a physician in the past year reported being offered assistance in quitting smoking (4). Among current smokers and former smokers who were trying to quit and had seen a health care provider in the past year, only 61.8% reported that they received advice to quit from those providers (5).

Experts at the National Institute on Alcohol Abuse and Alcoholism (NIAAA) and the National Institute on Drug Abuse confirm that addiction is a "brain disease" that should be included in a review of systems just like any other biologic disease process. A medical diagnosis of addiction requires medical intervention in the same manner that a diagnosis of diabetes mellitus requires nutritional counseling, therapeutic agents, or both.

Medical care can be compromised if physicians are unaware of a patient's alcohol or drug abuse and, thus, miss related diagnoses or medication interactions with illicit drugs or alcohol. If the problem is not identified, major health risks may go unrecognized. Furthermore, patients may be harmed when substance abuse is treated by a physician as a moral rather than medical issue. Women who abuse alcohol or illicit drugs are more likely than men to be stigmatized and labeled as hopeless (6). Many women are reluctant to report use for several reasons, including the belief that they could lose their children, partners, or jobs or be placed in jail.

Smoking

Tobacco use can impair fertility, adversely affect fetal and maternal health, and predispose women to chronic diseases, such as cancer, pulmonary disease, and cardiovascular disease (7, 8). Maternal complications of smoking include spontaneous abortion, ectopic pregnancy, premature rupture of membranes, placenta previa, and placental abruption. Fetal effects include intrauterine growth restriction, prematurity, and low birth weight. Recent evidence also shows that exposure to secondhand smoke can increase the likelihood of cardiovascular disease, sudden infant death syndrome, and other smoking-related conditions, such as asthma.

As mentioned earlier, only 61.8% of current smokers and former smokers who were trying to quit reported that they received advice to quit from their health care providers (5). Physician reports of their use of evidence-based interventions mirrors that of their patients. A recent study in Ohio showed that 62% of obstetrician–gynecologists believed smoking cessation advice would be of significant value to their pregnant patients. Almost all of them (98%) asked their pregnant patients about smoking, but fewer engaged in advising (66%), assessing (42%), assisting (29%), or arranging for follow-up visits or referrals (6%) (9). The best way to identify smokers, especially among pregnant women, is to provide screening using a series of nonjudgmental questions.

All reviews conducted since the mid-1990s report consistent evidence that counseling by a trained clinician in one or more face-to-face sessions is effective for assisting smokers in their attempts to quit smoking. Meta-analyses reported strong, consistent evidence that pharmacologic treatments for smoking cessation can help people quit smoking and some evidence that a

---

Resources

Substance Use

Alcoholics Anonymous
http://www.aa.org

American Society of Addiction Medicine
http://www.asam.org

Narcotics Anonymous
http://www.na.org

National Cancer Institute: Smoking Quitline
http://cancer.gov/cancertopics/smoking

Robert Wood Johnson Foundation
http://www.rwjf.org

Substance Abuse and Mental Health Services
 Administration
http://www.samhsa.org

combination of the nicotine patch and a self-administered form of nicotine replacement therapy is more effective than a single form of nicotine replacement (10).

Overall, strategies shown to be effective for improving success of attempts to quit smoking include counseling, pharmacotherapies either alone or in combination, or pharmacotherapies combined with psychologic counseling. Among these options, there is a direct relationship with increasing intensity of counseling, use of more than one pharmacotherapy, and combining counseling and pharmacotherapy (10). The first-line medications include bupropion SR, nicotine gum, nicotine inhaler, nicotine lozenge, nicotine nasal spray, nicotine patch, and varenicline. The second-line medications include clonidine and nortriptyline. There is insufficient evidence to recommend medications for certain populations; eg, pregnant women, smokeless tobacco users, light smokers, and adolescents (11). These strategies can be effective whether applied in clinical settings using a rubric like the 5 A's (Box 22) or applied by telephone (eg, a quit line service) upon referral from a physician.

Various guidelines and professional organizations recommend that these approaches to assisting smokers in their attempts to quit be used in all clinical encounters with women. Additionally, assistance should be tailored to the particular issues faced by women at each life stage. For example, preconception care recommendations issued by the Centers for Disease Control and Prevention outline the importance of pursuing smoking cessation as part of preconception care (12). Similarly, the role of tobacco smoking in chronic illnesses can be discussed with older women who have completed their childbearing. Although the 5 A's approach has been particularly studied in pregnant women, this concept is appropriate for pregnant and nonpregnant smokers alike (11).

Alcohol Abuse

Although light to moderate alcohol consumption in middle-aged or older adults has been associated with some health benefits, such as reduced risk of coronary heart disease, alcohol misuse can lead to health problems and other problems in women. Abuse of alcohol is a major health problem for American women of any socioeconomic status, race, ethnicity, and age.

Alcohol abuse carries higher risks of cardiac and hepatic complications for women than for men. The alcohol-associated mortality rate is 50–100 times higher, and there is an increased burden of mental and physical disability. For some women, alcohol use can increase their risk of certain cancers (especially breast cancer), osteoporosis, early menopause, irregular menses, infertility, and early pregnancy loss. Maternal alcoholism is one of the leading preventable causes of fetal neurodevelopmental disorders.

Box 22

Treating Tobacco Use and Dependence: The Five A's

Step 1. Ask   Systematically identify all tobacco users at every visit:

- Ask every nonpregnant patient the question, "Do you currently smoke cigarettes?"
- Ask every pregnant patient the recommended multiple choice question.

Step 2. Advise   In a clear, strong, and personalized manner, strongly urge every tobacco user to quit.

Step 3. Assess   Determine the willingness of every tobacco user to make an attempt to quit at this time (eg, within the next 30 days). For women who are unwilling to quit smoking, physicians may consider brief counseling designed to increase their motivation to quit. One counseling approach—the 5 R's—involves a discussion of any one or more of the following issues:

- Risk of adverse outcomes
- Rewards associated with quitting smoking both in terms of health and feeling and looking better
- Relevance of smoking to the woman and her pregnancy, her health, and her family
- Roadblocks that undermine quit attempts and how to work around them
- Repetition of quit attempts as an opportunity to learn more about how to quit and to increase the likelihood of quitting

Step 4. Assist   Aid the patient in quitting by developing a quit plan.

Step 5. Arrange   Schedule follow-up contact, either in person or by telephone.

Fiore MC, Jaen CR, Baker TB, Bailey WC, Benowitz NL, Curry SJ, et al. Treating tobacco use and dependence: 2008 update. Clinical Practice Guideline. Rockville (MD): U.S. Department of Health and Human Services; 2008. Available at: http://www.surgeongeneral.gov/tobacco/treating_tobacco_use08.pdf. Retrieved November 12, 2008.

Physicians have been slow to implement universal screening, and rates of detection and referral to treatment among nonpregnant women remain very low.

Routine use of standardized tools will improve detection rates.

Screening questions related to alcohol and drug use should be asked equally of men and women and regardless of race or economic status. Women may be screened with the use of questionnaires such as T-ACE, TWEAK, or the NIAAA quantity and frequency questions. These questionnaires are more accurate than other tests in detecting women's patterns and tolerance to alcohol and other substance abuse, which differ from those of men (Box 23) (13). Women are more likely to be hidden drinkers and frequently underreport alcohol use, especially during pregnancy.

Few laboratory studies are helpful in screening and diagnosing patients who abuse alcohol. A blood alcohol level is of limited value, because ethanol is eliminated rapidly; thus, this test cannot predict actual drinking behaviors. Liver function studies can be of some value. A complete blood count may reflect macrocytosis caused by the direct effect of ethanol or associated folate deficiency. Positive tests for anemia may reflect folate deficiency, gastrointestinal bleeding, or bone marrow suppression.

Pregnant women are more likely to be screened than nonpregnant women. However, although the vulnerability of the fetus is an important concern, much evidence suggests that pregnant and nonpregnant women alike who abuse alcohol or use illicit drugs have coexisting or preexisting conditions (eg, mental health disorders, domestic violence, stress, childhood sexual abuse, poverty, or lack of resources) that make them vulnerable. Universal screening questions, brief intervention, and referral to treatment are believed to reduce the likelihood of preterm birth and neonatal complications in current and future pregnancies and to improve parenting capabilities.

Positive screening results merit referral for intervention. Interventions are summarized in the NIAAA Treatment Improvement Protocol number 35 and are designed to increase motivation to change by respecting autonomy, supporting self-efficacy, and offering hope and resources (14).

Illicit Drugs

In 2001, 37.6% of adult females reported having ever used illicit drugs, 10.6% reported use in the past year, and 5.5% reported use in the past month (15). The most frequently used drug was marijuana, followed by nonmedical use of any psychotherapeutic drug (eg, pain relievers, tranquilizers, stimulants, and sedatives).

Illicit drug use has major physical and mental health consequences and is associated with increased rates of sexually transmitted diseases in women, including hepatitis and human immunodeficiency virus (HIV) infection, as well as depression, domestic violence, poverty, and appreciable prenatal and neonatal complications. Among pregnant women aged 15–17 years, the rate of use increased to 15% in 2001. Between 1992 and 1998,

the health care costs associated with drug abuse were estimated at more than $144 billion yearly, including $503 million associated with health care costs for drug-exposed newborns (16).

Toxicologic screening can be used to detect recent use of various nonalcoholic substances. Immunoassay procedures generally are used, but confirmatory testing reduces false-positive results. Many laboratories perform multiple tests as a "drug panel" aimed at commonly used illicit drugs to detect illicit drug exposure within the past 1–3 days. Patient consent should be obtained before any toxicologic screening, and clinicians should be familiar with any state reporting requirements regarding the use or abuse of substances during pregnancy.

Intervention for Users of All Substances of Abuse

The management of an effective overall therapeutic process in a primary care setting is probably not possible for most primary care providers. Physicians can, however, *S*creen for illicit drug use, offer a *B*rief *I*ntervention, and *R*efer their patients to specialized *T*reatment (SBIRT). The SBIRT process also is accepted as effective for the reduction of problem drinking and tobacco use by various public health agencies of the U.S. Department of Health and Human Services and many medical specialty societies. Several SBIRT models, such as the 5 A's, have been shown to be effective in improving outcomes of persons with problematic alcohol and nicotine use in general medical care settings (17). Evidence from a formal evaluation by the U.S. Preventive Services Task Force showed insufficient evidence to recommend for or against the use of SBIRT for illicit drug users because of the absence of sufficient numbers of studies.

Recovery from substance abuse is a long-term process. Better outcomes are seen in individualized programs that provide a greater range, frequency, and intensity of services. Four critical components of treatment should be pursued: 1) detoxification and relief of acute physical symptoms, 2) medications combined with counseling, 3) behavior therapies for skill building and problem solving to prevent relapse, and 4) assessment and treatment of coexisting mental and medical disorders.

Despite appreciable decreases in use and, in some cases, total abstinence from illicit drug, tobacco, or alcohol use during pregnancy, up to two thirds of women relapse after delivery. Providing support services (eg, transportation or childcare services) can aid in illicit drug treatment. Social service departments in many hospitals are an invaluable source of assistance and referral for patients with substance abuse problems. Many additional community and clinical resources are available for patient and professional use (see Resources).

Use of alcohol and illicit drugs among youth is prevalent. Individuals who begin drinking when they are aged 14 years are at least three times more likely to experience dependence than individuals who delay drinking until they are aged 21 years (18). Drinking at younger ages increases the likelihood of alcohol-related unintentional injuries, motor vehicle crash involvement after drinking, and unprotected sexual intercourse. Most adult smokers (98%) began smoking as adolescents or young adults; 83% of smokers started before they were

---

Box 23

Alcohol and Substance Use Screening Tools

T-ACE

T   Tolerance: How many drinks does it take to make you feel high?

More than 2 drinks is a positive response—score 2 points.

A   Have people **A**nnoyed you by criticizing your drinking?

If "Yes" —score 1 point.

C   Have you ever felt you ought to **C**ut down on your drinking?

If "Yes"—score 1 point.

E   **E**ye Opener: Have you ever had a drink first thing in the morning to steady your nerves or get rid of a hangover?

If "Yes"—score 1 point.

A total score of 2 or more points indicates a positive screen for pregnancy risk drinking.

Reprinted from the American Journal of Obstetrics and Gynecology, Vol 160, Sokol RJ, Martier SS, Ager JW, The T-ACE questions: practical prenatal detection of risk drinking, 863-8; discussion 868-70, Copyright Elsevier 1989.

TWEAK

T   Tolerance: How many drinks can you hold?

If 5 or more drinks, score 2 points.

W   Have close friends or relatives **W**orried or complained about your drinking in the past year?

If "Yes"—2 points.

E   **E**ye Opener: Do you sometimes take a drink in the morning when you get up?

If "Yes"—1 point.

A   **A**mnesia: Has a friend or family member ever told you about things you said or did while you were drinking that you could not remember?

If "Yes"—1 point.

K(C)   Do you sometimes feel the need to **C**ut down on your drinking?

If "Yes"—1 point.

The TWEAK is used to screen for pregnant at-risk drinking, defined here as the consumption of 1 oz or more of alcohol per day while pregnant. A total score of 2 points or more indicates a positive screen for pregnancy risk drinking.

Modified from Chan AW, Pristach EA, Welte JW, Russell M. Use of the TWEAK test in screening for alcoholism/heavy drinking in three populations. Alcohol Clin Exp Res 1993;17:1188-92.

NIAAA Questionnaire

- Do you drink? Do you use drugs?
- On average, how many days per week do you drink alcohol (beer, wine, or liquor)?
- On a typical day when you drink, how many drinks do you have?

Positive score: more than 14 drinks per week for men and more than 7 drinks per week for women.

- What is the maximum number of drinks you had on any given occasion during the past month?

Positive score: more than 4 for men and more than 3 for women.

National Institute on Alcohol Abuse and Alcoholism. Helping patients with alcohol problems: a health practitioner's guide. Bethesda (MD): NIAAA; 2003. Available at: http://www.niaaa.nih.gov/publications/Practitioner/PractitionersGuideFINAL.pdf. Retrieved January 7, 2004.

aged 18 years, and 16% of smokers started between the ages of 18 years and 24 years (7). Comprehensive anti-smoking programs have been shown to reduce youth initiation. They include the creation of smoke- and tobacco-free environments; legislation and other mechanisms to increase the unit price of tobacco products; the enforcement of tobacco laws and regulations, such as minimum age for purchasing cigarettes; and mass media education campaigns, especially when these programs are combined with other interventions, such as school- and community-based education programs, and increases in excise taxes on tobacco (10).

Confidentiality

A dilemma is created by state laws that require physicians to report the nonmedical use of controlled substances, especially by pregnant women. Although such laws have the goals of referring pregnant women for assessment and chemical dependency treatment if indicated and of protecting fetuses and newborns from harm, they may unknowingly result in pregnant women not seeking prenatal care or concealing drug use from their obstetricians.

Some physicians are reluctant to record information related to alcohol or substance use in medical records because of competing obligations. Because medical records may not be safe from inappropriate disclosure despite federal and state privacy protections, a patient may experience real harm, such as job loss unrelated to workplace performance, eviction from public housing, or termination of insurance. Concerns about protection of confidentiality and nonmaleficence can be addressed most appropriately by including only medically necessary, accurate information in the medical record and informing the patient about the purpose of any disclosure.

Prevention of Relapse

Current reviews show insufficient evidence to support the use of any specific intervention for helping smokers (including pregnant women) who have successfully quit for a short time to avoid relapse (19). The evidence is most supportive of interventions designed around strategies to identify and resolve tempting situations (19). Very little research focuses on other approaches, so research is inconclusive. Until more evidence is available to design specific interventions for relapse prevention, it may be more efficient to focus resources on supporting the initial cessation attempt rather than on additional relapse prevention efforts.

References

1. Melvin CL, Maibach E, Marx J. Marketing research to drive inteventions, program and policies to help pregnant smokers quit: a case study. The 2002 National Conference on Tobacco or Health [abstract]. San Francisco (CA): NCTH; 2002. Available at: http://ncth.confex.com/ncth/2002/techprogram/paper_4645.htm. Retrieved November 12, 2008.

2. Thorndike AN, Rigotti NA, Stafford RS, Singer DE. National patterns in the treatment of smokers by physicians. JAMA 1998;279:604–8.

3. Woller SC, Smith SS, Piasecki TM, Jorenby DE, Helberg CP, Love RR, et al. Are clinicians intervening with their patients who smoke? A "real-world" assessment of 45 clinics in the upper Midwest. Wis Med J 1995;94:266–72.

4. Goldstein MG, Niaura R, Willey-Lessne C, DePue J, Eaton C, Rakowski W, et al. Physicians counseling smokers. A population-based survey of patients' perceptions of health care provider-delivered smoking cessation interventions. Arch Intern Med 1997;157:1313–9.

5. Cokkinides VE, Ward E, Jemal A, Thun MJ. Under-use of smoking-cessation treatments: results from the National Health Interview Survey, 2000. Am J Prev Med 2005; 28:119–22.

6. Ehrmin JT. Unresolved feelings of guilt and shame in the maternal role with substance-dependent African American women. J Nurs Scholarsh 2001;33:47–52.

7. U.S. Department of Health and Human Services. Women and smoking: a report of the Surgeon General. Washington, DC: U.S. Government Printing Office; 2001.

8. U.S. Department of Health and Human Services. The health consequences of smoking: a report of the Surgeon General. Washington, DC: U.S. Government Printing Office; 2004.

9. Jordan TR, Dake JR, Price JH. Best practices for smoking cessation in pregnancy: do obstetrician/gynecologists use them in practice? J Womens Health (Larchmt) 2006; 15:400–41.

10. Ranney L, Melvin C, Lux L, McClain E, Morgan L, Lohr K. Tobacco use: prevention, cessation, and control. Evidence Report/Technology Assessment No. 140. AHRQ Publication No. 06-E015. Rockville (MD): Agency for Healthcare Research and Quality; 2006. Available at: http://www.ahrq.gov/downloads/pub/evidence/pdf/tobaccouse/tobuse.pdf. Retrieved November 12, 2008.

11. Fiore MC, Jaen CR, Baker TB, Bailey WC, Benowitz NL, Curry SJ, et al. Treating tobacco use and dependence: 2008 update. Clinical Practice Guideline. Rockville (MD): U. S. Department of Health and Human Services; 2008. Available at http://www.surgeongeneral.gov/tobacco/treating_tobacco_use08.pdf. Retrieved November 12, 2008.

12. Johnson K, Posner SF, Biermann J, Cordero JF, Atrash HK, Parker CS, et al. Recommendations to improve preconception health and health care—United States. A report of the CDC/ATSDR Preconception Care Work Group and the Select Panel on Preconception Care. CDC/ATSDR Preconception Care Work Group; Select Panel on Preconception Care. 2006;55(RR–6):1–23.

13. Chang G, Wilkins-Haug L, Berman S, Goetz MA, Behr H, Hiley A. Alcohol use and pregnancy: improving identification. Obstet Gynecol 1998;91:892–8.

14. Substance Abuse and Mental Health Services Administration. Enhancing motivation for change in substance abuse. Treatment Improvement Protocol (TIP) series; 35. Rockville (MD): SAMHSA; 1999. Available at: http://www. ncbi.nlm.nih.gov/books/bv.fcgi?rid = hstat5.chapter.61302. Retrieved November 12, 2008.

15. Substance Abuse and Mental Health Services Administration. Results from the 2007 National Survey on Drug Use and Health: national findings. Rockville (MD): SAMHSA; 2008. Available at: http://www.oas.samhsa.gov/nsduh/ 2k7nsduh/2k7Results.pdf. Retrieved November 12, 2008.

16. Office of National Drug Control Policy. The economic costs of drug abuse in the United States, 1992–2002 (Publication No. 207303). Washington, DC: Executive Office of the President; 2004. Available at: http://www.whitehousedrug policy.gov/publications/economic_costs/economic_costs. pdf. Retrieved November 12, 2008.

17. Kaner EF, Dickinson HO, Beyer FR, Campbell F, Schlesinger C, Heather N, et al. Effectiveness of brief alcohol interventions in primary care populations. Cochrane Database of Systematic Reviews 2007, Issue 2. Art. No.: CD004148. DOI: 10.1002/14651858.CD004148.pub.3.

18. Hingson RW, Heeren T, Jamanka A, Howland J. Age of drinking onset and unintentional injury involvement after drinking. JAMA 2000;284:1527–33.

19. Hajek P, Stead LF, West R, Jarvis M, Lancaster T. Relapse prevention interventions for smoking cessation. Cochrane Database of Systematic Reviews 2005, Issue 1. Art. No.: CD003999. DOI: 10.1002/14651858.CD003999.pub3.

Family Planning

Pratima Gupta and Philip D. Darney

In recent years a number of family planning methods have been introduced, thus expanding women's choices. Health care providers, including obstetrician–gynecologists, primary care physicians, and nurse practitioners, can work with women to determine the method that is best for them, given their preferences and their medical histories, future reproductive plans, and lifestyles.

Hormonal Methods

Hormonal contraceptives contain either estrogen plus a progestin or progestin alone. Changes in bleeding are the single most frequent, concerning, and obvious side effect of hormonal contraceptives. Thus, anticipatory guidance about the possibility, frequency, and duration of menstrual disturbances can decrease concern about, and dissatisfaction with, the method and can decrease the rate of early discontinuation of the method.

Progestin-Only Methods

Progestin-only methods of contraception include progestin-only contraceptive pills, injectable depot medroxyprogesterone acetate (DMPA), subdermal implants, and the levonorgestrel intrauterine system (see "Intrauterine Contraceptives"). Progestin-only methods should be considered for women in whom estrogen is contraindicated, including women with a history of thromboembolic disease or congenital heart disease; women who are older than 35 years and smoke; and women with hypertension, migraines with aura, or other risk factors.

Progestin-only methods may be used safely while breast-feeding, although they should not be used by women less than 6 weeks postpartum. Injectable DMPA and subdermal implants are long acting, highly effec-

tive, discreet, and reversible; for these reasons, individuals at high risk for unplanned pregnancy, such as adolescents, have used them successfully.

The noncontraceptive benefits of progestin-only methods include decreases in menstrual blood loss, anemia, menstrual cramping, ovulatory pain, and pain with endometriosis, as well as decreased risks of endometrial and ovarian cancer (1).

Progestin-only methods do not protect against sexually transmitted diseases (STDs) or human immunodeficiency virus (HIV) infection, although they may provide some protection against pelvic inflammatory disease (PID) by thickening cervical mucus. Menstrual disturbances are the main reason why women discontinue progestin-only contraception. Some women experience systemic side effects, such as breast tenderness, acne, and mood changes, including depression. Some of the systemic side effects of implants, such as acne and hirsutism, are associated with the decrease in levels of sex hormone-binding globulin caused by the decreased follicular production of estradiol (1). Weight gain is a common reason for discontinuing hormonal contraceptive use, but only injectable DMPA has been associated clearly with increasing weight (2).

Absolute contraindications to progestin-only methods are limited to pregnancy and current breast cancer. Use of a progestin-only method generally is not recommended for women who have had breast cancer without recurrence for less than 5 years, active hepatitis, severe cirrhosis, benign or malignant liver tumors, or pulmonary embolism and those who have current deep vein thrombosis. Discontinuing progestin-only methods should be considered in any woman who develops migraines with focal neurologic symptoms, ischemic heart disease, or stroke (3). Case–control studies by the World Health Organization showed no increased risk of thrombosis for depot medroxyprogesterone or implant users (4); however, the absolute safety of progestin-only methods with regard to the risk of thrombosis has not been studied prospectively. Large epidemiologic studies have not identified an increased risk of stroke, myocardial infarction, or venous thromboembolism with use of some progestin-only oral contraceptives. Thus, progestin-only oral contraceptives represent a reasonable contraceptive choice for women at high risk of, or with known, coronary artery disease, cerebrovascular disease, venous thromboembolic disease, hypertension, or other conditions in which use of contraceptive doses of estrogen are contraindicated (5).

PROGESTIN-ONLY PILLS (MINIPILLS)

Mechanism of Action and Efficacy. Progestin-only pills contain levonorgestrel, norethindrone, norgestrel, lynestrenol, desogestrel, or ethynodiol diacetate in small amounts to prevent conception through a combination of mechanisms: ovulation suppression in some cycles, thickening of cervical mucus to prevent sperm penetration, atrophy of the endometrium, and altered tubal ciliary function. The amount of progestin in progestin-only pills is approximately 25% of that in combined oral contraceptive pills.

Progestin-only pills must be taken at the same time each day to be effective. The hormone is eliminated within 24 hours, at which time the cervical mucus regains its normal permeability to sperm. As a result, progestin-only pills typically have higher failure rates than combined oral contraceptives. With perfect use, the first-year probability of pregnancy is 0.5%. With typical use, the failure rate is 8%, varying according to age, with younger women having more unintended pregnancies—an association seen with all contraceptives (6).

Advantages and Disadvantages. When progestin-only pills are discontinued, fertility returns immediately because ovulation is not usually suppressed and cervical mucus returns quickly to an estrogen-dominated state. Because ovulation is not reliably inhibited, the minipills are less effective than other methods of hormonal contraception unless they are taken with absolute regularity. If a minipill user becomes pregnant, there is a higher risk of ectopic pregnancy than in women using no or other methods of contraception. Women taking medications that stimulate hepatic enzymes (such as antiepileptics or rifampin) should not rely on progestin-only pills as their sole method of pregnancy prevention (3).

INJECTABLE DEPOT MEDROXYPROGESTERONE ACETATE

Mechanism of Action and Efficacy. Depot medroxyprogesterone acetate is given as a 1-mL, deep intramuscular injection every 12 weeks. Because DMPA is not a sustained-release system, its action relies on obtaining high serum levels of progestin. This high concentration of DMPA (150 mg of microcrystals) not only thickens the cervical mucus and alters the endometrium, as do other progestins, but also suppresses levels of follicle-stimulating hormone (FSH) and luteinizing hormone (LH) and blocks the LH surge, thereby preventing ovulation. The failure rate of DMPA in the first year of use in the United States is 0.3% with perfect use and 3% in the first year with typical use (1). A contraceptive level is maintained for at least 14 weeks, providing a 2-week reinjection margin to maintain maximum efficacy. A new formulation has been approved by the U.S. Food and Drug Administration (FDA) that allows the self-administration of a subcutaneous dose of 104 mg every 3 months, with efficacy and bleeding patterns like those of intramuscularly injected DMPA.

Advantages and Noncontraceptive Benefits. Injectable DMPA is highly effective, discreet, reversible, coitus independent, and easy to use. Although most women experience irregular bleeding and spotting during the first year of use, 70% of users experience amenorrhea after 2 years and 80%, after 5 years (1). This change is acceptable for many women and desired by some. Injectable DMPA decreases the risk of ectopic pregnancy, as well as the frequency of sickle cell crises and seizures (1). Adolescents taking DMPA have higher continuation rates and fewer unplanned pregnancies than do adolescents taking oral contraceptive pills (1).

Because serum concentrations of DMPA are high in women receiving DMPA injections every 3 months, the efficacy of this method is not influenced by weight or by the use of medications that induce hepatic enzymes (1). Depot medroxyprogesterone acetate can be used by lactating mothers (6 weeks postpartum or later) because negligible concentrations are found in breast milk immediately after delivery (1).

Side Effects, Risks, and Disadvantages. The most common side effect of DMPA is irregular bleeding and spotting, which decrease after the first 12 months of use, and eventual amenorrhea. Up to 25% of patients discontinue DMPA in the first year because of irregular bleeding. Users also may experience breast tenderness, weight gain, headaches, and depression (6). Because some women have a delay in ovulation and fertility of as much as 6–18 months after the last injection, this method is not recommended for women hoping to conceive in the following year (7).

Observations of reduced bone mineral density in patients currently taking DMPA have led to concerns that DMPA-induced bone loss might increase the long-term risk of fractures years after discontinuation of the drug, particularly in young women who have not yet attained their peak bone mass and in perimenopausal women who, upon discontinuation, may have reached menopause with no opportunity to regain their bone mass and who may be starting to lose bone mass (8). However, the available data do not show that DMPA increases the risk of osteoporotic fractures in later life (9). Despite the lack of a proven increase in fracture rate, in 2004, FDA issued a black box warning on DMPA package labeling stating that the use of DMPA may cause significant bone loss, that the bone loss increases with duration of use, and that it may not be completely reversible (10).

SINGLE-ROD ETONOGESTREL IMPLANT

A contraceptive implant containing 68 mg of etonogestrel (ENG), the active metabolite of desogestrel, in a single rod made of ethylene vinyl acetate was approved for use in the United States in July 2006. It is the only implantable contraceptive currently available in the United States. Etonogestrel is initially absorbed by the body at a rate of 60 micrograms per day, and the rate slowly declines to 30 micrograms per day after 2 years of use. The ENG implant can be removed at any time at the woman's discretion, but it will remain effective for at least 3 years.

Mechanism of Action and Efficacy. Progestin-containing implants have two primary mechanisms of action: inhibition of ovulation and restriction of sperm penetration through cervical mucus. The ENG implant suppresses ovulation by altering the hypothalamic–pituitary–ovarian axis and down-regulating the LH surge that is required to support the production, growth, and maturation of ovarian follicles. Antiestrogenic actions of the progestins affect the cervical mucus, making it viscous, scanty, and impenetrable by sperm. These ovarian and cervical mechanisms of action provide high contraceptive efficacy and occur before fertilization. No signs of embryonic development have been found among implant users (7).

Based on other similar methods, contraceptive failure rate can be estimated at less than 1%. Among participants who were overweight, blood concentrations of the ENG remained at levels adequate to prevent pregnancy, but not enough overweight subjects participated to demonstrate efficacy in this group. Administration of a low dose of progestin and maintenance of stable serum levels provide high efficacy, a long duration of action, a short fertility recovery time, and no serious cardiovascular effects.

Because the ENG implant is a progestin-only method, it can be used by most women who have contraindications to estrogen-containing contraceptives. The sustained release of low doses of progestin avoids the high initial dose delivered by injectables and the daily hormone surges associated with oral contraceptives. This implant can be used by most breast-feeding women and technically can be inserted immediately postpartum (1), although it should not be used during the first 6 weeks postpartum. There are no effects on breast milk quality or quantity, and infants grow normally (11). Another advantage of the implant method is that it allows women to plan their pregnancies precisely; return of fertility after removal is prompt, in contrast to the 6- to 18-month delay in ovulation that can follow DMPA injections (7).

One of the major advantages of the implant and other sustained-release methods is the high contraceptive efficacy. In addition, implant use has not been associated with changes in carbohydrate or lipid metabolism, coagulation, liver or kidney function, or immunoglobulin levels (1).

Disadvantages, Risks, and Side Effects. Implants require a minor surgical procedure by trained clinicians for insertion and removal. The cost-effectiveness of the method depends on long-term use; early discontinuation negates this benefit (12). Side effects associated with the ENG implant include menstrual irregularities, including infrequent bleeding, amenorrhea, prolonged bleeding, frequent bleeding, as well as weight gain, acne, breast pain, and headache. Bleeding irregularities are cited as the most common reason for discontinuation of the ENG implant. Despite side effects and dependence on clinicians to insert implants, most women using implantable contraception are satisfied with the method; they cite its long duration of use, convenience, and high efficacy.

Combined Hormonal Contraceptives

Combined hormonal contraceptives include combined oral contraceptive pills, the contraceptive vaginal ring, and the transdermal contraceptive system. These hormonal delivery methods have similar mechanisms of action, serum levels of estrogen and progestin, physiological effects, noncontraceptive benefits, and prescribing precautions. For guidelines on the use of hormonal contraception in women with coexisting medical conditions, see Table 10 and Boxes 24 and 25.

MECHANISM OF ACTION

Combined hormonal contraceptives contain an estrogen to control bleeding and a progestin to inhibit ovulation. The progestational agent suppresses LH to inhibit ovulation and causes cervical mucus thickening and

Table 10. Pharmacokinetic Combination Oral Contraceptive–Antiretroviral Drug Interactions

Antiretroviral Levels	Contraceptive Steroid Levels	Antiretroviral
Protease Inhibitors		
Nelfinavir	Decreased	No data
Ritonavir	Decreased	No data
Lopinavir/ritonavir	Decreased	No data
Atazanavir	Increased	No data
Amprenavir	Increased	Decreased
Indinavir	Increased	No data
Saquinavir	No data	No change
Nonnucleoside Reverse Transcriptase Inhibitors		
Nevirapine	Decreased	No change
Efavirenz	Increased	No change
Delavirdine	Probably increased	No data

World Health Organization. Medical eligibility criteria for contraceptive use. 3rd ed. Geneva: WHO; 2004. Available at: http://www.who.int/reproductive-health/publications/mec/mec.pdf. Retrieved November 12, 2008.

endometrial glandular atrophy. In addition to preventing breakthrough bleeding by stabilizing the endometrium, the estrogenic agent suppresses FSH to prevent the growth of a dominant follicle and potentiates the action of the progestin (1).

Advantages and Noncontraceptive Benefits

Combined hormonal contraceptives have excellent contraceptive efficacy, many noncontraceptive benefits, and high user satisfaction. They are safe for most women, can be used throughout the reproductive years, are rapidly reversible, can be discontinued without a medical visit, are coitus independent, and are, for the most part, well tolerated. These products decrease menstrual blood loss, dysmenorrhea, cycle irregularities, and iron-deficiency anemia. They are useful in the management of hyperandrogenic anovulation because they create a regular bleeding pattern and protect the endometrium against the effects of unopposed estrogen. In addition, combined hormonal contraceptives offer a noncontraceptive benefit for perimenopausal symptoms, such as hot flushes. Although they do not protect against STDs and HIV infection, these contraceptives, like progestin-only methods, reduce the risk of infection of the upper reproductive tract (uterus, fallopian tubes, and ovaries) by thickening cervical mucus. They decrease the risk of ovarian, endometrial, and possibly colon cancers. They also reduce acne and hirsutism, decrease pain with endometriosis, and decrease the risk of ectopic pregnancy (6).

Side Effects and Complications

Side effects of combined hormonal contraceptives can be caused by the estrogen or progestin component. Estrogen-related side effects are an uncommon source of signs and symptoms in current lower-dose formulations equivalent to pills containing less than 50 mg of ethinyl estradiol. Estrogenic side effects include nausea, bloating, increased breast size and tenderness, and leukorrhea. Rare complications include hypertension, arterial vascular disease (myocardial infarction and stroke), and venous thromboembolism (6).

The progestin in combined oral contraceptives suppresses endogenous production of testosterone and can decrease acne, oily skin, hirsutism, and libido. However, progestin in combined hormonal contraceptives can produce androgenic effects, including headache, emotional lability, depression, acne, weight gain, breast tenderness, increased low-density lipoprotein cholesterol levels, and decreased high-density lipoprotein cholesterol levels.

Carbohydrate metabolism is not affected by current low-dose formulations (6). Three more progestin-receptor-selective, less androgenic progestins are in use in the United States, and others are available elsewhere. They include norgestimate, desogestrel (both are nortestosterone derivatives), and drospirenone (a spironolactone derivative). Drospirenone has diuretic-like effects and should not be prescribed for women with renal or adrenal insufficiency or hepatic dysfunction; it requires additional monitoring of serum potassium for women taking certain medications (13). The use of combination oral contraceptives formulated with the progestin desogestrel is associated in some epidemiologic studies with a risk of venous thromboembolism 1.5–2 times higher than that associated with levonorgestrel oral contraceptives; however, the rate of venous thromboembolism is low with all lower-estrogen-dose contraceptives, ranging from 1 to 3 cases per 10,000 women per year of use (5).

TYPES OF HORMONAL CONTRACEPTIVES

Pills. Traditionally the use of combined oral contraceptive pills entails taking one active, hormonal pill daily for 21 days, followed by a pill-free or placebo interval of 1 week to allow a scheduled withdrawal bleed. Most combined oral contraceptives currently in use contain an estrogen dose equivalent to 35 mg or less of ethinyl estradiol, as well as 0.15–1 mg of progestin, depending on its potency.

Failures of combined oral contraceptives are usually attributable to missed pills or early discontinuation. First-year failure rates among women taking combined oral contraceptives are 0.1% with perfect use and 7.6% with typical use (6). Up to 60% of women taking combined oral contraceptives discontinue their use in the first year because of poor cycle control (breakthrough bleeding and spotting) and other side effects; of these women, most discontinue use in the first month. Breakthrough bleeding occurs in 35–62% of women sometime in their first four cycles of combined oral contraceptive use and in 15–40% in the first cycle, depending primarily on the estrogen content—usually the less estrogen, the more bleeding (6).

The advantages of combined oral contraceptives include the user's control of the method and its use as emergency contraception (although progestin–levonorgestrel alone is at least as effective with fewer side effects); disadvantages include the need for daily administration. There is no physiologic advantage to phased preparations, although some women have improved bleeding patterns at lower doses. The addition of either estrogen or progestin during the "pill-free" 7-day interval also can result in better cycle control at doses. Women with extended use of oral contraceptives can avoid menses altogether, but some irregular bleeding usually occurs. Any oral contraceptive can be taken continuously, but some are packaged for continuous use.

Combined Contraceptive Vaginal Ring. The combined contraceptive vaginal ring is a flexible, transparent ring 54 mm in diameter, made of ethylene vinyl acetate copolymer. The user places and removes the ring herself; there is no wrong way to insert it. Each ring is designed for one cycle of use, which is 3 weeks of continuous ring use followed by 1 week without the ring to provoke a scheduled withdrawal bleed. The ring releases 120 micrograms of etonogestrel (the active metabolite of desogestrel) and 15 micrograms of ethinyl estradiol per day. It is approved for 3 weeks of continuous use, but contraceptive levels of steroid are maintained in the blood for 5 weeks, and like oral contraceptives, the ring can be used continuously.

In addition to having the advantages of all combined hormonal contraceptives, the ring is convenient and discreet and provides good cycle control with sustained delivery of low-dose hormones (the area under the curve of hormone concentrations is smaller with the ring than with oral contraceptives or the patch). With perfect use, 0.3% of women will become pregnant in the first year of ring use (14). The pregnancy rate with typical use is unknown because the ring is too new to allow researchers to collect adequate data. The ring has been demonstrated to have high acceptability, high compliance, and high continuation rates (15). In a large, multicenter study, 4% of women who discontinued the ring did so because of foreign body sensations, coital problems, expulsion, and vaginal discomfort. Unlike other combined methods, the ring is very unlikely to cause irregular bleeding in the initial months of use. In a clinical trial, adverse events associated with the ring were uncommon and included headache, leukorrhea, and vaginitis (15).

Transdermal Contraceptive System. The transdermal contraceptive system is a 4.5-cm square patch that provides continuous circulatory levels of norelgestromin (the active metabolite of norgestimate) and ethinyl estradiol equivalent to 150 micrograms of norelgestromin and 20 micrograms of ethinyl estradiol per day. The area under the curve of the hormonal concentrations achieved by the patch is greater than with typical oral contraceptives. One patch is applied weekly for 3 consecutive weeks, followed by 1 week without its use to allow for a scheduled withdrawal bleed. The first-year pregnancy rate for perfect use is 0.3% (14); the rate for typical use is not yet determined.

Patch users have higher rates of compliance and more perfect use than do users of combined oral contraceptives (16). Patches maintain their adhesiveness for a week regardless of heat, moisture, activity levels, or site of application; detachment occurs in less than 2% of patients (17). Advantages of the patch, in addition to those of all combined hormonal contraceptives, include convenience, ease of use, and continuous delivery of low doses of estrogen and progestin. Application site reactions, breast discomfort, and dysmenorrhea are seen more commonly in initial cycles of patch use (17).

RISKS AND DISADVANTAGES

Venous Thromboembolism. Most medical concerns about combined hormonal contraceptives focus on the estrogen component and the associated risk of venous thromboembolism and arterial vascular disease. Many of the original precautions were based on risks observed with pills containing 50–100 micrograms of ethinyl estradiol or mestranol. These risks are greatly reduced with currently available lower-dose formulations, which have fewer metabolic and hemostatic effects (18). The increased risk of venous thromboembolism remains the greatest concern with combined hormonal contraceptives; this risk is increased 3 to 4 times with even the lowest-dose combined oral contraceptive but remains low, at 1–3 per 10,000 woman-years (5). The risk of deep vein thrombosis may be approximately 1.5–2 times higher with combined oral contraceptives containing the newer progestins (such as desogestrel and gestodene) than with those containing levonorgestrel. Overall, the risk of venous thromboembolism is lower with lower-dose formulations than it is with higher-dose formulations. The risk of arterial cardiovascular disease is increased in women taking combined hormonal contraceptives who have other risk factors, particularly smoking, hypertension, diabetes mellitus, and obesity.

The average overall ethinyl estradiol concentration (the area under the curve) in patch users is 60% higher than in women who take a 35-microgram ethinyl estradiol pill; however, peak ethinyl estradiol concentrations are 25% lower than in pill users (19). It is unclear whether this finding will be associated with a higher frequency of adverse events, such as thromboembolism. Two studies, both based on medical insurance claims, demonstrated conflicting reports in terms of the increased risk of venous thromboembolism and contraceptive patch use (20, 21). Although they are observational studies with a relatively small number of events, limitations in design, and conflicting results, one should assume there is a possibility of increased risk of venous thromboembolism in patch users compared with oral contraceptive users, given the only available data. This potential risk should be balanced against the benefits of this method for preventing pregnancy in women who may not be able to use other methods successfully.

Breast Cancer Risk. Users of combined oral contraceptives are slightly more likely than the general population to have a breast cancer diagnosis. This increased risk may be due to detection bias or to the promotion of a cancer that is already present. Current or past users (within the past 10 months) of combined oral contraceptives are more likely than nonusers to have localized disease. Women who have used combined oral contraceptives are at no increased risk of breast cancer 10 years after discontinuing their use and are as likely to die of breast cancer as are women who have not used combined oral contraceptives (22). Women with a family history of breast cancer do not increase their risk by taking combined oral contraceptives (23).

Obesity and Contraceptive Efficacy. The use of most hormonal contraceptives is associated with little or no effect on body weight. Weight fluctuations, particularly weight gain, in women tend to be due to increasing age and changes in lifestyle, irrespective of contraceptive use (24).

Whether elevated body weight reduces the effectiveness of combined hormonal contraceptives is controversial. Although several studies have shown an association between pregnancy rate and increasing body weight or increasing body mass index in women taking combined oral contraceptives (25), most trials do not include enough overweight women to draw meaningful conclusions. In addition, when adjustment is made for age, parity, education, income, and race or ethnicity, the differences in pregnancy rates often are not significant (26).

The effect of body weight on the efficacy of the ring is unknown; however, subanalysis of clinical trials of the ring demonstrates no excess pregnancies in obese women (27). Pooled data on the transdermal combination hormonal contraceptive patch demonstrate one third of the on-treatment pregnancies occurring in the heaviest one tenth of women (weight greater than 198 lb) (25). The efficacy of copper or levonorgestrel intrauterine device (IUD) or injectable DMPA is not decreased in obese women. Despite a few studies that have demonstrated slightly reduced contraceptive efficacy with excessive body weight, heavier women should not be restricted from taking combined hormonal contraception if these methods are the best available options: the risk of pregnancy is still significantly lower with these methods than with a barrier method or no method at all.

CONTINUOUS SUPPRESSION

Combined hormonal contraception can be prescribed for continuous use to achieve a number of different goals:

- To decrease the number of placebo days per cycle
- To reduce the number of placebo weeks or withdrawal weeks per year
- To eliminate withdrawal weeks entirely
- To reduce the incidence of breakthrough bleeding
- To reduce the incidence of some side effects of menstruation, such as headache

Combined oral contraceptives also are marketed in packaging specifically designed to facilitate continuous pill taking, providing for four pill-free intervals per year or for an entire year of pill taking. With the elimination of placebo pills, other monophasic combined oral contraceptives can be used in the same way to decrease the frequency of withdrawal bleeding (13). The combined contraceptive patch and ring also can be used continuously without a monthly withdrawal bleed. The primary disadvantage of continuous use is breakthrough bleeding, although some women may prefer it to menstrual-like symptoms.

Intrauterine Contraceptives

The precise mechanism of action of IUDs is not known, although it is likely that they work through several mechanisms. Intrauterine devices primarily prevent fertilization (28). When the uterus is exposed to a foreign body, a sterile inflammatory reaction occurs that is toxic to sperm and ova and prevents fertilization through the production of cytotoxic peptides, acrosomal enzyme activation, inhibition of sperm motility, reduced sperm capacitation and survival, and sperm phagocytosis (28). Copper ions increase this toxic effect. Serious complications of the IUDs are rare and include postinsertional PID, expulsions, perforations, and pregnancy complications (1). The IUD is more effective at preventing intrauterine pregnancies than at preventing ectopic pregnancies.

Ideal Candidates and Contraindications

The IUD is recommended for women who want a reversible, long-acting, highly-effective contraceptive method. Nulliparous women are candidates for IUD.

There are relatively few absolute contraindications to the copper or levonorgestrel IUD. Both are contraindicated in women with active, recent (within the last 3 months), or recurrent pelvic infection or STDs; undiagnosed abnormal vaginal bleeding that may indicate a serious condition; endometrial or untreated cervical cancer; pregnancy; or a severely distorted uterine cavity resulting from anatomic abnormalities. Both type of IUDs can be used with caution in women at increased risk for STDs or HIV infection or in women with limited access to care in the event of infection (3).

Advantages of intrauterine contraception generally outweigh the risks in women with uncomplicated valvular heart disease; nondistorting uterine abnormalities, including leiomyomas; and menorrhagia without anemia. In women with diabetes mellitus or migraine headaches, the copper IUD can be prescribed without restriction, and advantages generally outweigh risks with the use of the levonorgestrel system (3). The IUD may be used immediately after an uninfected vaginal or cesarean delivery, an abortion, or a miscarriage (1).

The use of intrauterine contraception for the following reasons is acceptable:

- Previous PID
- Past ectopic pregnancy or irregular menses
- Cervical intraepithelial neoplasia
- Benign ovarian tumors
- Obesity
- Breast cancer (the levonorgestrel IUD should be prescribed only after consultation with a gynecologic oncologist)
- Breast-feeding (at least 6 weeks postpartum)
- HIV infection

Types of Intrauterine Device

COPPER INTRAUTERINE DEVICE

Efficacy. The copper IUD is approved for 10 years of use but has been shown to be effective for at least 12 years. After prolonged continuous use, the cumulative pregnancy rate is 1.6% at 7 years, and 2.2% at 8 and 12 years (29). Overall, the failure rate is substantially less than 1 per 100 women per year, except in women younger than 25 years, who experience a slightly higher failure rate, most likely because they are more fertile than older women. (28). The long-term rates of failure for the copper IUD are comparable with those for typical sterilization operations.

Advantages and Noncontraceptive Benefits. Women who cannot use hormonal methods can use copper IUDs. After 5 years of continued use, the TCu-380A IUD is the most cost-effective method of contraception available (28). Intrauterine devices protect against ectopic pregnancy: copper IUD users are 90% less likely to have an ectopic pregnancy than women using no method, although a larger proportion of pregnancies with either IUD are ectopic. The copper IUD has no systemic side effects. Long-term use is associated with a high degree of safety. There is rapid return to fertility and no increased risk of infertility after IUD removal, even in nulliparous users. The copper IUD is associated with an apparent decreased risk of endometrial cancer and with no increased risk, and possibly a decreased risk, of cervical cancer (30).

Side Effects, Risks, and Disadvantages. The copper IUD may increase menstrual blood loss, cramping, intermenstrual spotting, and vaginal discharge. These side effects usually diminish after the first 3 months of use. Heavy menses and dysmenorrhea are the most frequent reasons for copper IUD removal in the first year (1).

LEVONORGESTREL INTRAUTERINE DEVICE

The U.S. Food and Drug Administration approved the hormone-releasing levonorgestrel IUD in 2000. It is composed of a T-shaped polyethylene frame with a collar attached to the vertical stem and containing 52 mg of levonorgestrel dispersed in polydimethylsiloxane. In vivo, it releases 15 micrograms of levonorgestrel daily (in vitro, 20 micrograms is released). The levonorgestrel system is approved for up to 5 years of use in the United States but has been shown to be effective up to 7 years (31). In addition to producing the foreign-body reaction seen with other IUDs, hormonal IUDs release progestin that causes endometrial decidualization, glandular atrophy, and thickened cervical mucus. The levonorgestrel IUD also produces serum concentrations of progestin that lead to partial inhibition of ovarian follicular development and ovulation, although most women have some ovulatory cycles. This system results in the lowest serum concentrations of progestin of any hormonal contraceptive but does not decrease estradiol levels below physiologic values. Levonorgestrel concentrations in the endometrium and myometrium are much higher than in the serum (1).

Efficacy. The levonorgestrel IUD is the most effective form of reversible contraception available (1), followed closely by the TCu-380A. With perfect use of the levonorgestrel system, the first-year probability of pregnancy is 0.1%; with typical use, the probability is 0.1–0.2%. With 7 years of continuous use, the cumulative pregnancy rate is 1.1% (6).

Advantages and Noncontraceptive Benefits. Like the copper IUD, the levonorgestrel IUD is highly effective, discreet, coitus independent, easy to use, and cost-effective if used for longer than 2 years. It does not interfere with lactation, protects against ectopic pregnancy, and is rarely associated with systemic side effects. In addition, it decreases menstrual blood loss, increases hemoglobin levels, and decreases dysmenorrhea (28). It is as effective as endometrial ablation for the treatment of menorrhagia (32) and is more effective than cyclic oral progestins (33). In women with anovulatory cycles and in perimenopausal and postmenopausal women taking estrogen, the levonorgestrel IUD can be used to protect the endometrium from the effects of unopposed estrogen by preventing hyperplasia (34).

Side Effects, Risks, and Disadvantages. Intrauterine levonorgestrel may cause irregular bleeding and spotting in the first several months of use. The main reason for its discontinuation is amenorrhea that is caused by endometrial decidualization and atrophy rather than anovulation. This side effect is experienced by 30% of women after 2 years of use (35). Menstrual problems, including amenorrhea, oligomenorrhea, and spotting, decline after 1 year and are less common among patients older than 30 years (36). Hormonal side effects (including headache and skin and hair changes) are the most common reasons for elective removal of the levonorgestrel IUD in the first 36 months of use, although removal because of these side effects is rare (31).

Contraindications and Precautions. There are few absolute contraindications to the use of intrauterine levonorgestrel. Recommendations against the use of progestin-only contraceptive methods apply to the use of the levonorgestrel IUD as well. The exception is insertion in women with breast cancer, which should be done only in consultation with a gynecologic oncologist.

Emergency Contraception

Postcoital contraception, also called *emergency contraception,* is used to prevent pregnancy after unprotected intercourse. The several methods of postcoital contraception currently available include taking oral levonorgestrel, combined oral contraceptives (including the Yuzpe regimen), or mifepristone or the insertion of a copper IUD (Table 11). Postcoital contraception is indicated when another method of contraception failed, when no contraception was used, or when intercourse was forced.

Although there is no harm associated with the repeated use of postcoital contraception, its routine use is not recommended as a contraceptive because its efficacy is lower than that of routine methods of contraception. In addition, the methods used for postcoital contraception afford no protection against STDs.

Emergency contraception can reduce the incidence of unintended pregnancy and induced abortion (1), but it is underused. In 1997, only 1% of U.S. women reported ever having used emergency contraception (1). The advance provision of emergency contraception, in the form of a prescription or a packet of pills, has been shown to increase its use; giving the patient the pill package was most likely to result in use (37). However, this U.S. study and another study from Scotland failed to show a decrease in unintended pregnancies associated with the use of emergency contraception, perhaps because it was not used frequently enough (37, 38).

Postcoital Oral Levonorgestrel

In 1999, the FDA approved levonorgestrel in 0.75-mg tablets for use as emergency contraception, and in 2006 it approved the over-the-counter availability of emergency contraception for individuals (men or women) aged 18 years and older; proof of age is required in the form of government-issued photo or nonphoto identification (39). Limited data suggest that adolescents use emergency contraception appropriately and tolerate the drug approximately as well as adults do (40).

Although the exact mechanism of pregnancy prevention is unknown, levonorgestrel is believed to inhibit ovulation, prevent fertilization, or interfere with implan-

Table 11. Postcoital Contraception

Method	Recommended Time From Unprotected Intercourse	Failure Rate per 100 Women*	Contraindications
None	N/A	8	N/A
Levonorgestrel	5 days	1	Pregnancy
Yuzpe regimen	5 days	2–3	Pregnancy and absolute contraindications to oral contraceptives
Mifepristone	5 days	Less than 1	Unknown
Copper IUD	5 days	Less than 0.1	Pregnancy and risk of sexually transmitted diseases

*For a single act of unprotected intercourse in the second or third week of the menstrual cycle
Abbreviation: IUD indicates intrauterine device.

tation of the fertilized ovum by altering the endometrium. Taking postcoital levonorgestrel reduces the risk of pregnancy from 8% to 1% for a single act of unprotected intercourse in the second or third week of the menstrual cycle, which is equivalent to an 88% reduction in risk (41).

There are almost no contraindications to postcoital levonorgestrel other than allergy to ingredients in the tablets, unexplained vaginal bleeding, and pregnancy, although the hormone will not harm the fetus if it is mistakenly taken when the woman is already pregnant. Side effects are fewer with levonorgestrel than with postcoital estrogen plus progestin (see "Yuzpe Regimen") and include nausea, abdominal pain, headache, dizziness, breast tenderness, and heavier or lighter bleeding with subsequent menses (41). Postcoital levonorgestrel has not been shown to have teratogenic effects. There is a slightly increased risk of ectopic pregnancy if postcoital levonorgestrel fails (1).

Postcoital levonorgestrel can be taken up to 5 days after unprotected intercourse. The efficacy of levonorgestrel decreases with time from exposure and is greatest when taken within 24 hours of unprotected intercourse. Two methods have been well studied and have similar efficacy and safety: 1) a 0.75-mg levonorgestrel tablet taken as soon as possible after exposure, followed by a second tablet 12 hours later, and 2) a single 1.5-mg dose of levonorgestrel (42).

Yuzpe Regimen

In 1982, A. A. Yuzpe developed a postcoital method that uses standard combined oral contraceptives in higher doses than the doses used for long-term contraception. The mechanism of action of the regimen is presumed to be similar to that of postcoital levonorgestrel. The Yuzpe

regimen has a failure rate of 2–3%. It reduces the risk of pregnancy by approximately 75% for a single act of unprotected intercourse in the second or third week of the menstrual cycle (1). The Yuzpe regimen is associated with more side effects, particularly nausea and vomiting, than is postcoital levonorgestrel. The regimen should be taken within 72 hours of unprotected intercourse but has proven efficacy through 5 days after exposure. Like levonorgestrel, the efficacy of the Yuzpe regimen decreases as the time from exposure increases.

Postcoital Copper Intrauterine Device Insertion

A copper IUD can be inserted up to the time of implantation—approximately 5 days after ovulation—for the prevention of pregnancy after unprotected intercourse. Most providers choose to provide the IUD up to 5 days from unprotected intercourse because it usually is difficult to determine the precise time of ovulation (43). This method should be considered for women who desire long-term contraception. The intrauterine presence of a foreign body and the copper ions are thought to prevent implantation. The levonorgestrel system, along with other long-acting hormonal methods, has not been studied for postcoital contraception and is not recommended for this use.

With a failure rate of less than 0.1%, postcoital copper IUD insertion is the most effective of any emergency contraception method available (6). Side effects are similar to those associated with routine insertion and include cramping, spotting, and increased transient menstrual bleeding. Women who have an IUD inserted for postcoital contraception should be considered appropriate candidates for IUD use; women who want to continue intrauterine contraception are the best candidates.

Sterilization

Surgical sterilization is popular worldwide; approximately 223 million couples use either tubal sterilization (180 million) or vasectomy (43 million) for contraception. In the United States, more than half a million women undergo sterilization annually. In 2002, it was the most common method of contraception in women older than 35 years (1). Although tubal sterilization is highly effective and death attributable to the procedure is rare, complications can occur. Proper patient selection and counseling, as well as careful attention to sterilization technique, maximize patient satisfaction and outcomes. For a detailed discussion, see "Sterilization" in the current edition of *Precis: Gynecology*.

References

1. Speroff L, Darney PD. A clinical guide for contraception. 4th ed. Philadelphia (PA): Lippincott Williams & Wilkins; 2005.

2. Westhoff C, Jain JK, Milsom I, Ray A. Changes in weight with depot medroxyprogesterone acetate subcutaneous injection 104 mg/0.65 mL. Contraception 2007;75:261–7.

3. World Health Organization. Medical eligibilty criteria for contraceptive use. 3rd ed. Geneva: WHO; 2004. Available at: http://www.who.int/reproductive-health/publications/mec/mec.pdf. Retrieved November 12, 2008.

4. Cardiovascular disease and use of oral and injectable progestogen-only contraceptives and combined injectable contraceptives. Results of an international, multicenter, case-control study. World Health Organization Collaborative Study of Cardiovascular Disease and Steroid Hormone Contraception. Contraception 1998;57:315–24.

5. Use of hormonal contraception in women with coexisting medical conditions. ACOG Practice Bulletin. No. 73. American College of Obstetricians and Gynecologists. Obstet Gynecol 2006;107:1453–72.

6. Hatcher RA, Trussell J, Cates W, Stewart F, Kowal D. Contraceptive technology. 19th revised ed. New York (NY): Ardent Media; 2007.

7. Croxatto HB. Clinical profile of Implanon: a single-rod etonogestrel contraceptive implant. Eur J Contracept Reprod Health Care 2000;5(suppl 2):21–8.

8. Westhoff C. Depot-medroxyprogesterone acetate injection (Depo-Provera): a highly effective contraceptive option with proven long-term safety. Contraception 2003;68: 75–87.

9. Kaunitz AM, Miller PD, Rice VM, Ross D, McClung MR. Bone mineral density in women aged 25-35 years receiving depot medroxyprogesterone acetate: recovery following discontinuation. Contraception 2006;74:90–9.

10. Food and Drug Administration. Depo-provera (medroxyprogesterone acetate injectable suspension): 2004 safety alerts for drugs, biologics, medical devices, and dietary supplements. Rockville (MD): FDA; 2004. Available at: http://www.fda.gov/medwatch/SAFETY/2004/DepoProvera_Label.pdf. Retrieved November 14, 2008.

11. Reinprayoon D, Taneepanichskul S, Bunyavejchevin S, Thaithumyanon P, Punnahitananda S, Tosukhowong P, et al. Effects of the etonogestrel-releasing contraceptive implant (Implanon) on parameters of breastfeeding compared to those of an intrauterine device. Contraception 2000;62:239–46.

12. Trussell J, Leveque JA, Koenig JD, London R, Borden S, Henneberry J, et al. The economoc value of contraception: a comparison of 15 methods. Am J Public Health 1995; 85:494–503.

13. Drey EA, Darney PD. Recent developments in hormonal contraception. Rev Endocr Metab Disord 2002;3:257–65.

14. Zieman M, Hatcher RA, Cwiak C, Darney PD, Creinin MD. Managing contraception 2007-2009. 9th ed. Tiger (GA): Bridging the Gap Foundation; 2007.

15. Roumen FJ, Apter D, Mulders TM, Dieben TO. Efficacy, tolerability and acceptability of a novel contraceptive vaginal ring releasing etonogestrel and ethinyl oestradiol. Hum Reprod 2001;16:469–75.

16. Dittrich R, Parker L, Rosen JB, Shangold G, Creasy GW, Fisher AC. Transdermal contraception: evaluation of three transdermal norelgestromin/ethinyl estradiol doses in a randomized, multicenter, dose-response study. Ortho Evra/Evra 001 Study Group. Am J Obstet Gynecol 2002; 186:15–20.

17. Audet MC, Moreau M, Koltun WD, Waldbaum AS, Shangold G, Fisher AC, et al. Evaluation of contraceptive efficacy and cycle control of a transdermal contraceptive patch vs an oral contraceptive: a randomized controlled trial. ORTHO EVRA/EVRA 004 Study Group. JAMA 2001; 285:2347–54.

18. Venous thromboembolic disease and combined oral contraceptives: results of international multicentre case-control study. World Health Organization Collaborative Study of Cardiovascular Disease and Steroid Hormone Contraception. Lancet 1995;346:1575–82.

19. Food and Drug Administration. Ortho Evra (norelgestromin/ethinyl estradiol) information. Rockville (MD): FDA; 2008. Available at: http://www.fda.gov/cder/drug/infopage/orthoevra/default.htm. Retrieved November 12, 2008.

20. Cole JA, Norman H, Doherty M, Walker AM. Venous thromboembolism, myocardial infarction, and stroke among transdermal contraceptive system users [published erratum appears in Obstet Gynecol 2008;111:1449]. Obstet Gynecol 2007;109:339–46.

21. Jick SS, Kaye JA, Russmann S, Jick H. Risk of nonfatal venous thromboembolism in women using a contraceptive transdermal patch and oral contraceptives containing norgestimate and 35 microg of ethinyl estradiol. Contraception 2006;73:223–8.

22. Wingo PA, Austin H, Marchbanks PA, Whiteman MK, Hsia J, Mandel MG, et al. Oral contraceptives and the risk of death from breast cancer [published erratum appears in Obstet Gynecol 2008;111:454]. Obstet Gynecol 2007;110: 793–800.

23. Marchbanks PA, McDonald JA, Wilson HG, Folger SG, Mandel MG, Daling JR, et al. Oral contraceptives and the risk of breast cancer. N Engl J Med 2002;346:2025–32.

24. Gallo MF, Lopez LM, Grimes DA, Schulz KF, Helmerhorst FM. Combination contraceptives: effects on weight. Cochrane Database of Systematic Reviews 2008, Issue 4. Art. No.: CD003987. DOI: 10.1002/14651858.CD003987. pub3.

25. Zieman M, Guillebaud J, Weisberg E, Shangold GA, Fisher AC, Creasy GW. Contraceptive efficacy and cycle control with the Ortho Evra/Evra transdermal system: the analysis of pooled data. Fertil Steril 2002;77:S13–8.

26. Brunner Huber LR, Hogue CJ, Stein AD, Drews C, Zieman M. Body mass index and risk for oral contraceptive failure: a case-cohort study in South Carolina. Ann Epidemiol 2006;16:637–43.

27. Westhoff C. Higher body weight does not affect Nuva Ring's efficacy [abstract]. Obstet Gynecol 2005;105(suppl): 56S.

28. Mechanism of action, safety and efficacy of intrauterine devices. Report of a WHO Scientific Group. World Health Organ Tech Rep Ser 1987;753:1–91.

29. Long-term reversible contraception. Twelve years of experience with the TCu380A and TCu220C. Contraception 1997;56:341–52.

30. Nelson AL. Contraindications to IUD and IUS use. Contraception 2007;75:S76–81.

31. Sivin I, Stern J. Health during prolonged use of levonorgestrel 20 micrograms/d and the copper TCu 380Ag intrauterine contraceptive devices: a multicenter study. International Committee for Contraception Research (ICCR). Fertil Steril 1994;61:70–7.

32. Hurskainen R, Teperi J, Rissanen P, Aalto AM, Grenman S, Kivela A, et al. Clinical outcomes and costs with the levonorgestrel-releasing intrauterine system or hysterectomy for treatment of menorrhagia: randomized trial 5-year follow-up. JAMA 2004;291:1456–63.

33. Lethaby AE, Cooke I, Rees M. Progesterone or progestogen-releasing intrauterine systems for heavy menstrual bleeding. Cochrane Database of Systematic Reviews 2005, Issue 4. Art. No.: CD002126. DOI: 10.1002/14651858. CD002126. pub2.

34. Varila E, Wahlstrom T, Rauramo I. A 5-year follow-up study on the use of a levonorgestrel intrauterine system in women receiving hormone replacement therapy. Fertil Steril 2001;76:969–73.

35. Ronnerdag M, Odlind V. Health effects of long-term use of the intrauterine levonorgestrel-releasing system. A follow-up study over 12 years of continuous use. Acta Obstet Gynecol Scand 1999;78:716–21.

36. Backman T, Huhtala S, Blom T, Luoto R, Rauramo I, Koskenvuo M. Length of use and symptoms associated with premature removal of the levonorgestrel intrauterine system: a nation-wide study of 17,360 users. BJOG 2000; 107:335–9.

37. Raine T, Harper C, Leon K, Darney P. Emergency contraception: advance provision in a young, high-risk clinic population. Obstet Gynecol 2000;96:1–7.

38. Raymond EG, Trussell J, Polis CB. Population effect of increased access to emergency contraceptive pills: a systematic review. Obstet Gynecol 2007;109:181–8.

39. Food and Drug Administration. Plan B: questions and answers. Rockville (MD): FDA; 2006. Available at: http://www.fda.gov/cder/drug/infopage/planB/planBQ andA20060824.htm. Retrieved November 12, 2008.

40. Harper CC, Rocca CH, Darney PD, von Hertzen H, Raine TR. Tolerability of levonorgestrel emergency contraception in adolescents. Am J Obstet Gynecol 2004;191:1158–63.

41. Randomised controlled trial of levonorgestrel versus the Yuzpe regimen of combined oral contraceptives for emergency contraception. Task Force on Postovulatory Methods of Fertility Regulation. Lancet 1998;352:428–33.

42. Polis CB, Schaffer K, Blanchard K, Glasier A, Harper CC, Grimes DA. Advance provision of emergency contraception for pregnancy prevention (full review). Cochrane Database Syst Rev 2007;CD005497. Review.

43. Zhou L, Xiao B. Emergency contraception with Multiload Cu-375 SL IUD: a multicenter clinical trial. Contraception 2001;64:107–12.

Urinary Tract Disorders

Linda Brubaker

Urinary tract symptoms, including urinary incontinence, are common among women. Approximately 10–30% of women between 15 years and 64 years and 25% of women older than 65 years experience urinary incontinence (1). Urinary tract infections and other disorders of the lower urinary tract can be appreciable problems for women. Because nearly all urinary tract symptoms can be relieved with various interventions, patients benefit greatly when their physician understands the prevention, pathophysiology, evaluation, and treatment of these common disorders. The obstetrician–gynecologist plays a pivotal role in the initial assessment and treatment of women with these conditions. Although these conditions are rarely life threatening, the symptoms significantly decrease the quality of life for affected women. The physician's role is to focus on the symptoms that are most bothersome and reduce their effect for the patient. In choosing treatment for one condition, the potential for exacerbating another condition must be considered. For example, surgery for minor stress incontinence may dramatically worsen urge incontinence.

Urinary Incontinence

Many women experience a low level of urinary incontinence at some point during their lives. The threshold for a woman's seeking treatment is generally related to how much the symptoms bother her and her willingness to accept treatment. Adherence to the following general principles will optimize urinary tract function for women:

- Obstetric and gynecologic care should avoid compromising the urinary tract whenever possible.
- During annual medical visits, the interval history should include routine screening for symptoms of pelvic floor disorders, including urinary and fecal incontinence.

Resources

Urinary Tract Disorders

American Urogynecologic Society
http://www.augs.org

American Urological Association
http://www.auanet.org

Interstitial Cystitis Association
http://www.ichelp.org

National Association for Continence
http://www.nafc.org

- When symptoms are found, a stepwise evaluation and treatment plan aimed at improving the individual woman's quality of life should be implemented, beginning with simple interventions.
- Follow-up or referral should be provided as needed.

Detection of Urinary Incontinence

Every obstetrician–gynecologist has patients with urinary incontinence. Physicians can detect this condition in their obstetric as well as their gynecologic patients by inquiring about it regularly. It is important for physicians to include urinary tract screening during annual visits and to positively reinforce symptom-reporting conversations that the patient initiates. A variety of simple questionnaires are available to help make office evaluation effective. These questionnaires can be completed by the patient before her visit with the physician. The Urogenital Distress Inventory Short Form (UDI-6) uses six questions for the patient to assess how much the current urogenital symptoms bother her (2). Selected questions relating to urinary incontinence are shown in Box 26.

Another potential screening questionnaire is the Patient Global Impression of Severity Scale, which asks the patient to report the severity of her urinary symptoms (3). This brief instrument is shown in Box 27.

A great deal of emphasis has been placed on appropriately diagnosing the two subtypes of urinary incontinence—stress incontinence and urge incontinence. Many women have elements of both subtypes. Because patients rarely convey their symptoms in medical terms, the physician should undertake simple initial steps to help her diagnose either of these incontinence subtypes after a simple office evaluation.

The term *genuine stress incontinence* is no longer current. The clinical diagnostic term is simply *stress incontinence*. The term *urodynamic stress incontinence* may be used when the finding is confirmed by urodynamic testing. Stress incontinence symptoms are reported as spurts of urine during increases in intraabdominal pressure, such as physical activity, coughing, or sneezing. Typically, this symptom occurs in vaginally parous women with mild to moderate loss of anterior vaginal support. Stress incontinence also may occur in nulliparous women who have some process that markedly increases the intraabdominal pressure (eg, chronic lung disease, severe straining during defecation, obesity, or unusual occupational weight lifting). Older paradigms that dichotomize urethral hypermobility and intrinsic sphincter deficiency are being replaced with the under-

---

Box 26

UDI-6 Short Form (Abridged)

Do you experience, and if so, then how much are you bothered by:

- Leakage related to feeling urgency
- Leakage related to activity, coughing, or sneezing

  0 = not at all

  1 = slightly

  2 = moderately

  3 = greatly

Short forms to assess life quality and symptom distress for urinary incontinence in women: the Incontinence Impact Questionnaire and the Urogenital Distress Inventory. Continence Program for Women Research Group. Uebersax JS, Wyman JF, Shumaker SA, McClish DK, Fantl JA. Neurourology & Urodynamics. 1995;14:131–9. Copyright ©1995. John Wiley & Sons, Inc. Reproduced with permission of John Wiley & Sons, Inc.

Box 27

Patient Global Impression of Severity (PGI-S) Scale

Check the one number that best describes how your urinary symptoms are now:

1. Normal
2. Mild
3. Moderate
4. Severe

Reprinted from American Journal of Obstetrics and Gynecology, Vol 189, Yalcin I, Bump RC, Validation of two global impression questionnaires for incontinence, Pages 98–101, Copyright 2003, with permission from Elsevier.

---

standing that urethral support and urethral sphincteric function are on a continuum. An individual woman may have elements of both contributing conditions. Some women have underlying conditions that compromise the neuromuscular integrity of the supportive tissues or the sphincter mechanism itself (eg, prior continence surgery, disk protrusion, urethral dilation, or sacral tumors). This subset of women may benefit from consultation with an incontinence specialist.

Many women also are affected by urge incontinence, often with the symptom complex of overactive bladder that is used to indicate an idiopathic process that results in urgency, usually with frequency symptoms, urge incontinence, or both. In some women, these symptoms are related to abnormalities with the bladder muscle itself, which can cause detrusor overactivity. However, cystometric evidence of detrusor overactivity is poorly correlated with symptoms of urge incontinence, urgency, and frequency. Because of the risk–benefit ratio for initial urge incontinence therapy, cystometric or urodynamic test results are not required to initiate empiric treatment of urge incontinence in most women.

In a subgroup of women, detrusor overactivity is caused by a well-recognized group of neurologic disorders (eg, Parkinson disease, multiple sclerosis, or stroke). When a neurologic process causes detrusor overactivity, the term *detrusor hyperreflexia* is used. The term *neurogenic bladder* is no longer current and should not be used.

Other, less common forms of urinary incontinence include genitourinary fistula, ectopic ureter, and urethral diverticulum. Symptoms that suggest these conditions include continuous urinary leakage or isolated suburethral masses. These lesions should be kept in mind during the evaluation.

INITIAL EVALUATION

The goal of initial evaluation for a woman seeking treatment of urinary incontinence is to ensure that there are no treatable pathologic conditions that may be contributing to the patient's symptoms, such as undiagnosed urinary tract infection, incomplete emptying (postvoid residual higher than 100), or prolapse beyond the hymen. Other conditions that would alter initial management might include unlikely fistulae or rare systemic neurologic diseases that present with urinary symptoms. In addition, the physician should clarify the patient's goals for her own treatment. The older paradigm of assuming that each woman's goal was complete continence is known to be incorrect. Patients may wish to see improvement of a certain symptom for particular social or professional situations (eg, less frequency). Clarification of the patient's goals enhances the possibility of treatment satisfaction (4–6).

PATIENT HISTORY

Obtaining a history of the function of the lower urinary tract is part of a complete pelvic floor assessment. Symptoms associated with the storage and emptying phases of the bladder cycle should be determined. Specific questions should gather information about irritative symptoms (eg, urgency and frequency), incontinence (ie, stress or urge), and voiding dysfunction (urinary retention or postvoid fullness). Examples of questions that work well in suggesting potential incontinence subtypes are given in Box 28.

The obstetric history should include questions regarding the onset of symptoms after delivery, use of instrumented deliveries, and repair of recognized anal sphincter lacerations. The surgical history should con-

---

Box 28

Questions to Determine Urinary Incontinence Subtypes

1. During the past 3 months, have you leaked urine (even a small amount)?

    Yes   No

2. During the past 3 months, did you leak urine:
(check all that apply)

    a. When you were performing some physical activity such as coughing, sneezing, lifting, or exercise?

    b. When you had the urge or the feeling that you needed to empty your bladder, but you could not get to the toilet fast enough?

    c. Without physical activity and without a sense of urgency?

3. During the past 3 months, did you leak urine most often:
(check only one)

    a. When you were performing some physical activity, such as coughing, sneezing, lifting, or exercising?

    b. When you had the urge or the feeling that you needed to empty your bladder, but you could not get to the toilet fast enough?

    c. Without physical activity and without a sense of urgency?

    d. Approximately equally as often with physical activity as with a sense of urgency?

Definitions of type of urinary incontinence are based on responses to question 3.

Response to Question 3	Type of Incontinence
a. Most often with physical activity	Stress only or stress predominant
b. Most often with the urge to empty the bladder	Urge only or urge predominant
c. Without physical activity or sense of urgency	Other cause or other cause predominant
d. Approximately equally with physical activity and sense of urgency	Mixed

Brown JS, Bradley CS, Subak LL, Richter HE, Kraus SR, Brubaker L, et al. The sensitivity and specificity of a simple test to distinguish between urge and stress urinary incontinence. Diagnostic Aspects of Incontinence Study (DAISy) Research Group. Ann Intern Med 2006;144:715–23.

---

tain details of any prior surgery for incontinence, including indications and the technique and materials used. History of pelvic cancer therapy should include the dates and findings of any cystoscopic examinations. It is helpful to identify reversible conditions that cause or contribute to urinary incontinence (Table 12). Because many medications have lower urinary tract side effects, current medication use should be reviewed in detail.

Unfamiliar medications should be verified. Diuretics and α-antagonists, two classes of medication commonly used to manage hypertension, may cause incontinence in susceptible women. When incontinence is related temporarily to the onset of medication use or to a dosage increase (such as with a diuretic), it may be reasonable to use alternative medications that have a lesser effect on the lower urinary tract.

A urinary diary may be helpful in the evaluation of incontinence (Fig. 12). This simple instrument allows the patient to record voided volumes, leakage episodes (and amounts), and type and volume of fluid intake. Although a 3- to 5-day diary is optimal, evaluation of the events of a single typical 24-hour period can be clinically very helpful. Healthy women may void up to 13 times in 24 hours and once a night. Reviewing this diary allows the physician to suggest simple behavioral interventions, such as fluid and medication adjustments. In addition, the physician can further assess the severity of the leakage and begin to formulate opinions on the etiology of the problem and the need for further evaluation.

PHYSICAL EXAMINATION

Beyond the goals of the standard gynecologic examination, including speculum and bimanual examination, the specific goal of the urogynecologic physical examination is to assess vaginal topography and describe the support of the urethrovesical junction. Components of the neurologic evaluation should include demonstration of intact perineal sensation and testing of the bulbocavernosus reflex, active rectal sphincter tone, and resting rectal sphincter tone. In addition, the physician can detect treatable local conditions (eg, hypoestrogenism, levator atrophy, and fecal impaction) that affect bladder control. Quantification of hypermobility of the urethrovesical junction by direct measurement (eg, the cotton swab test)

Table 12. Identification and Management of Reversible Conditions That Cause or Contribute to Urinary Incontinence

Condition	Management
Conditions Affecting the Lower Urinary Tract	
Urinary tract infection (symptomatic with frequency, urgency, dysuria)	Antimicrobial therapy
Atrophic vaginitis or urethritis	Oral or topical estrogen
Vaginal delivery	Behavioral intervention muscle training; no surgical therapy postpartum, because condition may be self-limiting
Stool impaction	Disimpaction; appropriate use of stool softeners, bulk-forming agents, and laxatives, if necessary; high-fiber intake, adequate mobility, and fluid intake
Drug Side Effects*	
Diuretics: polyuria, frequency, and urgency	With all medications, discontinuation or change in therapy as clinically possible; dosage reduction or modification (eg, flexible scheduling of rapid-acting diuretics) also may help
Caffeine: aggravation or precipitation of urinary incontinence	
Anticholinergic agents: urinary retention, overflow incontinence, and impaction	
Psychotropic agents:	
Antidepressants: anticholinergic actions and sedation	
Antipsychotics: anticholinergic actions, sedation, rigidity, and immobility	
Sedatives, hypnotics, or central nervous system depressants: sedation, delirium, immobility, and muscle relaxation	
Narcotic analgesics: urinary retention, fecal impaction, sedation, and delirium	
Alpha-adrenergic blockers: urethral relaxation	
Alpha-adrenergic agonists: urinary retention (present in many cold and diet over-the-counter preparations)	
Beta-adrenergic agonists: urinary retention	
Calcium channel blockers: urinary retention	
Alcohol: polyuria, frequency, urgency, sedation, delirium, and immobility	
Increased Urine Production	
Metabolic (hyperglycemia and hypercalcemia)	Better control of diabetes mellitus; therapy for hypercalcemia depends on underlying cause
Excess fluid intake	Reduction in intake of diuretic fluids (eg, caffeinated beverages)
Volume overload	
Venous insufficiency with edema	Support stocking, leg elevation, sodium restriction, and diuretic therapy
Congestive heart failure	Medical therapy
Impaired Ability or Willingness to Reach a Toilet	
Delirium	Diagnosis and treatment of underlying cause(s) of acute confusional state
Chronic illness, injury, or restraint that interferes with mobility	Regular toileting, use of toilet substitutes, and environmental alterations (eg, bedside commode or urinal)
Psychologic	Removal of restraints if possible; appropriate pharmacologic or nonpharmacologic treatment or both

*Many side effects are seen with over-the-counter drugs, the use of which may not be reported by some patients.

Time	Intake (amount and type of fluid)	Voluntary void	Leakage episode	Did urge to urinate precede leakage?

Figure 12. A sample urinary diary.

does not confirm any form of incontinence, and this test need not be performed on a routine basis. Vaginal support can be described using the pelvic organ prolapse quantification system (POPQ) (7) or other validated systems.

URINALYSIS AND POSTVOID RESIDUAL VOLUME

Sterile urine and a normal postvoid residual volume should be documented in all women who desire evaluation of their incontinence. This documentation can be done with ultrasonography or a small-gauge catheter within 10 minutes after voiding. The residual volume should be less than 100 mL. Postvoid residual volume determination is the most important test to detect overflow incontinence, a condition in which incontinence is a phenomenon secondary to primary urinary retention.

Infection should be treated and sterile urine demonstrated before further incontinence evaluation. If the residual volume is elevated, the test should be repeated on a separate visit. Persistently high residual volume should be evaluated; this evaluation should precede the complete incontinence evaluation. Patients with persistent infections, elevated postvoid residuals, or both may benefit from consultation with an incontinence specialist.

Initial Interventions

Resolution of the patient's main symptoms should be foremost in the physician's treatment plan. The initial impression and treatment recommendations should be discussed with the patient to determine what type of treatment she prefers. Her own experience with treatment and her knowledge of the experiences of family and friends may influence her treatment choice. In general, the initial intervention should be safe and reasonably effective. Additional testing may be required in selected patients with an unclear diagnosis and in those who have had unsuccessful initial therapy and are considering surgery, including repeat surgery.

Once the patient and physician agree to start treatment, simple initial interventions should include opti-

mizing the function of pelvic floor muscles and teaching behavioral interventions to reduce symptoms, such as fluid management and voiding habits. These nonsurgical techniques often are best facilitated by a nonphysician, such as a nurse continence advisor, a physical therapist, or both. Once these interventions have been initiated, it is prudent for the physician to check on their efficacy within 2–3 months. Estrogen therapy is not an effective treatment of stress incontinence, although it reduces the rate of urinary tract infection and sensory symptoms, such as urgency. If symptoms persist, further therapy may be required.

BEHAVIORAL THERAPIES

Behavioral therapies are helpful to virtually every patient with urinary incontinence. Many patients have adopted behavioral changes in their own attempts to control incontinence symptoms. The physician can save time and have a more direct effect by inquiring what the patient has already tried on her own.

Simple techniques, including adjustment of type and volume of fluid intake, may be discussed after review of the urinary diary. Older patients frequently have nocturnal diuresis. The diaries of these patients reflect several episodes of nighttime voiding, possibly with enroute urinary loss. However, the important diary clue is that the bladder volume is large, sometimes larger than the patient's first morning voided volume. The bladder is simply being overwhelmed with the nocturnal diuresis. Rather than the addition of a nighttime bladder medication, a late-afternoon supine rest can assist the diuresis. Rarely, taking a late-afternoon diuretic may be necessary.

The problem of large fluid intake, often to aid weight loss efforts, should be addressed. Inadequate hydration may be found in women who restrict fluid intake as a method of compensating for their incontinence symptoms. In addition, caffeinated beverages increase urinary urgency and frequency and may exacerbate incontinence episodes.

Timed voiding is effective for approximately 60% of women with urge incontinence. Based on the voiding diary, the physician and patient select a voiding interval that is slightly shorter than the current interval that results in leakage. The patient is instructed to void using a specific interval during waking hours. Over 6–8 weeks, the intervals are gradually lengthened until the patient is able to urinate without leakage at 3- to 4-hour intervals. This technique has appreciable advantages, including a lack of systemic side effects and minimal cost. It is an ideal initial intervention for many women. These patients learn a valuable technique that can be used again in the future should urge incontinence become bothersome. Written materials are most helpful for optimal patient understanding and compliance.

Muscle Training

Women with weakened pelvic floor muscles may benefit from muscle training. These protocols are helpful for patients with urge or stress incontinence. Important components of muscle rehabilitation are 1) strength and 2) appropriate timing of contraction of these muscles. The physician's role is critical in identifying muscle weakness and emphasizing the importance of muscle rehabilitation. Strength can be gained through a variety of exercise programs. There is little scientific evidence to recommend any specific muscle-training regimen; however, it is likely that general principles of muscle strengthening apply. Physical therapists and nurses may be helpful in initiating and supervising the rehabilitation program. Women with weak pelvic floor muscles may perform Kegel exercises on their own if they are able to isolate the muscles to generate contractions (Box 29). In unusual cases, the patient may need to exercise in a supine or hip-raised position. With improved strength, she may advance to exercising in the upright position. Women with profound weakness or apparent paralysis generally require a supervised exercise program.

Once sufficient strength has been generated, the woman must learn to use these strengthened muscles correctly to inhibit urinary urge and reduce incontinence episodes. She must learn to contract these muscles firmly in advance of a cough, sneeze, or similar anticipated "stress." Likewise, this maneuver can inhibit an urge and allow time to get to the toilet without leakage. Strength without timing or timing without strength will give clinically unsatisfactory results. The patient's dedication to the activity is likely to diminish with time. The physician plays an important role in reinforcing concepts and providing encouragement to the patient.

Electrical Stimulation

Electrical stimulation with a transvaginal probe reduces urge incontinence in approximately 50% of affected women (8). Like timed voiding and muscle training, this treatment is free of systemic side effects. The main

> **Box 29**
>
> ### Kegel Exercises
>
> Kegel exercises (pelvic muscle exercises) help improve urinary control in 40–75% of patients with mild to moderate symptoms. The patient performs the exercise by contracting the pubococcygeus muscle, thus improving the tone of the voluntary external urethral musculature. Exercises are indicated in patients with stress or urge incontinence. The success of pelvic muscle exercises depends on the patient's ability to identify the correct muscles for the exercise and her commitment to performing the exercises. Simple written or verbal instructions often are insufficient to teach patients how to perform pelvic muscle exercise properly.
>
> The correct method also can be taught during a routine pelvic examination. While the examiner identifies the muscle by direct palpation, the patient is asked to contract the muscle, and verbal feedback can be provided to ensure appropriate performance of the exercise. Women who are unable to isolate their pelvic muscles or who cannot contract these muscles may need biofeedback or electrical stimulation.
>
> Muscle training should be individualized based on ability. Commonly, patients may be instructed to perform 10–20 10-second pelvic floor contractions three or more times per day. A minimum of 30 contractions per day for at least 6 weeks usually is required to achieve a detectable beneficial effect. Older women may need a longer training period. These exercises should be performed indefinitely to prevent the relapse of incontinence.

drawback is the cost of rental or purchase of the device, which may be an out-of-pocket expense for many patients. Several devices approved by the U.S. Food and Drug Administration (FDA) are available, and treatment can be home based or, less commonly, office based.

Typically, a transvaginal probe is used once or twice daily for 15–20 minutes. Symptom relief generally occurs within 6–8 weeks and may persist with reduced (eg, three-times weekly) stimulation. Women with pacemakers should avoid this therapy unless other options are not available. Implanted neurostimulators may be considered for women with severe, refractory urge incontinence.

Vaginal Devices

Pessaries that are modified for incontinence, called *continence dishes* and *continence rings*, provide additional suburethral pressure and are safe and reasonably effective (Fig. 13). Ongoing studies (ClinicalTrials.gov) will soon report the results of a randomized study comparing continence pessaries, pelvic muscle and behavioral training, and the concomitant use of these two therapies (9).

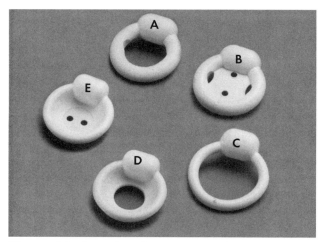

Figure 13. Examples of pessaries used to treat incontinence. **A.** Ring with knob. **B.** Ring with support and knob. **C.** Incontinence ring. **D.** Incontinence dish. **E.** Incontinence dish with support. (Courtesy of Cooper Surgical, Inc., Trumbull, CT.)

PHARMACOTHERAPY

The FDA has approved no medication for the treatment of stress urinary incontinence. However, there are several FDA-approved medications for treatment of urge incontinence. Medications for detrusor overactivity are typically anticholinergic agents. Thus, the side effect profile for these agents includes dry mouth and worsening constipation. Narrow-angle glaucoma is an absolute contraindication to the use of this class of medications, and these medications should be used cautiously in women with appreciable cardiovascular disease. Oxybutynin chloride is available in generic formulations. Medication can be started in very low doses and be self-titrated over 6–8 weeks with written instructions. Other FDA-approved medications include tolterodine, darifenacin, solifenacin, and trospium (10). Brand-name formulations are most costly but are more convenient with daily dosing, which appears to increase patient compliance. It is important for the prescribing physician to set realistic expectations regarding symptom control. When patients experience effective use of this class of medications, improvement, rather than complete continence, is typical.

Further Evaluation

Women with refractory symptoms after initial therapy may require further evaluation, especially before the initiation of any invasive therapy, such as surgery or bulking agents. Poor follow-up is a shortcoming of incontinence treatment. The physician may assume, incorrectly, that patients who do not return have experienced satisfactory relief from their incontinence. Lay organizations have gathered appreciable information that challenges this assumption, indicating that incontinent women often feel dissatisfied with the efficacy and range of incontinence treatment options.

STRESS TEST

Before considering surgery for stress incontinence, the physician should objectively reproduce the sign of transurethral urine loss. Any positive stress test (momentary transurethral loss of urine when the intraabdominal pressure is increased) is strong evidence of stress incontinence. The urogynecologic stress test shares one characteristic of the cardiac stress test: both tests must be made progressively more "difficult" to have a meaningful negative result. Thus, a negative result on a urinary stress test performed when the patient is supine or has an empty bladder does not rule out stress incontinence. However, when the test is performed when the patient has a full bladder and coughs repetitively while standing, a negative result is meaningful and should be documented in the chart as a "negative standing, full-bladder stress test."

In general, a negative stress test result when the patient is standing and has a full bladder should preclude the recommendation of surgery to correct incontinence. When surgery is planned for repair of pelvic organ prolapse, the physician should perform the stress test while repositioning the vaginal walls to the anticipated postoperative position. If appreciable incontinence is present, a continence procedure can be considered.

SIMPLE URODYNAMIC TESTING

Simple cystometry demonstrates the activity of the detrusor muscle, documents urodynamic stress incontinence, and provides information about bladder capacity. Single-channel (bladder only) and dual-channel (bladder and abdominal) cystometry techniques are used. This test does not require specific urogynecologic equipment. Simple manometric systems can suffice. Three important aspects of bladder function—compliance, detrusor activity, and sensation—can be assessed by this simple test.

Further Therapy

Patients with refractory symptoms may benefit from further therapy, such as surgery, neuromodulation, and botulinum A injections. Certain patients with refractory symptoms also may benefit from consultation with an incontinence specialist who offers a full range of advanced therapies.

SURGERY

Continence surgery can be offered to women whose stress incontinence is appreciable, bothersome, and objectively confirmed. The selection of specific continence procedures is beyond the scope of this manuscript. Interested readers are referred to the most recent Cochrane reviews addressing this evolving area in incontinence therapy (11). Concomitant prolapse surgery can be performed at the same time as stress incontinence surgery.

NEUROMODULATION

Implanted sacral electrodes have been demonstrated to reduce urge incontinence. This treatment may be beneficial in women whose symptoms are refractory to less invasive treatments (12).

BOTULINUM A INJECTIONS

Experimental evidence suggests a possible role for botulinum A toxin in the treatment of refractory urge incontinence (13). This treatment may cause transient urinary retention, and physicians must detect this adverse effect.

Urinary Tract Infections

At least one third of all women experience a urinary tract infection in their lifetimes. The well-recognized clinical scenario of a healthy woman who reports the sudden onset of dysuria and urinary urgency and frequency is typical (14). These symptoms may be reported by telephone contact. If it is an isolated, nonrecurring event for an otherwise healthy woman, management is straightforward. Empiric treatment is cost-effective, and urinalysis or culture and sensitivity testing are not needed. Short-course (1- to 3-day) antibiotic regimens can be prescribed after drug allergies and interactions have been verified (15). Urinary analgesics, either nonprescription or prescription, may offer prompt relief of symptoms even before the onset of action of the antibiotic (16).

To establish that it is an uncomplicated, isolated event, several important questions should be asked. Generally, simple urinary tract infections are not associated with recurrence or relapse. Thus, asking about previous episodes, their frequency, the response to therapy, and any contributing events will help detect recurring or relapsing infections. Refractory symptoms after a short course of antibiotics, recurrent symptoms within 2 weeks of treatment, or more than three infections in a 12-month period should raise suspicion of an underlying disorder (Fig. 14). In these more complicated situations, proper diagnosis and treatment are aided by urine culture and sensitivity testing (17).

Some women report a relationship between their symptoms and sexual activity (18). When these episodes are documented to be infectious by serial cultures, postcoital administration of antibiotics is the best-documented effective technique. A single postcoital dose of an inexpensive urinary tract antibiotic has excellent efficacy in reducing the total number of infections. Anecdotal reports suggest that the propensity for coitus-related infections may be related to the woman's sexual partner. Thus, the physician might consider discontinuing this antibiotic regimen if the woman changes sexual partners. Spermicide and diaphragm use increase the risk of urinary tract infection. Users with symptoms should be encouraged to use alternative methods of contraception.

If the physician suspects a disorder beyond a simple lower urinary tract infection, additional evaluation with urine cultures and sensitivity testing may be warranted. Involvement of the upper urinary tract may be signaled by flank pain or fever. Women with asymptomatic bacteriuria are more likely to develop upper urinary tract infection during pregnancy.

Recurrent and Persistent Infections

The diagnosis of recurrent or relapsing infection requires sequential urine cultures. The most common organism found (80%) is *Escherichia coli*. Other organisms include staphylococci; group D streptococci; and *Klebsiella, Enterobacter, Proteus,* and *Pseudomonas* species. Although empiric treatment can begin before the first culture result is available, it is imperative to obtain a urine sample before treatment. Recurrent infections are characterized by positive results of urine cultures. These infections are appropriately treated with an antibiotic to which the uropathogen is susceptible and should be monitored up to approximately 2 weeks after therapy to document that the urine is sterile.

Recurrence is documented by a repeat episode with the same symptoms. Typically, the culture shows that the same organism, although often a different serotype is present. The diagnosis of recurrent infection should be supported by several (three is ideal) episodes of culture-positive infection, effective treatment, and a negative result of posttreatment culture. In an asymptomatic woman, a colony count of more than 10^5 is indicative of infection. However, in a symptomatic patient, colony counts of more than 10^2 are compatible with the diagnosis of infection. It is helpful to have a flow sheet in the office chart to document the date and result of each episode, the antibiotics used, the results, and the duration of treatment. A subgroup of women has relapsing infections, which are related to the presence of the same infecting organism (19).

Some women have persistent infections. In this group, initial culture results are positive and an appropriate antibiotic is prescribed, but the posttreatment culture results remain positive. This sequence should raise suspicion of an anatomic problem that allows the harboring of the infectious etiology. Several possibilities include a urinary tract stone, a foreign body, or a urinary tract anatomic abnormality. These conditions must be ruled out by imaging studies of the upper tracts and diagnostic cystoscopy. Prolonged use of suppressive antibiotics can be instituted only after culture docu-

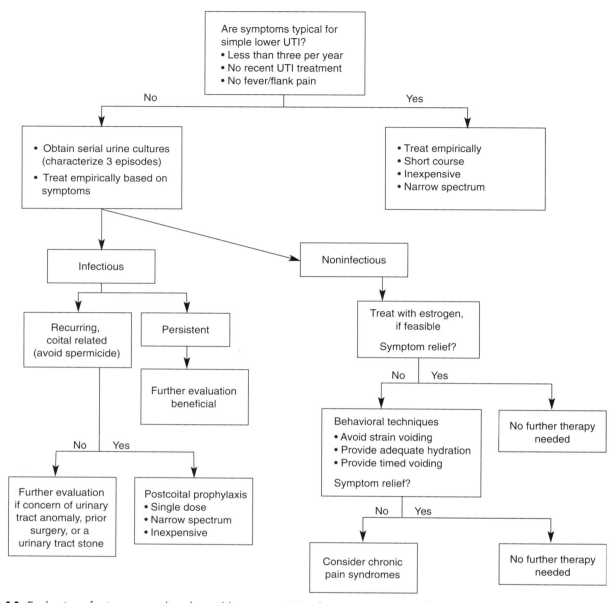

Figure 14. Evaluation of urinary tract disorders. Abbreviation: UTI indicates urinary tract infection.

mentation of persistent infection that is not attributable to other treatable conditions. Long-duration antibiotic regimens typically consist of a single daily dose for 3–6 months. If the woman is symptom-free during this interval, she and the physician should mutually decide whether continuation of the regimen is clinically prudent, taking into account the frequency and severity of previous episodes, as well as the cost, inconvenience, and side effects of daily antibiotic use.

Noninfectious Problems

Some women report recurrent infection in the presence of negative results of urine cultures (20). These symptoms generally are similar to those of a standard episode of lower urinary tract infection and are called sensory

disorders, which does not indicate an underlying pathology per se. In many such cases, urinalysis shows leukocytes and blood in the urine. Sometimes the cause is an infection that escapes detection because it is caused by a nonpathogenic organism or one that requires special testing (eg, *Chlamydia* or *Mycoplasma* species). Herpes infection and other vulvovaginal infections can produce symptoms of cystitis with pain on urination.

When these possibilities have been ruled out, chronic conditions, such as painful bladder, bladder diverticula, or foreign bodies can be considered and ordinarily will require referral to a specialist (21). This decision for further evaluation, rather than continuation of empiric therapy, avoids the misadventures associated with continuing ineffective antibiotic therapy, use of urethral dilatation, or repetitive dietary changes of no proven value. Estrogen deficiency is believed by some to cause the new onset of irritative symptoms. Urogenital estrogen deficiency has been associated with irritative symptoms of an infectious and a noninfectious sensory nature and may respond well to appropriate estrogen therapy. Symptoms that persist after estrogen therapy may be related to underlying pain disorders in the pelvis, systemic pain disorders (fibromyalgia), or other bladder disorders, such as painful bladder syndrome (formerly, interstitial cystitis) or detrusor overactivity.

Many women who have sensory disorders of the lower urinary tract, and in whom no cause can be found after complete evaluation, adopt behavioral changes that may inadvertently maintain or worsen their symptoms (22). Typically, these women report a symptom of postvoid fullness; that is, a need to urinate again shortly after a voluntary void that seemed to be complete at the time. The bladder-voiding cycle does not function optimally when low volumes of urine are voided. Thus, they often use physiologically inappropriate mechanisms such as Valsalva voiding. This "strain voiding" technique is commonly used to "be sure that the bladder is empty." This goal is unrealistic and physiologically unnecessary. It is not the presence of a small or even a normal amount of urine in the bladder that causes the symptoms. Rather, an inappropriate sensory signal is driving the urge to urinate. Behavioral techniques that discourage strain voiding and encourage standardized intervals between voiding (eg, no less than 1 hour apart) often are helpful in breaking this dysfunctional voiding cycle.

Behavioral interventions must be individualized. Often, the type and volume of fluid intake must be modified. Some women markedly restrict their fluid intake, making their urine concentrated. It is believed that highly concentrated urine may exacerbate sensory disorder symptoms in some women. Certainly, this behavior increases the tendency toward low-volume voids. Other women drink predominantly acidic substances, commonly cranberry juice, in the erroneous belief that infection is the basis for their symptoms. This behavior may increase irritative symptoms. The physician can play an important educational role in uncovering these behaviors and recommending reasonable alternatives.

In some women, these disorders become established as part of a chronic pain syndrome. A variety of names for this syndrome have been used; they include urethritis, urethral syndrome, chronic cystitis, chronic trigonitis, and interstitial cystitis. Urethral syndrome is associated with symptoms of dysuria and frequency without a demonstrable cause. The leukocyte esterase test result is negative, and a low bacteria count (approximately 1,000 per milliliter) is found on quantitative cultures. Chlamydial infection and gonorrhea should be ruled out by nucleic acid amplification testing of the cervix. If pyuria is found and cultured colonies reach or exceed 10^2 per milliliter, antibiotic therapy is indicated.

Painful bladder syndrome has received special attention. Although this term is no longer accepted nomenclature, the entity is still recognized. This severe form of lower urinary tract pain predominantly affects women. It is widely recognized that many patients have other concomitant pain syndromes, and there are questions as to whether the primary pain disorder is within the bladder itself. Differing opinions on etiology result in differing treatment approaches. Some experts suggest that findings related to the bladder wall are secondary. Lay organizations and support groups have formed with the express hope of improving diagnosis and treatment of women with this condition. These women may benefit from referral to a physical therapist skilled in the treatment of underlying pelvic myofascial pain.

Most primary care physicians can play an important role in supervising the overall care of women with chronic pain. When the results of a thorough evaluation have been normal and appropriate consultation has yielded no answer, the patient can benefit from continued sympathetic support. Cure may not be realistic, but symptom control with the techniques used for other painful, chronic conditions can provide relief in many cases. Because they are desperate, these patients often undergo multiple invasive, ineffective treatments, including a variety of surgical interventions.

Early evidence suggests that these pain syndromes respond to several forms of body work, including physical therapy, acupuncture, and osteopathic manipulation (23). Treatment of underlying skeletal or musculoskeletal problems may be beneficial, has low risk, and may be considered.

Common lower urinary tract disorders are treated by the obstetrician–gynecologist. Documentation of an infectious or noninfectious etiology is essential. The general schemes for assessment are outlined in Figure 14. Interpretation of the result of sequential urine cultures and appropriate triage maximize the efficacy of treatment and lead to cost-efficient evaluations. The symptoms of sensory disorders may mimic those of infectious disorders; however, the treatment algorithms differ appreciably. Noninvasive treatments, an understanding of chronic pain syndromes, and appropriate consultation offer optimal symptom control.

References

1. Abrams P, Cardozo L, Khoury S, Wein A, editors. Incontinence: proceedings from the Second International Consultation on Incontinence. Plymouth, U.K.: Health Publication Ltd; 2002.

2. Uebersax JS, Wyman JF, Shumaker SA, McClish DK, Fantl JA. Short forms to assess life quality and symptom distress for urinary incontinence in women: the Incontinence Impact Questionnaire and the Urogenital Distress Inventory. Continence Program for Women Research Group. Neurourol Urodyn 1995;14:131–9.

3. Yalcin I, Bump RC. Validation of two global impression questionnaires for incontinence. Am J Obstet Gynecol 2003;189:98–101.

4. Elkadry EA, Kenton KS, FitzGerald MP, Shott S, Brubaker L. Patient-selected goals: a new perspective on surgical outcome. Am J Obstet Gynecol 2003;189:1551–7; discussion 1557–8.

5. Hullfish KL, Bovbjerg VE, Steers WD. Patient-centered goals for pelvic floor dysfunction surgery: long-term follow-up. Am J Obstet Gynecol 2004;191:201–5.

6. Mahajan ST, Elkadry EA, Kenton KS, Shott S, Brubaker L. Patient-centered surgical outcomes: the impact of goal achievement and urge incontinence on patient satisfaction one year after surgery. Am J Obstet Gynecol 2006;194: 722–8.

7. Bump RC, Mattiasson A, Bo K, Brubaker LP, DeLancey JO, Klarskov P, et al. The standardization of terminology of female pelvic organ prolapse and pelvic floor dysfunction. Am J Obstet Gynecol 1996;175:10–7.

8. Brubaker L. Electrical stimulation in overactive bladder. Urology 2000;55:17–23; discussion 31–2.

9. Richter HE, Burgio KL, Goode PS, Borello-France D, Bradley CS, Brubaker L, et al. Non-surgical management of stress urinary incontinence: ambulatory treatments for leakage associated with stress (ATLAS) trial. Pelvic Foor Disorders Network. Clin Trials 2007;4:92–101.

10. Andersson KE. Antimuscarinics for treatment of overactive bladder. Lancet Neurol 2004;3:46–53.

11. Maher C, Baessler K, Glazener CM, Adams EJ, Hagen S. Surgical management of pelvic organ prolapse in women. Cochrane Database of Systematic Reviews 2007, Issue 3. Art. No.: CD004014. DOI: 10.1002/14651858.CD004014.pub3.

12. Groenendijk PM, Lycklama a Nyeholt AA, Heesakkers JP, van Kerrebroeck PE, Hassouna MM, Gajewski JB, et al. Urodynamic evaluation of sacral neuromodulation for urge urinary incontinence. Sacral Nerve Stimulation Study Group. B J U Int 2008;101:325–9.

13. Brubaker L, Richter HE, Visco A, Mahajan S, Nygaard I, Braun TM, et al. Refractory idiopathic urge urinary incontinence and botulinum A injection. Pelvic Floor Disorders Network. J Urol 2008;180:217–22.

14. Stamm WE. Criteria for the diagnosis of urinary tract infection and for the assessment of therapeutic effectiveness. Infection 1992;20 Suppl 3:S151–4; discussion S160–1.

15. Stamm WE. Controversies in single dose therapy of acute uncomplicated urinary tract infections in women. Infection 1992;20 Suppl 4:S272–5.

16. Stamm WE, Hooton TM. Management of urinary tract infections in adults. N Engl J Med 1993;329:1328–34.

17. Saint S, Scholes D, Fihn SD, Farrell RG, Stamm WE. The effectiveness of a clinical practice guideline for the management of presumed uncomplicated urinary tract infection in women. Am J Med 1999;106:636–41.

18. Hooton TM, Roberts PL, Stamm WE. Effects of recent sexual activity and use of a diaphragm on the vaginal microflora. Clin Infect Dis 1994;19:274–8.

19. Gupta K, Sahm DF, Mayfield D, Stamm WE. Antimicrobial resistance among uropathogens that cause community-acquired urinary tract infections in women: a nationwide analysis. Clin Infect Dis 2001;33:89–94.

20. Latham RH, Stamm WE. Urethral syndrome in women. Urol Clin North Am 1984;11:95–101.

21. Karram MM, Siddighi S. Lower urinary tract infection. In: Bent AE, Cundiff GW, Swift SE, editors. Ostergard's urogynecology and pelvic floor dysfunction. 6th ed. ed. Philadelphia (PA): Lippincott Williams & Wilkins; 2007. p. 148–69.

22. FitzGerald MP. Chronic pelvic pain. Curr Womens Health Rep 2003;3:327–33.

23. Weiss JM. Pelvic floor myofascial trigger points: manual therapy for interstitial cystitis and the urgency-frequency syndrome. J Urol 2001;166:2226–31.

Sexuality and Sexual Dysfunction

Rosemary Basson

Sexual problems are reported by approximately 40% of U.S. women in community studies and by up to 90% of women seeking gynecologic care. These problems rarely occur as single disorders. For example, difficulty with arousal and desire is common, as is the lack of orgasm and arousal. With time, chronic dyspareunia typically becomes associated with low desire and low arousability.

Women view their sexuality as an important quality-of-life issue that frequently is affected by reproductive events (1, 2). Thus, the obstetrician–gynecologist's role in assessing sexual dysfunction, initiating treatment, and making appropriate referrals is crucial. Moreover, gynecologic disease and therapeutic interventions can affect sexual response. Management of sexual problems by obstetrician–gynecologists may include the following components:

- Providing basic, detailed information about sexual response cycles and underlying physiology
- Assessing factors that contribute to low desire, low arousal, or lack of orgasm so that both partners can make appropriate changes
- Assessing and managing chronic dyspareunia or apareunia (often associated with unconsummated relationships)
- Prescribing medication or hormone therapy
- Advising caution regarding the lack of safety data on some products claiming to help sexual dysfunction

Sexual Response Cycle

The sexual response cycle in women is complex, and events do not always occur in a predictable sequence, as they usually do in men. A model of women's sexual response is shown in Figure 15 (3). This model depicts the many sexual motivations, sexual stimuli, and psychologic and biologic factors that govern the processing of those stimuli (ie, that determine the woman's arousability).

Women's motivations for sexual activity vary (4). To increase the emotional closeness with her partner is a common motivation (4). If a woman experiences sexual arousal and the stimuli continue, provided the woman remains focused and the sexual arousal is enjoyed, she then may sense sexual desire—she now wants to continue the experience for the sake of the sexual sensations. A psychologically and physically positive outcome heightens emotional intimacy with her partner, thereby strengthening her motivation. Any spontaneous desire (ie, sexual thinking, conscious sexual desire experienced ahead of the sexual engagement, or fantasizing) may augment this inherently responsive cycle. Spontaneous desire is particularly common early in relationships or when partners have been apart, is sometimes related to the menstrual cycle, and is extremely variable among women. Community studies suggest that for women in long-term relationships, spontaneous desire is particularly rare.

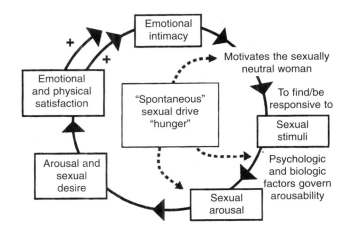

Figure 15. Blended intimacy-based and sexual drive-based cycles. (Basson R. Female sexual response: the role of drugs in the management of sexual dysfunction. Obstet Gynecol 2001;98:350–3.)

Women's Sexual Arousal

Arousal includes a variety of physiological processes and emotional experiences. Women are not always aware of the physiological events involved in their own sexual arousal. Events that may be part of arousal include mental sexual excitement; vulvar and vaginal congestion; pleasure from stimulation of the engorging vulva or the anterior vaginal wall and underlying Halban's fascia; increased and modified lubrication; relaxation of vaginal nonvascular smooth muscle; pleasure from stimulation of nongenital areas of the body; and other somatic changes, such as increased blood pressure, heart rate, muscle tone, respiratory rate, and temperature. Subjective arousal can be impaired by a number of psychologic factors.

The genital congestion of arousal, although present, may not be recognized consciously or may be recognized only minimally; it may not be interpreted as sexual or may not be enjoyed despite sexual interpretation. Even a frankly dysphoric emotional response may occur. Throbbing, tingling, and feelings of urgency for more genital contact and vaginal entry are far less consistent for sexually healthy women than are the equivalent sensations in men. These feelings have not been found to correlate with subjective sexual arousal. Similarly, in healthy women, the correlation between laboratory-based objective measurement of genital congestion in response to an erotic stimulus and subjective arousal varies greatly. The genital congestion is prompt, is reflexive, and occurs within 30 seconds to a maximum of 2 minutes, whereas subjective arousal (to the same stimulus) may take 10 minutes (5). Unlike in men, genital congestion is prompt on viewing sexual behavior between the nonpreferred gender and also on viewing nonerotic but "sexual" images (eg, primates mating) (6). Most women who ultimately receive the diagnosis of female sexual arousal disorder report minimal or no sexual arousal and, sometimes, negative emotions during the erotic stimulus. However, testing shows increases in genital congestion similar to those of sexually healthy women (7).

Sexual Dysfunction

Classification

Table 13 shows definitions of the types of disorders that are currently used for establishing the diagnosis of female sexual dysfunction by the *Diagnostic and Statistical Manual of Mental Disorders*, Fourth Edition, and the American Foundation for Urologic Disease. The definitions also note whether any of the following descriptors are involved:

1. Factors from the woman's past that may have caused psychosexual maldevelopment

2. Contextual factors that appear to provide logic for the dysfunction

3. Medical and psychiatric factors

Also, the degree of distress (mild, moderate, or severe) and the degree of dysfunction (lifelong or acquired, situational or generalized) should be noted.

Coexisting Etiologic Factors

Several factors should be taken into account when assessing a patient with sexual dysfunction. These factors include mood and personality issues, effects of medications, and interpersonal relationships.

MOOD AND PERSONALITY FACTORS

A growing body of data shows that women seeking help for desire and arousal disorders and chronic dyspareunia show certain psychologic and personality traits more commonly than do sexually healthy women. Specifically, in addition to strong links to present or past clinical depression, women with low desire more frequently report evidence of mood instability and low self-esteem; they are more worried, anxious, and introverted. Of women with chronic dyspareunia associated with provoked vestibulodynia, a definite subgroup shows marked psychologic distress, including negative affect, a marked fear of negative evaluation by others, and a tendency to be hypervigilant for harm to self and to catastrophize when thinking about their pain. This internal stress may alter immune and neurologic systems.

MEDICATION EFFECTS

Taking medications, including selective serotonin reuptake inhibitors and other antidepressants, β-blockers, and antiandrogens, as well as long-term codeine or other opiate use, may compound or cause sexual dysfunction. Additionally, a subgroup of women taking oral or transdermal contraceptives, regardless of the androgenicity of the progestin involved, consistently report lowered desire and arousability, possibly as a result of the suppression of endogenous ovarian androgen production and binding of androgen to the increased sex hormone-binding globulin (SHBG).

INTERPERSONAL RELATIONSHIPS

Studies of women in menopause showed that women's positive feelings for their partners protected them from the experience of bothersome menopausal symptoms (8, 9) that were shown to reduce the sexual response indirectly. These studies and others of women of various ages also showed that feelings for the partner had the strongest influence on sexual desire and sexual responsiveness. The best predictors of sexual health included the nonsexual aspects of the relationship, sexual attitudes, and emotional well-being.

Table 13. Definitions of Female Sexual Dysfunction

DSM-IV-TR Definition	Revised Definition by the American Foundation for Urologic Disease International Consensus Committee 2003	Comments
Hypoactive sexual desire disorder: persistent or recurrently deficient (or absent) sexual fantasies and desire for sexual activity. The judgment of deficiency is made by the clinician taking into account factors that affect sexual functioning, such as age and context of the person's life.	Sexual desire/interest disorder: absent or diminished feelings of sexual interest or desire, absent sexual thoughts or fantasies, and a lack of responsive desire. Motivations (here defined as reasons/incentives) for attempting to become sexually aroused are scarce or absent. The lack of interest is beyond a normative lessening with life cycle and relationship duration.	The evidence is that minimal spontaneous sexual thinking or desiring of sex ahead of sexual experiences does not necessarily constitute disorder, (given the data on women in sexually satisfactory established relationships). Lack of desire triggered during the sexual encounter; ie, "responsive" desire, is integral to the revised diagnosis.
There is no DSM-IV-TR definition addressing lack of arousal.	Combined arousal disorder: absent or markedly reduced feelings of sexual arousal (sexual excitement and sexual pleasure) from any type of stimulation and absent or impaired genital sexual arousal (vulval swelling and lubrication).	There is no sexual excitement (in the mind) and no awareness of reflexive genital vasocongestion. (Research shows that usually the reflex congestion has occurred.)
There is no DSM-IV-TR definition addressing lack of subjective arousal.	Subjective arousal disorder: absent or markedly reduced feelings of sexual arousal (sexual excitement and sexual pleasure) from any type of stimulation. Vaginal lubrication and other signs of physical response still occur.	There is sexual excitement (in the mind) but the patient is aware of adequate lubrication—usually because intercourse is painless.
Female sexual arousal disorder: Persistent or recurrent inability to attain or to maintain an adequate lubrication/ swelling response of sexual excitement until completion of the sexual activity.	Genital arousal disorder: absent or impaired genital sexual arousal—minimal vulvar swelling or vaginal lubrication from any type of sexual stimulation and reduced sexual sensations from caressing genitalia. Subjective sexual excitement still occurs from nongenital sexual stimuli.	The presence of subjective arousal (sexual excitement) from nongenital stimuli; eg, erotica, stimulating the partner, receiving breast stimulation, or kissing; is key to this revised diagnosis.
Female orgasmic disorder: Persistent or recurrent delay or absence of orgasm following a normal sexual excitement phase.	Female orgasmic disorder: despite the self-report of high sexual arousal or excitement, there is either lack of orgasm, markedly diminished intensity of orgasmic sensations, or marked delay of orgasm from any kind of stimulation.	Women with arousal disorders frequently do not experience orgasm. Their correct diagnosis is one of an arousal disorder.

Data from American Psychiatric Association. Diagnostic and statistical manual of mental disorders: DSM-IV-TR. 4th ed., text revision. Washington, DC: American Psychiatric Association; 2000 *and* Basson R, Leiblum S, Brotto L, Derogatis L, Fourcroy J, Fugl-Meyer K, et al. Definitions of women's sexual dysfunction reconsidered: advocating expansion and revision. J Psychosom Obstet Gynaecol 2003;24:221–9.

Hormonal Factors

ESTROGEN EFFECTS

Although estrogen supplementation is not believed to influence sexual desire directly, it is thought that testosterone acts within the brain cell by way of its conversion to dihydrotestosterone and estradiol. None of the larger studies has shown a relationship between women's sexual function and hormone levels, including levels of testosterone, other than the consistent finding that low estrogen levels are associated with dyspareunia.

Postmenopausal estrogen deficiency usually causes observable vulvar vaginal atrophy. However, vaginal dryness and dyspareunia may or may not occur. Of note, the increase from baseline in vaginal blood flow in postmenopausal women in response to an erotic stimulus is not impaired (7). The clinical relevance of this finding is that women should ensure that they are mentally sexually excited by the sexual interaction (ie, that it is sufficiently erotic for them) before intercourse is attempted. However, when the baseline flow is markedly reduced, dyspareunia is likely.

Systemic estrogen therapy may be considered for recently menopausal women with sleep disturbance, mood symptoms, or vasomotor symptoms. When the primary problem appears to be dyspareunia associated with vaginal atrophy, vaginal estrogen is prescribed.

Androgen Deficiency

Testosterone supplements have been approved in Europe and elsewhere for low sexual desire subsequent to surgical menopause. Although there is strong consensus in the scientific community that androgens are needed for women's sexual response, the scientific study of physiologic supplementation is just beginning. Furthermore, published safety data are for only 6 months, whereas women's sexual lives usually continue indefinitely unless there is no available sexual partner.

Endogenous Androgens

Uncertainty remains regarding androgen production by postmenopausal ovaries. Most likely the production is variable (10). Adrenal output of precursors of androgen and estrogen, including androstenedione, dehydroepiandrosterone, and dehydroepiandrosterone sulfate, decreases by approximately two thirds between the mid 30s and early 60s (11).

Women who undergo premenopausal bilateral oophorectomy experience an acute decrease in testosterone levels. Sexual dysfunction may or may not occur. Of note, three recent studies confirmed that women who choose elective oophorectomy for benign pathologic conditions do not report the onset of sexual dysfunction when monitored for 1 and 3 years (12–14).

Because androgen production of most middle-aged and older women and estrogen production of all postmenopausal women are intracellular, many variables affect the final androgen activity. These variables include the amount of precursor hormone, the activity of enzymes to convert the precursors to estrogen and testosterone, the numbers and activities of cofactors, and variable androgen receptor sensitivity. Therefore, identifying patients with androgen deficiency is challenging.

There is no accepted threshold value for androgen below which symptoms of sexual dysfunction usually occur, and the measurement of androgen levels as part of the evaluation of sexual symptoms is not recommended. In fact, two large community studies found no correlation between testosterone levels and sexual symptoms (15, 16).

Perimenopausal Factors

Sexual dysfunction may be more common during the perimenopause than in the postmenopause (8, 9). Sexual difficulties in the perimenopause may be the result of high estrogen levels, which can cause breast soreness and reluctance to allow their stimulation; low estrogen levels, which can cause dyspareunia; or the fluctuation in estrogen levels, which can cause hot flushes and irritability and, thus, reduce sexual motivation. The ongoing decline in androgen precursors may add to difficulties with arousal and desire. Oral contraceptives to regulate menses may further compound the problem by increasing SHBG. These causes may be combined with psychosexual factors, including a woman's knowledge of her imminent infertility, and with contextual changes within her family, her sexual relationship, and perhaps her career and focus of life. Moreover, if emotional intimacy has waned, sexual contacts may be avoided and her needed stimuli deliberately not be put into place, so there will be minimal motivation or response.

Evaluation and Management

In providing therapy and prognosis for sexual dysfunction, it is important to establish clearly whether the sexual dysfunction is situational or generalized. If a woman's sexual response is healthy in some circumstances, it suggests that major physical organic factors are not involved. It is, therefore, very important to ask about sexual response to masturbation, viewing or reading erotica, and being around persons other than the regular partner, even when physical sexual interaction is not involved.

Women's Sexual Desire and Interest Disorder

The woman's interest in or enthusiasm for the idea of or request for sexual activity should be evaluated. When this interest or enthusiasm seems to be low or absent, the following factors should be considered:

- Mood
- Interpersonal issues
- Lack of useful sexual stimuli
- Lack of useful sexual context
- Psychologic issues within the woman herself (eg, past negative experiences or abuse, negative self-image, and feelings of shame or guilt)
- Coexisting arousal disorder (the woman may be motivated to seek sexual stimuli but has found that they do not arouse her)
- Expectation of a negative outcome (eg, dyspareunia or a partner's sexual dysfunction or poor sexual skills)
- An emotionally negative outcome

The questions provided in Box 30 may be helpful in the assessment of low sexual desire.

It is useful to construct, preferably with the couple, a model of the variable female sexual response that clarifies the usual requirement of emotional intimacy, the

Questions Helpful in Assessing Low Sexual Desire

1. How long have you had these concerns with respect to your sexual desire?

2. Do you sometimes have sexual thoughts, sexual daydreams, and fantasies (even though you may not act on them)?

3. At present, would you have sexual feelings of arousal from something that was potentially erotic to you (eg, a picture, book, movie, or dancing)?

4. Many women self-stimulate; is that something you still do from time to time?

5. What would your answers have been to the above questions previously?

6. A large proportion of women's desire, especially in long-term relationships, appears to be receptive or responsive. In other words, women can go happily through their day not really sensing any sexual need per se. However, if they are not too distracted or depressed and are not feeling distant from their sexual partner, they can respond to their partner or to other sexual stimuli. So I need to ask you about the circumstances when you consider being sexual, or when your partner is instigating sexual activity, and you lack desire. Can you describe these circumstances to me?

7. For many women, feeling emotionally close and able to trust their partner is as important as feeling that their partner is physically sexually attractive. How is the emotional intimacy with your partner—the trust, ability to be honest, and ability to share feelings (the hopes and the fears)?

8. Can you slowly respond to your partner's sexual touch, even if initially you have no sexual need yourself? Does the touching gradually become more pleasant and arousing? If so, would you then sense some desire to continue? This later desire; ie, not there at the beginning, is normal for many women. As you touch your partner, do your feelings change? Does anything negative happen (the situation is not what you want or intercourse is attempted too soon or there is pain; eg, with penetrating the vagina)? Can you stay focused on the experience? Are you able to guide your partner as to what pleases you? Is there anything being done to you that is discomforting? Does your partner have any sexual difficulties?

presence of useful sexual stimuli, and an appropriate context to trigger desire, in addition to the expectation of a rewarding physical and emotional outcome. The various interruptions in the woman's cycle then can be addressed. Issues, such as an excessive focus on the act of intercourse, a partner's sexual dysfunction, or lack of

sexual skill and knowledge, can be addressed. A referral to a psychiatrist or a psychologist may be needed when deep-seated intrapsychologic issues are preventing the woman from experiencing sexual desire in response to sexual stimuli or result in her experiencing dysphoric arousal. Alternatively, there may be an obvious need for relationship counseling if it becomes clear that interpersonal issues are precluding the intimacy necessary to drive the woman's cycle. Some of the more common psychologic factors precluding arousal can be addressed in the obstetrician–gynecologist's office; these factors include the avoidance of nonsexual distractions, insufficient privacy, sexual self-monitoring rather than focusing on enjoyment, and the woman's focusing on the partner's pleasure simultaneously with her own instead of "taking turns."

Any biologic factors limiting the effectiveness of stimulation should be addressed. They include depression; medications (including antidepressants); hyperprolactinemia (usually, irregular or absent menstrual cycle); fatigue from a sleep disorder, shift work, or disturbed nights; or decreased androgen activity. There is no pharmacologic treatment for hypoactive desire, but a few clinical trials are studying medications with action on different serotonin, dopamine, and melanocortin receptors.

Female Sexual Arousal Disorders

It is important to evaluate the following components of sexual arousal:

- Mental sexual arousal
  - —from reading, viewing, or hearing erotica
  - —from stimulating the partner
  - —from receiving sexual stimulation to nongenital and genital areas
  - —from deliberate sexual fantasy or recall of sexual memories
- Direct awareness of genital congestion, such as lubrication, tingling, and throbbing in response to such stimuli (more common in younger women)
- Indirect evidence of genital congestion: does direct massaging of vulval structures with her fingers, her partner's fingers, her partner's body, oral stimulation, a dildo, or penile vulval contact cause progressively intense sexual sensations?
- Cognitive and affective evaluation
  - —What are her thoughts? (Is she distracted, feeling sexually substandard, or worried that the outcome would be negative? Is she aware that the situation can expose her to sexually transmitted diseases or undesired pregnancy or, on the contrary, will confirm her infertility? Is she feeling that she is being used or that her feelings and desires are not being considered?)

—What are her emotions? (Is there sadness, embarrassment, guilt, awkwardness, or displeasure [eg, from the giving of stimulation to the partner]? Is she attracted to the partner?)

Any factors impairing subjective arousal, including fatigue, depression, medication (eg, selective serotonin reuptake inhibitors), loss of ovarian androgen after oophorectomy or chemotherapy, or loss of adrenal and ovarian androgen from pituitary or hypothalamic disease, should be addressed. The loss of estrogen (especially in the vagina) and vaginitis also should be considered. Therapy also should address a lack of required sexual stimuli and context, along with psychologic factors impairing subjective arousal.

There is no pharmacologic treatment for lack of subjective sexual arousal per se. However, when decreased androgen activity is suspected, investigational androgen therapy may be considered (see "Androgen Therapy for Hormonal Factors").

When lack of genital congestion, loss of pleasure from genital stimulation, loss of lubrication, experience of dryness, and discomfort with intercourse are associated with a lack of estrogen, local estrogen is recommended. When loss of genital congestion or loss of pleasure from direct stimulation is caused by autonomic nerve damage as a result of radical hysterectomy, multiple sclerosis (17), or diabetes mellitus (18), the off-label use of phosphodiesterase inhibitors can be considered if there are no contraindications, such as concomitant use of nitrates, symptomatic hypotension, or cardiac failure with hypovolemic states.

Female Orgasmic Disorder

The unsatisfactory components of the sexual experience should be documented in detail:

- Is the orgasm absent, delayed, or reduced in intensity?
- Does the patient really have an arousal disorder? If so, an evaluation should be performed as described for that disorder.
- Does the patient fear letting go of control? If so, is this fear logical (what is the degree of trust and safety)? What does the patient fear may happen?

Simultaneous increase in the number and intensity of stimuli (mental imagery and fantasy and visual, tactile, auditory, and written stimuli) may be helpful. Stimulation with vibrators is useful for women with and without nerve damage. Deep-seated issues involving control and trust may require psychologic intervention.

Dyspareunia

It is important to ask whether vaginal entry (ie, with a finger, penis, speculum, or tampon) is possible at all.

Women are hesitant to admit that intercourse has never occurred. The physician should establish whether the woman experiences sexual arousal when the attempted intercourse begins and progresses. Also, the physician should identify exactly when the woman experiences pain:

- With very partial entry of the penile head
- With attempted full entry of the penile head
- With penile movement
- With deep thrusting
- With the man's ejaculation
- With the patient's subsequent urination
- For hours or minutes after intercourse attempts

The assessment of dyspareunia involves a very careful introital, vaginal, and pelvic physical examination (19).

The goals of therapy include addressing biologic and psychosexual issues involved in the etiology and maintenance of the pain. Also, psychosexual issues resulting from repeatedly painful outcomes should be addressed.

To manage chronic dyspareunia, the following actions are recommended:

- Tell the patient to omit intercourse from the sexual experience to break the cycle of pain.
- Address the concomitant lack of desire and arousal.
- Manage specific pathologies; eg, deficient posterior fourchette or endometriosis.
- Refer the patient for pelvic physiotherapy or teach "reverse Kegel" exercises in conjunction with the woman's use of a series of conical vaginal inserts to address pelvic muscle hypertonicity.
- Prescribe topical estrogen for vulvar vaginal atrophy.
- For provoked vestibulodynia and dysesthetic vulvodynia, administer low-dose tricyclic antidepressants or antiseizure drugs, beginning at a low dose with a slow increase of dose to avoid side effects.
- For provoked vestibulodynia, administer 2% sodium cromoglycate; it is clinically superior to hydrocortisone, and stronger steroids carry a risk of a rebound effect. The medication must be placed exactly on the sites of allodynia, preferably with a syringe without a needle and under direct vision using a mirror. This therapy is investigational, as is the use of quercetin, a flavonoid. Both therapies inhibit the release of proinflammatory substances, including histamine and tryptase, from mast cells, which typically are present in biopsies of women with vestibulodynia. Nightly application of 5% lidocaine to the vestibule may be effective. When there is a history of recurrent candidiasis, administer fluconazole, 50 mg weekly, for 3–6 months.

- Manage fungal, trichomonal, or bacterial vaginitis as appropriate.
- Consider techniques to alter the mind's reaction to pain and stress, such as mindfulness or hypnosis (20).

Vaginismus

When screening for vaginismus, a number of issues should be clarified before determining a therapy:

- How does the patient feel about vaginal entry of the partner's or her own finger, a tampon, a physician's finger, or a speculum?
- If fear is present, can the patient describe exactly what she fears?
- Has there been any previously attempted internal examination? If so, it should be discussed.
- Does the woman have symptoms suggesting that the muscle tightening is secondary to other pathologic conditions, typically provoked vestibulodynia? Symptoms might include the following:

  —Vulval burning with partner ejaculation

  —Dysuria after attempts at vaginal entry

  —Vulval discomfort for minutes or hours after an intercourse attempt

  —Variable vulvodynia unrelated to intercourse attempts

Finally, it should be established whether the woman is experiencing symptoms atypical of vaginismus, such as lack of fear, lack of awareness of tensing the rest of the body, or marked diligence in trying to insert a finger or tampon despite difficulties with intercourse. (One would then suspect factors other than reflexive muscle tightening, eg, anatomic entities, erectile dysfunction of the partner, or lack of sexual skills or information.)

Typically, physical examination of a patient with vaginismus has been impossible because of reflexive muscle tightening. The recommended steps follow.

INITIAL VISIT

- Strongly suggest to the woman that she and her partner omit any attempts at vaginal entry, even with a finger, during their sexual experiences. Encourage the couple to resume or continue sexual experiences that are pleasurable and that do not carry the fear of a possible attempted entry.
- Explain that a future partial examination will involve inspection only.
- Encourage homework like the following before the next visit:

  —For a few minutes daily, the woman lies on the couch or bed or in the tub and touches as close to the introitus as possible.

  —Gentle spreading of the labia with her fingers is added.

  —Imagery is added; the woman imagines that she can allow the physician to inspect the vulva as she opens the labia.

SECOND VISIT

- Perform a simple inspection of the genitalia with the woman sitting up, using a mirror and in control. She spreads the labia.
- Homework continues with more touching of the introitus, encouraging entry past the hymen with her finger. Encourage her to "push down" or "bear down" as she inserts her finger to open the introitus.

THIRD VISIT

- Follow the steps for the second visit, as well as encourage the woman to put her or the examiner's (gloved) finger through the introitus as she bears down. Then encourage her to tighten and relax her muscles around the finger.
- Perform a simple digital examination only at this stage.
- Prescribe for the woman a series of vaginal inserts, preferably conical. She may need assistance with the first one in the office to achieve the correct angle of insertion and to receive guidance to bear down as she gently places the insert. At home, she uses the inserts daily by leaving them in place for 10–15 minutes while her mind is distracted, eg, while reading a book.

FOURTH VISIT

- Help the woman move from total control of vaginal entry to sharing the control with her partner. Encourage both partners to gently place the insert in her vagina and to try this maneuver on some occasions when they are being sexually active with nonpenetrative sex; they should briefly place the insert together under the conditions of physiological arousal. The insert then can be removed as the couple continues their nonpenetrative lovemaking.
- Advise the couple that when they are ready to attempt intercourse (after they have used the larger inserts), the first occasion should be with the woman holding her partner's penis "like an insert" and inserting it into her vagina (with both her hands around the base of his penis).

Androgen Therapy for Hormonal Factors

Five randomized controlled trials have shown benefit when transdermal testosterone, 300 micrograms per day (but not 150 micrograms per day or 450 micrograms per day) is administered to postmenopausal women with low sexual desire. Four trials involved women with bilateral oophorectomy. Recruited women were experiencing one to three "sexually satisfying events" per month. Using the pooled data, women receiving testosterone reported 1.9 more sexually satisfying events per month than they had at baseline, compared with 0.9 more among those receiving placebo (21). In most, but not all, studies, scores from a validated questionnaire showed a more significant increase in sexual desire and response and a decrease in distress in women using a testosterone patch than in women receiving a placebo. No trials have recruited women who report no sexually satisfying events per month but remain sexually active for reasons of affection and partner need. Such women find that despite their willingness to become aroused, neither their minds nor their bodies are responsive to formerly effective sexual stimuli.

The application of testosterone cream to the vulva has not been studied in randomized controlled trials. Dehydroepiandrosterone treatment for women has been the subject of a few small trials. One study of 24 women with primary and secondary adrenal insufficiency reported benefit, but five further trials were not confirmatory.

Data on the long-term safety of androgen supplementation are minimal. Uncertainty remains regarding the relationship between increased testosterone levels and cardiovascular risk (22), as well as the risk of breast cancer (23).

Replacing testosterone without estrogen is nonphysiologic; the safety of systemic estrogen therapy beyond 3–4 years is in question. Testosterone given premenopausally could result in masculinization of a female fetus, vulnerability to polycystic ovary syndrome in female offspring, menstrual irregularity, and insulin resistance.

No formulations of testosterone have been approved for use by women in the United States, and no long-term safety data are available. Although methyltestosterone is prescribed off label for sexual benefits, scientific evidence of benefit is seen only with doses that reduce high-density lipoprotein cholesterol. Liver toxicity has been reported with higher dosages in men. Dehydroepiandrosterone, considered a food additive, is not regulated for purity. Testosterone is available in a form that has been compounded for delivery in a transdermal cream, as a sublingual lozenge, and for oral administration, but these formulations are not approved by the U.S. Food and Drug Administration.

More scientific research is needed to understand fully the indications, benefits, and risks of androgen therapy. However, despite the guidelines from the Endocrine Society (24), some physicians well experienced in managing postmenopausal sexual dysfunction advocate a therapeutic trial under some circumstances. Other diagnoses that frequently affect sexual response should be excluded first. The most common are depression; psychodynamic factors that reduce arousability and desire,

either within the woman herself or between the two partners; and contextual factors that suggest that her low desire and arousal are adaptations rather than a disorder.

Testosterone therapy is not indicated when symptoms are limited to minimal or absent innate, spontaneous sexual wanting. An ability to feel some desire and a wish to continue a sexual experience once it has begun (ie, experiencing sexual desire after and with arousal) appears to be normal for many women (21, 25). Thus, investigational testosterone therapy should be considered only when sexual manifestations can be related to the following:

- Reduced arousal to nonphysical erotic stimuli
- Reduced arousal to nongenital physical stimuli
- Reduced arousal to genital stimuli given in an appropriate erotic or intimate context
- Absent or markedly reduced orgasms from the patient and her partner

Androgen activity may be augmented with the following methods:

- One of the following changes in hormone administration can be made to decrease SHBG, increase luteinizing hormone, or increase corticotropin, all of which can lead to increased androgen activity:
  - —Switch from oral to transdermal estrogen after menopause
  - —Discontinue use of hormonal contraceptives
  - —Discontinue systemic oral estrogen hormone therapy and use vaginal estrogen, if needed
  - —Avoid the use of systemic corticosteroids
- Physicians experienced in managing postmenopausal sexual dysfunction consider the investigational (unapproved) use of compounded testosterone administered as a cream, gel, sublingual lozenge, or oral capsule, along with continued systemic estrogen therapy. The optimal dosage of these forms of testosterone is not known, but the dosage should not be supraphysiologic. Patients should be counseled that safety data are limited (26).
- If methyltestosterone combined with estrogen is determined to be the best choice for a patient, advise the patient that high-density lipoprotein cholesterol levels should be monitored at least annually.

References

1. Nusbaum MR, Gamble G, Skinner B, Heiman J. The high prevalence of sexual concerns among women seeking routine gynecological care. J Fam Pract 2000;49:229–32.

2. Nappi RE, Verde JB, Polatti F, Genazzani AR, Zara C. Self-reported sexual symptoms in women attending menopause clinics. Gynecol Obstet Invest 2002;53:181–7.

3. Basson R. Female sexual response: the role of drugs in the management of sexual dysfunction [published erratum appears in Obstet Gynecol 2001;98:522]. Obstet Gynecol 2001;98:350–3.

4. Meston CM, Buss DM. Why humans have sex. Arch Sex Behav 2007;36:477–507.

5. Kukkonen TM, Binik YM, Amsel R, Carrier S. Thermography as a physiological measure of sexual arousal in both men and women. J Sex Med 2007;4:93–105.

6. Chivers ML, Bailey JM. A sex difference in features that elicit genital response. Biol Psychol 2005;70:115–20.

7. van Lunsen RH, Laan E. Genital vascular responsiveness and sexual feelings in midlife women: psychophysiologic, brain, and genital imaging studies. Menopause 2004;11:741–8.

8. Dennerstein L, Lehert P, Burger H, Dudley E. Factors affecting sexual functioning of women in the mid-life years. Climacteric 1999;2:254–62.

9. Avis NE, Stellato R, Crawford S, Johannes C, Longcope C. Is there an association between menopause status and sexual functioning? Menopause 2000;7:297–309.

10. Fogle RH, Stanczyk FZ, Zhang X, Paulson RJ. Ovarian androgen production in postmenopausal women. J Clin Endocrinol Metab 2007;92:3040–3.

11. Labrie F, Belanger A, Belanger P, Berube R, Martel C, Cusan L, et al. Androgen glucuronides, instead of testosterone, as the new markers of androgenic activity in women. J Steroid Biochem Mol Biol 2006;99:182–8.

12. Teplin V, Vittinghoff E, Lin F, Learman LA, Richter HE, Kuppermann M. Oophorectomy in premenopausal women: health-related quality of life and sexual functioning. Obstet Gynecol 2007;109:347–54.

13. Aziz A, Brannstrom M, Bergquist C, Silfverstolpe G. Perimenopausal androgen decline after oophorectomy does not influence sexuality or psychological well-being. Fertil Steril 2005;83:1021–8.

14. Farquhar CM, Harvey SA, Yu Y, Sadler L, Stewart AW. A prospective study of 3 years of outcomes after hysterectomy with and without oophorectomy. Am J Obstet Gynecol 2006;194:711–7.

15. Davis SR, Davison SL, Donath S, Bell RJ. Circulating androgen levels and self-reported sexual function in women. JAMA 2005;294:91–6.

16. Santoro N, Torrens J, Crawford S, Allsworth JE, Finkelstein JS, Gold EB, et al. Correlates of circulating androgens in mid-life women: the study of women's health across the nation. J Clin Endocrinol Metab 2005;90:4836–45.

17. Dasgupta R, Wiseman OJ, Kanabar G, Fowler CJ, Mikol DD. Efficacy of sildenafil in the treatment of female sexual dysfunction due to multiple sclerosis. J Urol 2004;171:1189–93; discussion 1193.

18. Caruso S, Rugolo S, Agnello C, Intelisano G, Di Mari L, Cianci A. Sildenafil improves sexual functioning in premenopausal women with type 1 diabetes who are affected by sexual arousal disorder: a double-blind, crossover, placebo-controlled pilot study. Fertil Steril 2006;85:1496–501.

19. Basson R, Schultz WW. Sexual sequelae of general medical disorders. Lancet 2007;369:409–24.

20. Pukall C, Kandyba K, Amsel R, Khalife S, Binik Y. Effectiveness of hypnosis for the treatment of vulvar vestibulitis syndrome: a preliminary investigation. J Sex Med 2007;4:417–25.

21. Basson R. Clinical practice. Sexual desire and arousal disorders in women. N Engl J Med 2006;354:1497–506.

22. Wild RA. Endogenous androgens and cardiovascular risk [editorial]. Menopause 2007;14:609–10.

23. Key T, Appleby P, Barnes I, Reeves G. Endogenous sex hormones and breast cancer in postmenopausal women: reanalysis of nine prospective studies. Endogenous Hormones and Breast Cancer Collaborative Group. J Natl Cancer Inst 2002;94:606–16.

24. Wierman ME, Basson R, Davis SR, Khosla S, Miller KK, Rosner W, et al. Androgen therapy in women: an Endocrine Society Clinical Practice guideline. J Clin Endocrinol Metab 2006;91:3697–710.

25. Cain VS, Johannes CB, Avis NE, Mohr B, Schocken M, Skurnick J, et al. Sexual functioning and practices in a multi-ethnic study of midlife women: baseline results from SWAN. J Sex Res 2003;40:266–76.

26. Braunstein GD. Safety of testosterone treatment in postmenopausal women. Fertil Steril 2007;88:1–17.

Abuse and Violence Against Women

Harise Stein and Paul D. Blumenthal

Psychologic, physical, and sexual abuse, occurring as isolated events or repeatedly within relationships, may have appreciable and lifelong effects on the health and well-being of women. With a lifetime prevalence of 23–60% for abuse, more women experience abuse and violence than they do breast cancer, diabetes mellitus, or hypertension (1, 2). Abuse is found in every socioeconomic and demographic group.

Physicians are in a unique position to provide women with perhaps their only opportunity for safe, private disclosure of abuse. This responsibility is reinforced by guidelines of the American College of Obstetricians and Gynecologists and state and federal regulations.

Abuse and Violence Across the Life Cycle

Childhood

Child abuse can include neglect and emotional, physical, and sexual harm. It is believed that 12–25% of female children are sexually abused, usually by a family member (3, 4). In 2005 there were more than 3.5 million reports of child abuse in the United States, and 1,460 children—four per day—died of abuse or neglect (5). Recognizing the extent of this problem, in 2005 the American Board of Pediatrics created a new board-certifiable pediatric subspecialty in child abuse.

In addition to being abused directly, children can be harmed during accidental involvement in parental altercations, while trying to protect a parent from violence, through neglect from abused mothers who are depressed or withdrawn, or simply by observing violence in the home. Children in abusive homes may develop psychologic, cognitive, behavioral, and social problems. Possible indicators of abuse include poor school performance, aggression, regression, sleep disturbances, and physical symptoms, such as headache and stomachache.

Resources

Abuse and Violence Against Women

Family Violence Prevention Fund
http://www.endabuse.org

National Coalition Against Domestic Violence
http://www.ncadv.org

National Center for Posttraumatic Stress Disorder
http://www.ncptsd.va.gov

Abuse at an early age also can cause measurable physiological changes in brain function and structure, especially in the prefrontal cortex, limbic areas, and hypothalamic–pituitary–adrenal axis. These regions of the brain are involved with emotion, pain control, memory, and learning. Decreased myelination and connectivity of neurons can predispose these children to health challenges during childhood and adulthood; the challenges include decreased cognitive performance, anxiety, depression, and substance abuse (6).

A large, long-term, prospective Kaiser study (the Adverse Childhood Experiences Study) is examining the effects of adverse childhood experiences, such as emotional, physical, and sexual abuse; neglect; and abuse of the child's mother. Results have shown a strong direct correlation between the number of adverse childhood experiences and several adult medical conditions, including depression, smoking, alcoholism, chronic obstructive pulmonary disease, ischemic heart disease, liver disease, obesity, and cancer (7).

It is important to note that girls who see or experience abuse may have difficulties trusting others that can extend to health care providers. They also may perceive that women are not valued and that abuse is a normal interpersonal interaction. They may accept or tolerate violence in later adult relationships or become violent themselves.

Adolescence

Young women face the highest rates of partner abuse and rape. They may have to contend with in-person and online sexual harassment by school peers, date or acquaintance rape that may be facilitated by surreptitiously administered drugs, and Internet predators. Teenagers who are in abusive relationships are more likely to get pregnant, contract sexually transmitted diseases (STDs), become depressed or suicidal, cut or harm themselves, have an exacerbation of eating disorders, use alcohol or other addictive substances, and drop out of school. Up to 25% of pregnant teenagers are in abusive relationships, a much higher rate than adults. Among 15- to 24-year-olds, homicide, usually by a partner, is the second leading cause of nonaccidental death for young white women and is the leading cause of nonaccidental death for young African-American women (2).

Adulthood

DOMESTIC VIOLENCE OR INTIMATE PARTNER VIOLENCE

Domestic violence refers to violence perpetrated in the context of a family or an intimate relationship. Family members may include parents, siblings, and other blood relatives, as well as legal relatives, such as stepparents, in-laws, and guardians. Violence that occurs between current or former partners is referred to as intimate partner violence. This term also applies to male abuse by female partners and to violence between partners in lesbian, gay, bisexual, and transgendered relationships. Domestic violence or *intimate partner violence* affects at least one woman in four during her lifetime (2).

Domestic violence is a leading cause of nonfatal injury in women and of emergency department visits. In addition, women who have been in abusive relationships show increased health care use for at least 5 years after their abuse ends (8).

Abuse is defined as a pattern of coercive behaviors, assaultive behaviors, or both used to gain power and control in a relationship. This pattern often begins with psychologic abuse and then can progress to include physical, sexual, and economic harm. Attacks are calculated, repetitive, and unpredictable; can be progressively more frequent and severe over time; and occur in a cyclic pattern. Economic abuse can include sabotaging a woman's educational or professional goals to limit her independent earning power.

Abusers also sabotage medical care (9). To ensure that the patient will cancel or not show up for her appointment, they may interfere with physician office communication; hide car keys, wallets, and insurance information; and use physical assault to cause obvious bruising. When evaluating whether to discharge a patient from a practice for multiple no-shows, the physician should consider why she may have missed her appointments.

Sexual abuse is common in abusive relationships. In addition to causing trauma, many abusers refuse to practice safe sex and sabotage birth control methods, leading to unwanted pregnancies and STDs (2).

RAPE

In the United States, at least one in six women has been raped in her lifetime. Many of these rapes are not reported (4). Rape may occur outside an intimate relationship, in an attack by a stranger or as a "date rape," in which some consensual sexual foreplay may have occurred but coitus was forced. Women who have experienced rape have high rates of depression and posttraumatic stress disorder (PTSD), which can affect their gynecologic care. Posttraumatic stress disorder flashbacks can be triggered by vaginal ultrasonography, office procedures, mammography, surgery, and obstetric delivery. See Box 31 for information on the management of patients with signs of possible abuse and PTSD.

Stalking is a series of malicious behaviors intended to instill fear of harm. It has been reported in 1 in 12 women throughout her lifetime, as well as in up to 40% of college students. Stalking has been characterized as "psychologic rape," and its victims have high rates of anxiety disorders, depression, PTSD, sleep disorders,

---

Box 31

Possible Signs of Abuse or Posttraumatic Stress Disorder During Pelvic Examinations or Procedures and How to Reassure the Patient

Signs
- High anxiety
- Reluctancy to get undressed
- Avoidance of eye contact
- Tearfulness
- Tight grip on the sides of the examination table
- Keeping legs together
- Withdrawal to touch
- Increased pelvic floor muscle tension
- Exaggerated startle response
- Staring or "spacing out"

Management
- Sit so you are at same height or lower than patient
- Ask if there is anything you can do to make examination easier for her
- Explain what you are going to do beforehand
- Show and explain equipment you are going to use
- Ask permission to touch
- Frequently ask how the patient is doing
- If the patient becomes very anxious:
  - tell her she is safe
  - reorient her to time and place
  - remind her of importance of examination
  - give her control to stop the examination when she wants
  - arrange comfort measures (warm blanket or cool cloth)

---

and suicidal tendencies. The most dangerous time for a woman is when she is leaving a relationship, because most homicides related to intimate partner violence are committed by a stalking former partner (10).

Older Age

The most frequent type of elder abuse is neglect, particularly self-neglect, but elder abuse also can include physical, sexual, and economic harm. Is it estimated that 2–10% of elders are abused (11). Neglect and abuse can be found in a home environment that includes family members and caregivers or in an institutional setting, such as a nursing home. Older women may present with physical manifestations of neglect, such as dehydration, malnutrition, contractures, and bedsores. Other signs may include poor hygiene, damage to glasses (from assault), evidence of underdosing or overdosing of medication (as a means of control), and social withdrawal.

Older women often fail to disclose their abusive situation for a variety of reasons, including having been threatened by their caregiver with the withholding of needed medication, especially pain medication, or of being sent to a nursing home; fear of losing their independence; shame at the way their adult children have treated them; and difficulty to disclose sexual abuse. Abuse may be particularly difficult to evaluate in elders with cognitive or communication impairment.

Special Groups

Pregnant Women

In some cases, physical abuse actually starts during pregnancy, when abusive partners resent the shift of focus away from themselves. Because abusive relationships occur in at least 4–8% of pregnancies, this problem is more common than many medical conditions that receive routine screening. Effects of abuse on pregnancy are considerable; they include maternal homicide, usually by a partner, which is the leading cause of nonaccidental death during pregnancy (Box 32) (2, 12).

Box 32

Possible Effects of Abuse on Pregnancy

Woman

- Delayed, sporadic, or no prenatal care
- Poor compliance with health instructions
- Poor weight gain
- Eating disorders
- Anemia
- Urinary tract infections and pyelonephritis
- High blood pressure
- Smoking and alcohol or substance abuse
- Sexually transmitted diseases and human immunodeficiency virus (HIV)
- Depression and posttraumatic stress disorder
- Death by homicide

Fetus or Newborn

- Miscarriage
- Direct fetal injury
- Bleeding and abruption
- Premature labor
- Premature rupture of membranes
- Low birth weight
- Hypoxia
- Uterine rupture
- Perinatal death
- Decreased maternal bonding
- Decreased likelihood to be breast-fed

Of women who are physically abused during pregnancy, 25–50% are kicked or punched in the abdomen (2). Blows to the abdomen may not leave immediately obvious marks on the skin. Thus, because most women are too ashamed or afraid to report abuse, life-threatening injuries, such as concealed abruption or ruptured spleen, may go undiagnosed by medical personnel. When abuse is known or suspected, careful inspection of the placenta after delivery may reveal signs of old or new abruption. Verification of placental trauma in pathology reports can aid patients in assault or custody disputes.

Abused women also may experience postpartum depression, leading to decreased bonding with their child. They may be less likely to breast-feed, because it upsets their partner or because of a personal aversion due to past sexual abuse (13).

Lesbians and Bisexual and Transgendered Women

Partner abuse in lesbians and bisexual and transgendered women occurs at the same or higher rates as in heterosexual couples and with the same dynamics. However, this group of women may face additional partner manipulation in the form of the threat of "outing" and stigmatization from health care and advocacy personnel (14).

Disadvantaged Women

Disadvantaged women, including some rural women, homeless women, and women in minority groups, such as African-American and Native-American women, may be more vulnerable to abuse because of economic, educational, and social factors. Lifetime estimates of domestic violence among Native-American women are as high as 60–90%. Because of previous experiences with racism, women in minority groups may be less likely to seek help from health care workers or law enforcement personnel (2).

Immigrants

Cultural differences may cause challenges for the physician, as well as for newly arrived and first-generation patients. For example, some immigrants may come from a patriarchal background in which wife beating, female circumcision, or female genital mutilation are considered normal. Additional barriers for immigrants include language difficulties, lack of legal documentation, and a lack of awareness of legal rights and available community resources. In addition, immigrants may have experienced torture, sex trafficking, or rape as an instrument of war and, thus, may require especially sensitive medical and gynecologic care.

Dependent or Disabled Women

Dependent adults may be unable to comprehend abuse or may be physically unable to protect themselves from it. They may be physically or economically dependent on their partner, family members, or caregivers, making it difficult to leave them. Because shelters are rarely able to take care of women with special needs, they may have few options to consider. The risk of violence from a partner may be 40% higher for disabled women than for other women, and sexual abuse, usually by a caregiver, is significantly higher for dependent women than for other women (2). Because the gynecologic needs of dependent adults often are underserved, consequences of abuse, such as STDs, may be overlooked. Cognitive and communication impairment also may complicate disclosure and abuse identification.

Chronically Ill Women

Women with chronic illnesses, particularly cancer, realistically may be unable to contemplate leaving their partners. Women in these circumstances may be more financially or emotionally vulnerable, especially in relation to medical insurance or the strain of treatment. Shelters are not equipped to accommodate women with medical problems. Abusers may continue or escalate the pattern of isolation from family and friends during critical periods of illness and undermine treatment and recovery. Isolated and dying elderly women may be neglected by family members, with financial abuse as a motivating factor (15).

Health Effects of Abuse

Psychologic Effects

Abuse, violence, and neglect can have profound psychologic consequences and are associated with high rates of anxiety, depression, and PTSD (16). Exacerbated eating disorders, emotional eating, and obesity also are significantly associated with a history of abuse (17).

Women have PTSD at twice the rate of men. Posttraumatic stress disorder can occur months or even years after a traumatic event and is cumulative with ongoing trauma. Women may not make the connection between their experience and their symptoms. Consequently, PTSD can lead to an extensive variety of sequelae, such as sleep disorders, cancellation of pelvic or other examinations because of flashback experiences, fear of dental examinations or operations, and use of smoking and alcohol or other substance abuse as a coping mechanism (18).

Physical Effects

A number of immediate and long-term gynecologic conditions can result from abuse. In addition to fertility control issues and genital infections, patients may experience ovulatory dysfunction and sexual health and sexuality problems (19). In addition, surgical wound healing is impaired in individuals who are anxious, depressed, or in difficult marital relationships (20).

In a drug trial for premenstrual dysphoric disorder, enrolled women reported a lifetime history of attempted sexual attack (95%) and completed sexual attack (81%). Of these women, 83% had never disclosed this information to a physician, and 65% had PTSD from the event (21). Abused women with premenstrual dysphoric disorder may have dysregulation of the autonomic nervous system and may respond differently to premenstrual syndrome medical treatment (22).

Clinical and laboratory studies have shown that depression, anxiety, and PTSD lower the pain threshold. In these cases, neurochemical changes in peripheral and central brain-processing areas cause patients to be more sensitive to pain. Although the relationship between abuse and chronic pelvic pain is recognized, other pain syndromes also can be affected, including headaches, which are commonly reported by abused patients (23). Secondary pain can result from increased muscle tension that may be caused by anticipatory anxiety about being hit.

A history of abuse in women has been correlated with a variety of bladder signs and symptoms, including frequency, incontinence, and interstitial cystitis. In one study that controlled for age and parity, the prevalence of incontinence was 72% in a support group for women with a history of childhood sexual abuse, compared with 22% in a group of women with no abuse ($P<.001$) (24).

Of the 10 factors in the Healthy People 2010 prevention agenda designed to focus on health promotion, seven can be linked strongly to abuse and violence against women. These factors include overweight and obesity, tobacco use, substance abuse, responsible sexual behavior, mental health, injury and violence, and access to health care.

Responsibilities of the Physician

Screening

The American College of Obstetricians and Gynecologists recommends abuse screening of new patients and of existing patients at annual, family planning, or preconception visits, as well as at prenatal visits (once each trimester) and the postpartum visit. It is advisable also to screen during certain clinical situations, such as unplanned pregnancy and a new STD diagnosis. A range of screening strategies is available, including indirect and direct oral questions and written screening instruments. It is imperative that screening take place in privacy and that nonfamily interpreters be used. Studies show that women are supportive of abuse screening (2).

In selecting a screening method, the two most important criteria are 1) whether the method is efficient for the office (so it will be performed regularly) and 2) whether the physician feels comfortable asking those specific questions so that the patient will feel comfortable responding. Screening questions need to be presented as "routine" so that the patient does not feel singled out. Avoid questions with the words *victim*, *abused*, or *battered*, which are stigmatizing. Because it may take years for a patient to trust her physician enough to disclose abuse, screening at least annually should be ongoing. Box 33 lists a few sample screening options. The Centers for Disease Control and Prevention maintains a compendium of intimate-partner violence assessment tools (25).

Equally or even more important than asking about abuse is how a health care practitioner responds to an affirmative answer. It is crucial that the response be supportive and nonjudgmental (Box 34). A single positive communication with a health care provider about this subject makes it 3.9 times more likely that the patient will accept an intervention and 2.6 times more likely that she will leave the relationship (26). Asking "Why don't you just leave?" is perceived very negatively by abused women, who are ashamed, frightened, and often struggling with overwhelming obstacles to leaving. These obstacles may include cultural, religious, financial, and immigration issues, as well as traumatizing threats toward the woman and her children.

A negative answer presents an educational opportunity. The practitioner should respond, "I just want you to know that if something like this ever does come up, this is a safe place to talk about it and get help." This sows the seed for future trust and potential disclosure. However, patient disclosure may not necessarily be the only goal; the patient may begin to feel empowered and contemplate change solely in response to physician concern in asking about this topic. In addition, a physician who routinely educates teenagers about healthy relationships can have an effect early on in a woman's life.

Efficiency

One barrier to obstetric–gynecologic screening for abuse is concern about the time required. Physicians who realize that it is not their job to "fix" the patient's life and who manage abuse as they would any other medical problem—take a history, be supportive, and refer—can handle screening for abuse in a compassionate, but efficient, manner. Physicians have access to extensive local and national support.

In the average obstetrician–gynecologist's office setting, most patients will take less than 10 seconds to screen. Usually, visits are not designated screening visits (but the physician is alert to signs), the nonabused patients answer "no" to screening, and most abused patients also answer "no" to screening.

By setting up their offices with patient materials, resources, links to ancillary support, and staff training, physicians can ensure that even an affirmative response

---

Box 33

Sample Screening Questions

Asking Indirectly

- How are things going at home?
- What is your relationship like with your partner (caregiver)?

Asking Directly

- I don't know if this is a problem for you, but because so many patients I see are dealing with abusive relationships I've started asking about it routinely. Does a partner or anyone at home, hurt, hit, or threaten you?

Options for Older Patients or Dependent Adults

- Does anyone make you sign papers you don't understand?
- Are you afraid of anyone at home?
- Does anyone touch you without your consent?
- Does anyone fail to take care of you when you need help?

If an Injury is Present

- Sometimes when I see an injury like this, it is because someone else caused it. Did someone do this to you?

Written Screen WAST-Short (Validated)*

1. In general, how would you describe your relationship?
   __ A lot of tension? __ Some tension?
   __ No tension?
2. Do you and your partner work out arguments with
   __ great difficulty? __ with some difficulty?
   __ with no difficulty?

*Data from Chen PH, Rovi S, Washington J, Jacobs A, Vega M, Pan KY, et al. Randomized comparison of 3 methods to screen for domestic violence in family practice. Ann Fam Med 2007;5:430–5.

Box 34

Responding to an Affirmative Answer

- I believe you.
- It took courage for you to tell me.
- This is not your fault.
- No one deserves to be treated this way.
- I'm sorry you have been hurt.
- It's against the law.
- Help is available to you.

can be smoothly incorporated into the office flow. A sign at the front desk stating that office policy is to initially room patients alone can help create a private time to talk to the patient or administer a written screen. When injuries are present, if there are legal reporting requirements, or if the practitioner desires to spend extra time, compensation is available through appropriate coding.

Assessment

Clues about an abusive relationship can be found not only by asking questions but also by assessing the patient's overall situation by observation (Box 35). What is the patient's partner or caregiver like? How do they interact? Does the partner or caregiver refuse to leave the patient's side, or does that person answer questions for her? Does the patient seem afraid? In these situations, physicians and staff members can arrange strategies to divide the pair and talk to the patient privately; eg, they might ask the patient for a urine sample or ask the partner or caregiver to clarify an insurance issue at the desk.

Are there any physical findings on the skin that suggest abuse? Soft tissue injuries of the head and neck and defensive injuries on the forearms are the most common injuries (27). Bruises—especially in various stages of healing or in a pattern (eg, in the shape of the loop of a cord)—are the most common type of reported injury. Burn injuries from cigarettes, hot objects, caustic substances, or immersion are more common in children and elders, as are signs of restraints on wrists, ankles, axilla, or corners of the mouth.

Practitioners should know how to handle the disclosure or suspicion of sexual assault in their localities.

Box 35

Red Flags of Past or Present Abuse

- "Nothing works"
- Very complicated or illogical clinical picture
- Symptoms out of proportion to findings
- Chronic pain syndromes
- Multiple visits with vague complaints
- High use of care of multiple specialties
- Depression
- Eating disorders or obesity
- Substance abuse
- Multiple no show or cancelled visits
- Multiple emergency room visits for "accidents"
- Delay in seeking care for an injury
- Injuries that do not fit history or history that keeps changing

---

Many states have a county system of forensic nurses in teams who are responsible for rape examinations. If the assault is recent, even a cursory speculum examination can negate subsequent evidence collection. Women who have been sexually assaulted need evaluation and prophylaxis for pregnancy and STDs, including human immunodeficiency virus (HIV) infection, as well as psychological counseling and follow-up.

Strangulation injuries often are overlooked. Of women who have restraining orders on their partners or who are in shelters, 50–65% have been strangled to unconsciousness at least once; the rate for abused women at home is unknown. It takes only 10 seconds of applied external pressure to the neck to cause unconsciousness and only minutes to cause death. Any woman with other abuse-related injuries should be asked specifically about strangulation, because 50% of the time there are no immediately visible signs on the neck. In extreme cases, a woman may have a stroke or increased laryngeal swelling over the following 24 hours, and die of asphyxiation (28, 29).

Referring

Once a patient is identified as being in an abusive situation, she needs appropriate counseling in addition to medical support. This counseling may be accomplished through immediate referral to a social worker or psychologist or by arranging for the patient to talk to a local shelter hotline from the physician's office. Many community women's shelters provide not only safe housing but also group, individual, child, financial, and legal counseling. Health care practitioners who choose to counsel the patient themselves need to keep in mind the stages-of-change model; unless the situation is urgent, these practitioners should tailor their questions and comments to the patient's level of awareness and motivation—precontemplation, contemplation, preparation, action, and maintenance (2).

Reporting and Documentation

Legally mandated reporting requirements for the various forms of abuse and neglect vary from state to state. Practitioners should know the requirements for their states, know how local law enforcement will respond to a report, and keep reporting forms and phone numbers readily available (see Resources).

Thorough and legible documentation can aid patients in legal and custody disputes. A body map is more effective and efficient for detailing injuries than a written description, and a picture is very effective as evidence (Box 36).

A patient may need to be assured that her disclosure will not be discussed with her partner or caregiver. However, it will help maintain trust to let a patient know up front the legal limits of confidentiality, such as

---

Box 36

Documentation of Abuse

Detailed documentation of abuse and violence is crucial in establishing forensic evidence and can significantly enhance a woman's right to initiate criminal and civil prosecution and to protection. The following minimal key elements should be included:

- Duration, frequency, and severity of abuse in patient's own words
- Physical findings, documented by a body map or photograph
- Safety assessment
- Written and printed patient education materials given to the patient
- Referrals made
- Any required reporting forms or contacts
- Provisions for follow-up

---

mandated reporting requirements. Practitioners need to consider the pros and cons of listing abuse as a diagnosis for billing purposes.

Patient Safety

Abused patients need a safety assessment. These risks can be evaluated with a few brief questions by the physician or someone appropriately trained. In addition, because most women underestimate their level of danger, providing information about danger risks is important. Office time can be saved with preprinted materials.

If the practitioner is in a state with mandated reporting and the patient's case is reported to the police, her abuser may be arrested immediately but be out on bail within 2 hours. This time is extremely dangerous for the patient, and she should be counseled about a safety plan by the physician, a trained staff member, a social worker, the police, or the local community hotline before she leaves the office or hospital. This counseling should include advice about getting a restraining order.

Staff Training and Patient Materials

Most patients do not disclose abuse-related issues even when asked. It is, therefore, important to provide informational materials. The information should be placed in locations, such as restrooms, where patients can read them privately, in a format that can be folded up and hidden. Make sure these materials are language and gender appropriate for the patient population. Office posters let the patient know the practitioner cares about this issue.

Office staff members who are trained to be aware of warning signs can alert the physician to potential abuse or neglect. Warning signs may include arguments in the waiting room, arm bruises detected when measuring blood pressure, frequent canceled appointments, lack of payment or follow-up by caregivers of elderly or dependent patients, or symptoms of confusion in an elderly patient who lives alone. Providing advanced training to a particular staff member can create a vital resource for abused patients, as well as time-saving assistance for the physician.

New Developments

Emphasis on Health Effects of Abuse in Adults and Children

Recent research has focused on the health effects of abuse beyond the stereotypical black eye and broken arm. A large Kaiser study found that one of the leading reasons a patient accepted an intervention was that a health care practitioner pointed out the effects on her health. By becoming aware of these health effects, practitioners can keep their patients informed and motivated to change. Another major motivator to change is realizing how an abusive situation affects children. Asking women how they think their children are being affected may help them decide to leave an abusive relationship (30).

National Teen Dating Abuse Helpline

In the spring of 2007, a 24-hour National Teen Dating Abuse Helpline was established, operating in all languages. The hotline provides message boards and live chat with trained counselors during the evening hours. Teenagers particularly appreciate being able to use the hotline to rehearse how to talk to their partners (see Box 37).

Box 37

National Hotlines

Domestic Violence
1-800-799-SAFE (7233)
[TTY 1-800-787-3224]
www.ndvh.org

Teen Dating Abuse
1-866-331-9474
[TTY 1-866-331-8453]
www.loveisrespect.org

Sexual Assault
1-800-656-HOPE (4673)
www.rainn.org

Stalking Resource Center
1-800-FYI-CALL (394-2255)
www.ncvc.org/src

Technology

THE CONS

Cell phones and e-mail have become methods of control, with abusive partners messaging or calling many times a day and demanding that a woman answer immediately or face the consequences that evening. In addition, there are hundreds of web sites and groups on the Internet where abusers can share information about tracking their partners' movements in real time by using hidden global positioning system units in women's cars, tapping telephone lines, using wireless video cameras for monitoring activities, turning cell phones into listening devices, using identity theft for harassment and stalking, and even using illegal spyware to record every keystroke a woman types on her computer at home or at work (31). Patients in abusive relationships are advised to use computers at a friend's house or at the library when dealing with sensitive subjects.

THE PROS

Technology has been helpful in abuse screening. Language-specific questions delivered by way of headphones or computer touch screens, some especially adapted for adults with disabilities, are under investigation. In an online safety assessment that is being developed, women can answer questions about the history of their relationships and receive a safety score with recommendations.

References

1. Pleis JR, Lethbridge-Cejku M. Summary health statistics for U.S. adults: National Health Interview Survey, 2006. Vital Health Stat 2007;(10):1–153. Available at: http://www.cdc.gov/nchs/data/series/sr_10/sr10_235.pdf. Retrieved November 12, 2008.

2. Gunter J. Intimate partner violence. Obstet Gynecol Clin North Am 2007;34:367–88, ix–x.

3. Kellogg N. The evaluation of sexual abuse in children. American Academy of Pediatrics Committee on Child Abuse and Neglect. Pediatrics 2005;116:506–12.

4. Tjaden P, Thoenes N. Extent, nature, and consequences of rape victimization: findings from the National Violence Against Women Survey. Washington, DC: National Institute of Justice; 2006. Available at: http://www.ncjrs.gov/pdffiles1/nij/210346.pdf. Retrieved November 12, 2008.

5. U.S. Department of Health and Human Services, Administration on Children, Youth and Families. Child maltreatment 2006. Washington, DC: U.S. Government Printing Office; 2008. Available at: http://www.acf.hhs.gov/programs/cb/pubs/cm06/cm06.pdf. Retrieved November 12, 2008.

6. Hagele DM. The impact of maltreatment on the developing child. N C Med J 2005;66:356–9.

7. Anda RF, Felitti VJ. Adverse childhood experiences (ACE) Study: bridging the gap between childhood trauma and negative consequences later in life. Atlanta (GA); San Diego (CA): Centers for Disease Control and Prevention; Health Presentations; Available at: http://www.acestudy.org. Retrieved November 12, 2008.

8. Rivara FP, Anderson ML, Fishman P, Bonomi AE, Reid RJ, Carrell D, et al. Healthcare utilization and costs for women with a history of intimate partner violence. Am J Prev Med 2007;32:89–96.

9. McCloskey LA, Williams CM, Lichter E, Gerber M, Ganz ML, Sege R. Abused women disclose partner interference with health care: an unrecognized form of battering. J Gen Intern Med 2007;22:1067–72.

10. Amar AF. College women's experience of stalking: mental health symptoms and changes in routines. Arch Psychiatr Nurs 2006;20:108–16.

11. National Center for Elder Abuse. Elder abuse: prevalence and incidence: fact sheet. Washington, DC: NCEA; 2005. Available at: http://www.ncea.aoa.gov/ncearoot/Main_Site/pdf/publication/FinalStatistics050331.pdf. Retrieved November 12, 2008.

12. Silverman JG, Decker MR, Reed E, Raj A. Intimate partner violence victimization prior to and during pregnancy among women residing in 26 U.S. states: associations with maternal and neonatal health. Am J Obstet Gynecol 2006; 195:140–8.

13. Klingelhafer SK. Sexual abuse and breastfeeding. J Hum Lact 2007;23:194–7.

14. Freedberg P. Health care barriers and same-sex intimate partner violence: a review of the literature. J Forensic Nurs 2006;2:15,24, 41.

15. Jayawardena KM, Liao S. Elder abuse at end of life. J Palliat Med 2006;9:127–36.

16. Falsetti SA. Screening and responding to family and intimate partner violence in the primary care setting. Prim Care 2007;34:641–57, viii.

17. Noll JG, Zeller MH, Trickett PK, Putnam FW. Obesity risk for female victims of childhood sexual abuse: a prospective study. Pediatrics 2007;120:e61–7.

18. Nakell L. Adult post-traumatic stress disorder: screening and treating in primary care. Prim Care 2007;34:593,610, vii.

19. Kalantaridou SN, Makrigiannakis A, Zoumakis E, Chrousos GP. Stress and the female reproductive system. J Reprod Immunol 2004;62:61–8.

20. Bosch JA, Engeland CG, Cacioppo JT, Marucha PT. Depressive symptoms predict mucosal wound healing. Psychosom Med 2007;69:597–605.

21. Golding JM, Taylor DL, Menard L, King MJ. Prevalence of sexual abuse history in a sample of women seeking treatment for premenstrual syndrome. J Psychosom Obstet Gynaecol 2000;21:69–80.

22. Girdler SS. PMDD spotlight: women with histories of abuse: a clinically meaningful subgroup? Medscape Ob/Gyn Womens Health 2007. Available at: http://www.medscape.com/viewarticle/565755. Retrieved November 12, 2008.

23. Meltzer-Brody S, Leserman J, Zolnoun D, Steege J, Green E, Teich A. Trauma and posttraumatic stress disorder in

women with chronic pelvic pain. Obstet Gynecol 2007; 109:902–8.

24. Davila GW, Bernier F, Franco J, Kopka SL. Bladder dysfunction in sexual abuse survivors. J Urol 2003;170:476–9.

25. Thompson MP, Basile KC, Hertz MF, Sitterle D. Measuring intimate partner violence victimization and perpretration: a compendium of assessment tools. Atlanta (GA): Centers for Disease Control and Prevention, National Center for Injury Prevention and Control; 2006. Available at: http:// www.cdc.gov/ncipc/dvp/Compendium/IPV%20 Compendium.pdf. Retrieved November 12, 2008.

26. McCloskey LA, Lichter E, Williams C, Gerber M, Wittenberg E, Ganz M. Assessing intimate partner violence in health care settings leads to women's receipt of interventions and improved health. Public Health Rep 2006;121:435–44.

27. Sheridan DJ, Nash KR. Acute injury patterns of intimate partner violence victims. Trauma Violence Abuse 2007; 8:281–9.

28. Wilbur L, Higley M, Hatfield J, Surprenant Z, Taliaferro E, Smith DJ Jr, et al. Survey results of women who have been strangled while in an abusive relationship. J Emerg Med 2001;21:297–302.

29. Smith DJ Jr, Mills T, Taliaferro EH. Frequency and relationship of reported symptomology in victims of intimate partner violence: the effect of multiple strangulation attacks. J Emerg Med 2001;21:323–9.

30. McCaw B, Bauer HM, Berman WH, Mooney L, Holmberg M, Hunkeler E. Women referred for on-site domestic violence services in a managed care organization. Women Health 2002;35:23–40.

31. Southworth C, Finn J, Dawson S, Fraser C, Tucker S. Intimate partner violence, technology, and stalking. Violence Against Women 2007;13:842–56.

Headache

Stephen D. Silberstein

Headache is one of the 10 most common reasons why a patient visits a physician's office. As a primary care provider, the obstetrician–gynecologist faces the task of differentiating common, benign headache disorders from more serious causes of headache. Although most patients have no serious underlying organic pathologic condition, physicians often perform many unnecessary tests and diagnostic procedures when assessing headache. Community surveys reveal that up to 80% of women report headache episodes during any given month and that headache prevalence declines with age. Applying the International Headache Society classification to a sample of 15,000 households (2,000 or more subjects), the American Migraine Study found that more than 23 million people in the United States experience migraine, with more than 11 million experiencing moderate to severe symptoms (1). Of these individuals, 4.5 million have one or more episodes of migraine with moderate to severe disability each month. Most of these patients are women (2).

Diagnosis

Headache can be classified as primary or secondary disorders. Primary headache is not directly related to underlying disease, whereas secondary headache is attributable to an underlying disorder. Historically, physicians and medical students have been admonished to "first rule out brain tumor" when a patient's principal symptom is headache. In general, this advice is not sound, because intracranial causes of headache are more rare than extracranial causes. In the diagnosis of headache, sensitivity, specificity, and predictive value are best for history, are good for examination, and are poor for chemical, electrical, and radiographic tests.

Resources

Headache

American Headache Society
http://www.americanheadachesociety.org

Migraine Research Foundation
http://www.migraineresearchfoundation.org

National Headache Foundation
http://www.headaches.org

National Institute of Neurological Disorders and Stroke
http://www.ninds.nih.gov

Some tests have less to offer than is popularly supposed. Skull and sinus radiographic studies seldom help, even when injury or acute infection is suspected. Electroencephalography is very helpful for seizure diagnosis, but poor for headache diagnosis. Computed tomography (CT) of the head is overused and seldom revealing. Magnetic resonance imaging and CT are at their best when central nervous system symptoms or signs are part of the headache syndrome. Both modalities are too expensive and their positive predictive value too low to warrant their use as diagnostic tests early in the workup of headache when specific neurologic symptoms or findings are absent. Table 14 identifies characteristics that can be used to assess a patient's headache history more specifically. Box 38 summarizes danger signs in the diagnosis of headache.

Classification and Treatment

The International Headache Society classification can be simplified to two major categories. The first category is primary headache (benign headache disorders), which includes migraine with or without aura, tension-type headache (episodic or chronic), and cluster headache. The second category is secondary headache—headache that is attributable to another disorder, such as post-traumatic and drug-rebound (medication overuse) headache. This section focuses on the more common primary headache disorders: tension-type headache and migraine, including menstrual-related migraine. Because cluster headaches are rare in women, they are not included. Some Internet information sources are listed in Resources.

Tension-Type Headache

The pain of tension-type headache usually is described as dull, aching, and not exacerbated by movement; characteristically it does not have the pulsatile or throbbing components that are associated with migraine. The tension-type headache usually is bilateral; the temporal and occipital regions are affected most commonly thus giving tension-type headache the so-called hatband distribution. The tension-type headache can be episodic (fewer than 15 days per month) or chronic (more than 15 days per month).

The pathophysiology of tension-type headache is not clear. It was assumed that tension-type headache is the result of increased muscle tension, although studies of resting muscle tension reveal more abnormalities in migraine. Because tension-type headache exhibits fea-

Table 14. Primary Headache Characteristics

Characteristic	Type of Headache and Etiology					
	Migraine	TTH	Cluster	TMJ	Temporal Arteritis	Tumor
Usual age at onset (years)	15–25	Variable	20–30	20–40	Older than 60	Any
Childhood history	Common	15%	Rare	No	No	No
Family history	Yes	+/–	Rare	No	No	No
Sex distribution	Females more affected than males	Females more affected than males	Males far more affected than females	Females more affected than males	+/–	Males and females affected equally
Aura	+Classic	No	No	No	No	No
Pain character	Throbbing	Aching	Stabbing	Aching	Aching	Aching
Pain distribution	+/– Unilateral	Diffuse	Retro-orbital	Ear	Temporal	Variable
Pain duration	Hours to days	Hours to constant	20–40 minutes	Variable	Constant	Progressive
Associated symptoms	Nausea, photophobia, and phonophobia	Depression	Horner lacrimation coryza	Jaw click and tenderness	Malaise and high ESR	Focality

Abbreviations: ESR indicates erythrocyte sedimentation rate; TMJ, temporomandibular joint; TTH, tension-type headache.

tures similar to those of myofascial pain (dull, aching, and diffuse), it is assumed that tension-type headache has myofascial origins. The often-used self-therapy of trapezius muscle massage and temporal muscle massage also suggests myofascial origins (3). Tension-type headache and myofascial pain may be due to central sensitization. Recent studies suggest that nitric oxide may play a role in the pathophysiology of tension-type headache, although the exact pathogenesis through the activation of vascular endothelium is not clear (4).

Although tension-type headache may manifest at any time in life, often it begins in childhood and progresses with varying frequency through adulthood. Typically, the pattern is not progressively more severe. Tension-type headache often is associated with episodes of emotional stress.

Tension-type headache usually can be diagnosed clinically, and therapy can be initiated with simple analgesics once organic disease has been ruled out by history and focused physical examination. Because depression often is associated with chronic tension-type headache (as well as with migraine), this disorder should be assessed with the expectation that the headache may improve as the depression is treated.

Treatment of tension-type headache begins with the use of appropriate over-the-counter medications and lifestyle changes. Nonsteroidal antiinflammatory drugs (NSAIDs) and acetaminophen are the most commonly used medications. The more recently developed NSAIDs

(cyclooxygenase-2 inhibitors) have been used for headache treatment. Although the cyclooxygenase-2 inhibitors have antiinflammatory action, current evidence does not suggest greater effectiveness.

Amitriptyline is the most thoroughly researched medication for preventive treatment of chronic tension-type headache. Its efficacy has been confirmed in clinical tri-

---

Box 38

Danger Signs in Headache Diagnosis

- Sudden onset
- Onset after age 50 years
- New or different headache
- "Worst" headache
- Accelerating pattern
- Onset with exertion, sexual activity, coughing, or sneezing
- Focal neurologic symptoms or signs not explained by prodrome or aura (eg, ataxia, numbness in extremities, sensory loss, and visual or neurologic changes)
- Abnormal medical evaluation (eg, fever, stiff neck, rash, hypertension, weight loss, tender or poorly pulsatile temporal arteries, lymphadenopathy, and recurrent nasal drainage or discharge)
- Papilledema

als (5). It is used in doses of 10–75 mg before bedtime. Other agents, such as low-dose selective serotonin reuptake inhibitors, have been effective in small clinical trials (5).

Migraine

Migraine is an episodic headache disorder that usually lasts 4–24 hours. It may be initiated by a prodrome and preceded by an aura (see Box 39). The headache, of moderate to severe intensity, may be unilateral or bilateral. It is typically, but not always, throbbing. Patients with migraine usually are photophobic and phonophobic and have nausea and sensitivity to movement. Vomiting and diarrhea are less common.

A condition previously termed *common migraine* is now called *migraine without aura*, and a condition previously termed *classic migraine* is now called *migraine with aura*. Types of auras (the complex of focal neurologic symptoms preceding an attack) include the following: 1) homonymous visual disturbances (most common; includes fortification spectra [bright, scintillating lights in a zigzag pattern moving across the field of vision], photopsia [sparks or flashing lights], and visual obscurations [visual illusions or distortions]); 2) unilateral paresthesias or numbness; 3) unilateral weakness; and 4) aphasia or unclassifiable speech difficulty. *Status migrainosus* refers to a bout of migraine that lasts longer than 72 hours. It may be associated with nausea, vomiting, and dehydration.

Menstrual-related migraine, a specific subset of migraine, is defined by the International Headache Society classification as attacks of migraine without aura that occur on days −2 to +3 of menstruation in at least two out of three menstrual cycles and additionally at other times of the cycle. The headache most commonly develops on days −1 to 1 of the menstrual cycle (the day before and the first day of bleeding) (6).

Women with migraine should keep a migraine diary. This diagnostic tool identifies ongoing patterns of attack, behaviors, food and beverage intake, and stressful situations that might be associated with migraine attacks. A typical menstrual calendar with expanded room for identification of behaviors and associations that might predispose the patient to migraine attacks can be used. By recognizing patterns that indicate menstrual migraine the physician can help patients initiate early treatment or avoid adverse behaviors. The diary also can serve as a tool to determine the efficacy of treatment.

The pattern and predictability of menstrual-related migraine render it amenable to focal therapies. Menstruation is a "built-in" migraine diary for patients with menstrual-related migraine and can alert the patient to the need for early treatment. In addition, the patient can be made aware of behaviors that may predispose her to worsening attacks and, thus, can avoid those behaviors when she is particularly susceptible.

MIGRAINE PATHOGENESIS

Migraine in women is related to a complex cyclic interaction among the pain control centers, the trigeminal nerve, and circulating levels of estrogen. When the trigeminal nerve is activated, neuropeptides are released, causing vasodilation and extravasation that result in a "sterile" inflammatory response. The inflammatory response further stimulates the trigeminal nerve to transmit impulses back to the brain, where they are perceived as pain. Estrogen withdrawal lowers the trigeminal nerve's response threshold.

Menstrual-related migraine occurs at the time of the greatest fluctuation in estrogen levels. It is due to estrogen withdrawal in susceptible women. Women taking combined oral contraceptives often have episodes of migraine headache during the steroid-free week, and postmenopausal women taking estradiol cypionate injections frequently have estrogen-withdrawal migraine. Estrogen withdrawal acts to decrease the nervous system pain control system.

This mechanism also may explain why pregnancy, with its sustained high estrogen levels, usually brings relief from the syndrome. Migraine symptoms may be relieved with menopause, but menopausal women with a history of menstrual-related migraine may have an exacerbation of symptoms if cyclic hormone therapy (HT) is instituted.

Episodes of headache, particularly migraine, become less frequent with age (6). However, HT may exacerbate migraine symptoms or minimize the natural improvement that is part of normal aging (6). Treatment can be particularly difficult when patients require HT but have an exacerbation of headache symptoms when it is used. Changing the form of estrogen (eg, changing from conjugated estrogens to a transdermal delivery system) often is effective. Similarly, to avoid wider fluctuations in estrogen levels, the patient can divide the daily dose and take one half in the morning and the other half in the evening. Other treatments for migraine during

---

Box 39

Migraine Triggers

- Too much or too little sleep and jet lag
- Carbon monoxide (from cigarettes)
- Environmental changes, including excessive heat, noise, or low atmospheric pressure
- Sensory stimuli, such as bright or flickering lights or strong odors
- Certain foods or beverages: monosodium glutamate, nitrites, and alcohol
- Menstruation

menopause may be similar to those used for young women, although the clinician should be cautious in the use of vasoactive substances (triptans) in old women. The physician must rule out the presence of appreciable cardiovascular (CV) disease before prescribing these medications, because triptans may be contraindicated for patients with known CV disease or treated hypertension.

Of particular concern to the clinician is a new-onset headache that occurs during the postmenopausal years and may be evidence of an underlying organic pathologic condition. Although migraine prevalence decreases with age, other problems, such as intracranial pathologic conditions and temporal arteritis, occur more commonly as women age (2).

Migraine Treatment

Menstrual-related migraine is due to declining estrogen levels. Two transdermal patches containing 0.05 mg of estrogen or one long-acting (7-day) transdermal patch containing 0.1 mg of estrogen applied the day before expected menstruation can be used for prevention. This approach effectively provides continuous estrogen levels throughout the cycle. A patient may also benefit from the short-term use of NSAIDs or frovatriptan around the period of vulnerability (7). For the postmenopausal patient, continuation of estrogen on a regular, uncycled schedule is the obvious alternative.

It is unclear why patients who already take a continuous estrogen preparation with intermittent cyclic progestins continue to have "menstrual migraines," because they do not experience a drop in estrogen levels. However, empiric treatment of this group of patients can include additional 0.05-mg transdermal patches after progestin withdrawal and expected menstruation. Alternatively, the preventive medications listed in Box 40 may be applied, depending on the patient's general health and CV status. Vasoactive abortive therapy should be used cautiously in old patients and may be contraindicated for patients with ischemic heart disease.

For reproductive-aged women who take oral contraceptives and experience menstrual migraine in the pill-free interval, additional transdermal or oral estrogen may be indicated to alter the effect of the sudden drop in synthetic estrogens that occurs after the final active tablet is taken. Long-cycle contraception can be effective for these women. Even though these women have endogenous estrogen levels, their ovaries remain relatively inactive because of the effects of oral contraceptives. Therefore, oral contraceptive withdrawal creates an artificial drop in the relatively high estrogen levels in these women.

Nonhormonal migraine management generally falls into three categories: acute, preventive, and rescue therapy. Patients who experience disabling migraine attacks need to be treated with triptans (almotriptan, sumatriptan, eletriptan, frovatriptan, naratriptan, rizatriptan, and zolmitriptan) (6). Preventive therapy is used for women with frequent disabling attacks of migraine. Short-term miniprophylactic treatment of migraine generally is considered for patients who have predictable attacks, such as patients with menstrual migraine. Treatment may be given either as prophylaxis for migraine (Box 40) or as acute treatment of headache (Table 15). Rescue treatment with opioids is appropriate for patients whose bouts of headache are refractory to the common therapies described here or for patients with medical complications that contraindicate the use of these medications.

A special category is the treatment of the pregnant woman with migraine. Most medications cross the placental barrier and, therefore, may affect the fetus

---

Box 40

Preventive Treatment of Migraine

β-Blockers
- Propranolol
- Nadolol
- Metoprolol
- Timolol

Calcium Channel Antagonists
- Verapamil

Nonsteroidal Antiinflammatory Drugs
- Aspirin
- Fenoprofen
- Flurbiprofen
- Ketoprofen
- Naproxen

Antidepressants
- Nortriptyline
- Amitriptyline
- Doxepin
- Imipramine
- Protriptyline
- Desipramine

Antiepileptic Drug
- Divalproex
- Topiramate

Other
- Riboflavin
- Butterbur

Data from Silberstein SD. Headaches and women: treatment of the pregnant and lactating migraineur. Headache 1993;33:533–40.

Table 15. Medications for Acute Treatment of Headache

Drug	Route	Key Points
Acetaminophen	Oral	Useful for mild to moderate attacks
NSAIDs	Oral	First-line therapy for most patients with mild to moderate migraine
	IM	
	Rectal	
Ergotamine tartrate	Rectal	Although available in other forms, rectal administration is associated with greater bioavailability and less vomiting
Dihydroergotamine	IM, IV	Useful for prolonged attacks refractory to other treatment
	Intranasal	First-line therapy
Sumatriptan	Subcutaneous	Rapid onset of action, but short half-life often leads to recurrence and necessity for second injection
	Oral	Slower onset, but relieves moderate to severe recurrent headache in 4 hours in up to 80% of patients
	Intranasal	
Almotriptan, eletriptan, frovatriptan, naratriptan, and rizatriptan	Oral	Long acting; relief likely from single dose
Zolmitriptan	Oral	Fast-acting relief from single dose
	Intranasal	
Opioids	Oral	Usefulness limited to patients in whom other therapies fail or who are intolerant of other therapies
	IM	
	Intranasal	
Corticosteroids	IM	Useful for prolonged attacks
	Oral	Refractory to other treatment

Abbreviations: IM indicates intramuscular; IV, intravenous; NSAID, nonsteroidal antiinflammatory drugs.

adversely. Because of these potential risks, medication use should be limited during pregnancy. Fortunately, most women with migraine report improvement during pregnancy, but migraine-abortive medications may be indicated for the pregnant woman whose headache continues to be severe and resistant to nonpharmacologic techniques (5). Simple analgesics, such as acetaminophen alone, acetaminophen with codeine, other opioids alone, or analgesics with caffeine, may be used. Ergotamine and ergot alkaloids are contraindicated during pregnancy. Triptans should be considered only on an individualized basis according to headache severity or refractoriness to other treatment. To date, no deleterious effects of triptans on the fetus have been documented, but these medications cannot be considered perfectly safe. If they are needed, clear informed consent should be obtained and the use of the medication in pregnancy entered into the manufacturer's registry.

Secondary (Organic) Headache

Organic headache, although rare, is particularly problematic in older patients. Any component of the patient's presentation and physical findings that suggests an organic pathology should be pursued aggressively and referral to an appropriate specialist made. These components include signs or symptoms of meningeal irritation, focal neurologic findings suggesting an intracranial lesion, extreme degrees of acute hypertension, and a history of the "worst" headache the patient has ever experienced. Women older than 50 years who have a sudden onset of new headache symptoms should be evaluated to rule out organic lesions.

Special attention should be given to elderly patients with symptoms that are consistent with temporal arteritis, such as jaw claudication, generalized aches, and swollen, tender cranial arteries. In the presence of these symptoms or other danger signs (Box 38), immediate referral or consultation should be obtained.

References

1. The International Classification of Headache Disorders: 2nd edition. Headache Classification Subcommittee of the International Headache Society. Cephalalgia 2004;24 Suppl 1:9–160.

2. Kaniecki R. Headache assessment and management. JAMA 2003;289:1430–3.

3. Ashina M, Bendtsen L, Jensen R, Sakai F, Olesen J. Muscle hardness in patients with chronic tension-type headache: relation to actual headache state. Pain 1999;79:201–5.

4. Ashina M, Bendtsen L, Jensen R, Olesen J. Nitric oxide-induced headache in patients with chronic tension-type headache. Brain 2000;123 (Pt 9):1830–7.

5. Silberstein SD. Tension-type headache. In: Noseworthy JH, editor. Neurological therapeutics principles and practice. 2nd ed. London: Informa Healthcare; 2006. p. 141–61.

6. Silberstein SD. Sex hormones and headache. Philadelphia (PA): Current Medicine Group; 2007.

7. Silberstein SD, Elkind AH, Schreiber C, Keywood C. A randomized trial of frovatriptan for the intermittent prevention of menstrual migraine. Neurology 2004;63:261–9.

Mental Health Issues

Zachary N. Stowe

Commonly encountered psychiatric disorders in women include eating disorders, mood disorders associated with reproductive life events, and cognitive decline. The clinician should be aware that in women, and in psychiatry in general, comorbidity is the rule, not the exception; this situation often complicates definitive diagnosis and response to treatment. The risk factors for the disorders and initial interventions are shown in Table 16.

Eating Disorders

Over the past several decades, eating disorders have received increased attention in research, clinical, and media arenas. Most investigators agree that eating disorders exist on a continuum of less harmful symptoms, such as dieting and low self-esteem, to more severe disorders that meet formal diagnostic criteria, including: 1) anorexia nervosa, 2) bulimia nervosa, or 3) eating disorder not otherwise specified. Anorexia nervosa and bulimia nervosa are psychiatric disorders that primarily afflict adolescent girls and women at a peak age of reproductive functioning. Overall, females make up 90% of the patients who have eating disorders, and the prevalence of eating disorders in women of childbearing potential is estimated to be approximately 4% (1). Early detection of subthreshold symptoms of these disorders offers the opportunity for interventions that potentially reduce the risk of the development of more serious eating disorders.

Resources

Mental Health Issues

American Psychiatric Association
http://www.psych.org

American Psychological Association
http://www.apa.org

Mental Health America
http://nmha.org

National Institute of Mental Health
http://www.nimh.nih.gov

National Mental Health Information Center
http://mentalhealth.samhsa.gov

North American Society for Psychosocial
   Obstetrics and Gynecology
http://www.naspog.org

Dieting

Rigorous dieting may lead to psychiatric morbidity, such as anxiety, depression (2), and most powerfully, clinically significant eating disorders. Dieting has demonstrated a profound effect on later risk of developing eating disorders, with severe dieters and moderate dieters being 18 and 5 times more likely, respectively, than nondieters to develop a clinically significant eating disorder over a 3-year period. Risk factors include 1) low self-esteem, 2) high stress levels, 3) body image distortions, and 4) a history of physical and sexual abuse. Patients often engage in unhealthy dieting behaviors. Because serious nutrient and mineral deficiencies, as well as dizziness and fainting, may result from these behaviors, they should be explored during the medical history.

Diet Pills, Vomiting, and Laxative Use

Prescription and over-the-counter diet pills are widely available. High school–aged females and males interviewed for a study reported current diet pill use rates of 4% and 2%, respectively (3).

Self-induced vomiting (purging) and laxative use for weight control have received considerable attention. The *sorority girl diet*, a term coined by the lay press, has serious potential health consequences; the onset of this diet typically precedes secondary education. A significant number of adolescents in grades 6–8 are reported to use self-induced vomiting, laxatives, or both to control or lose weight after eating large amount of food (4). A prospective study of individuals aged 9–12 years at baseline found that although less than 1% of boys and girls reported purging (vomiting or laxative use) at the beginning of the study, the onset of puberty brought about an increase in the purging rate among females but not males (5). Purging behavior is associated with increased rates of psychosocial problems and behavioral risk factors among females.

Effective treatments for eating disorders are limited, and most effective interventions are multifaceted. The widespread adverse effect of eating disorders—unhealthy weight loss strategies—place youth at risk for stunted growth, delayed puberty, nutrient deficiencies, illness, comorbid anxiety and depression, and death.

Effect of Eating Disorders on Reproductive Events

Eating disorders can affect menstrual cycle functioning. In addition, females with an eating disorder are less likely than those without an eating disorder to take oral

Table 16. Risk Factors and Interventions for Psychiatric Disorders

Disorder or Reproductive Event	Subtypes	Risk Factors*	Intervention
Eating disorders	Anorexia nervosa Bulimia Eating disorder not otherwise specified	Preoccupation with body image and inappropriate dieting behaviors	Referral
Pubertal mood disorders		Early onset puberty and family history of depression	Referral
Menstrual cycle	Premenstrual syndrome		Exercise program and support
	Premenstrual mood dysphoric disorder	History of depression, or anxiety, or both	SSRIs; calcium 1,200 mg per day; magnesium, 200–400 mg per day; and GnRH agonists[†]
	Premenstrual exacerbation	Preexisting psychiatric illness	Appropriate to primary illness
Pregnancy		History of depression, unplanned pregnancy, ambivalency about pregnancy, and use of antidepressant proximate to conception	Previously effective treatment and medication with reproductive safety data (new and improved medications typically have limited data)[‡]
Postpartum mood disorders	Maternity blues		Support
	Postpartum depression	History of depression, depression or anxiety in pregnancy, or both	Antidepressants (SSRIs more effective than TCA), and structured psychotherapy (CBT, IPT)
	Postpartum psychosis	History of psychosis and history of bipolar disorder	Emergent referral
Perimenopause		History of depression, hot flushes	Antidepressants (SSRIs more effective than TCA) and estrogen
Dementia and cognitive decline	Alzheimer disease Vascular dementia Mixed dementia	Cardiovascular disease, diabetes, cerebrovascular disease, and history of depression	Referral

*Risk factors across most disorders include a history of physical and sexual abuse, recent stressful life events represent significant risk factors.

[†]American College of Obstetricians and Gynecologists. Premenstrual syndrome. ACOG Practice Bulletin 15. Washington, DC: ACOG; 2000.
[‡]Use of psychiatric medications during pregnancy and lactation. ACOG Practice Bulletin No. 92. American College of Osbtetricians and Gynecologists. Obstet Gynecol 2008;111:1001–20.
Abbreviations: CBT indicates cognitive behavioral therapy; GnRH, gonadotropin releasing hormone; IPT, interpersonal psychotherapy; SSRI, selective serotonin reuptake inhibitor; TCA, tricyclic antidepressant.

contraceptives. Women with active bulimia were found to be 7.5 times more likely to report unplanned pregnancies than women without eating disorders (76% compared with 10%, respectively) (6). The same study found that bulimic symptoms improved as the pregnancies progressed for most subjects, yet 57% of the group had worsened symptoms after delivery. The prevalence of hyperemesis in women who have an active eating disorder is very high compared with the prevalence in the community at large. Patients have been noted to even acknowledge that a side benefit of hyperemesis is that it prevented excess weight gain (7). Obstetric outcome studies in women with an eating disorder have produced discordant results. Most investigators agree

that a history of an eating disorder increases the risk of postpartum depression (Box 41).

Depressive Symptoms and Major Depression

More than 30 million people in the United States experience clinical depression each year (8), and most of these patients are female. The rate of depression in women is typically twice that of men; eg, variability in the lifetime female-to-male ratios ranges from 1.6 in Beirut and Taiwan to 3.1 in West Germany (9). The identification and treatment of depression in women in the nonpsychiatric clinic setting has garnered increased attention over the past decade, particularly with respect to the effect of reproductive life events on mood disorders.

Women are at greatest risk for the first episode of major depression during the childbearing years (10). The identification of depression often is complicated by the overlap between the symptoms of depression and many signs and symptoms typically considered to be the normal sequela of reproductive life events, such as menstruation, pregnancy, the postpartum period, and the transition to menopause. The challenge of an accurate diagnosis calls to question the validity of applying the same diagnostic criteria to women during these life events (11). The adverse consequences of depression—marital instability, poor obstetric outcomes, delayed child development, and heightened risk of other medical illnesses—underscore the need to expand efforts for early identification and intervention.

Depressive Disorders Specific to Women

Disorders During Menarche

Before puberty, the prevalence of depression is similar for males and females, if not more common in prepubescent boys than in girls. By age 15 years, females are twice as likely as males to have had an episode of major depression, and this trend persists over the next four decades of life (12). By young adulthood (age 15–24 years), the lifetime prevalence of major depression in the United States is 20.6% for females but only 10.5% for males (13).

Along with the morphologic and biochemical changes of puberty, adolescents often experience appreciable social role transitions, including major shifts in school environment and in relationships with parents, peers, and intimate partners (12). Female adolescence is clearly a time when biologic and psychosocial changes intermingle; eg, morphologic changes, such as breast development and increased body fat, have a psychoso-

cial effect on self-image and perception by others (12). Thus, depressive vulnerability of women at this time is likely to be influenced by pubertal timing, age, self-image and morphologic changes, and psychosocial support (10). For example, body shape changes at the time of puberty generally are welcomed by young men but are more likely to be experienced as distressful by young women, at least in industrialized cultures (14).

Pubertal timing also may be an important factor. Young girls who have secondary sex characteristics earlier than their peers are more likely to experience depression during adolescence and more likely to have difficulties with body image (15). In fact, girls who mature early or late have been found to experience higher rates of major depression than girls who mature "on time" (30% versus 22% and 34% versus 22%, respectively) (16).

The high incidence of depression in peripubertal girls, particularly in girls with early development, at Tanner stage III, or both, warrants close attention to the possibility of clinical depression. Moreover, information about the increased rate of depression with puberty and risk factors would be a valuable aspect of training for parents, middle school teachers, and guidance counselors. Because puberty marks the onset of the marked difference in prevalence of depression based on sex, further research may elucidate other biologic markers of mood disorders, risk factors, or preventive measures.

Menstrual Cycle and Mood

Alterations in mood over the course of the menstrual cycle can be classified into three categories: 1) premenstrual syndrome (PMS), or premenstrual tension syndrome, a common syndrome with a myriad of symptoms reported in the literature; 2) premenstrual dysphoric disorder (PMDD), a more severe fluctuation in mood that requires prospective monthly charting for accurate diagnosis; and 3) premenstrual exacerbation, the exacerbation of a preexisting psychiatric illness during the luteal phase.

Women with PMDD experience a set of symptoms that have appreciable overlap with the symptoms of major depression, including social impairment, occupational impairment, or both. Approximately 3–6% of women fulfill the criteria for PMDD, with the peak incidence in the mid-30s (17). In contrast to menstrual cycle-related onset and cessation, premenstrual exacerbation of an undiagnosed psychiatric illness is common. In a prospective diagnostic assessment, 38.1% of women responding to advertisement for a PMDD clinical treatment study were found to actually have undiagnosed major depression, bipolar disorder, or panic disorder (18). The incidence of premenstrual exacerbation lacks systematic investigation, although the clinician should be aware that some psychiatric disorders may present as premenstrual symptoms. As a general rule, many medical conditions appear to worsen during the luteal phase relative to the follicular phase; they include asthma, epilepsy, migraine headache, depression, substance abuse, and sleep disorders. With respect to mood disorders, the potential for premenstrual exacerbation underscores the need to assess the presence of symptoms during the follicular phase to make an accurate diagnosis.

The risk factors for PMDD were examined in a large community study in which premenstrual symptoms of 4,164 women aged 36–44 years were analyzed. The study showed the following results:

1. There was a strong association between PMDD and a previous history of depression.
2. Less educated women were more likely to report appreciable PMDD symptoms.
3. Women working outside the home were more likely to fulfill the diagnostic criteria for PMDD.
4. Current cigarette smokers were approximately four times as likely to fulfill the criteria for PMDD as nonsmokers (19). Studies have reported that women with PMDD report more stressful life events and are more affected by stressors. In particular, women with PMDD are more likely to have histories of sexual abuse (20).

The menstrual cycle phase-specific presentation of PMDD supports some relationship to sex steroids. Notably, women with PMDD often report that their symptoms are alleviated by ovariectomy or by treatment with an ovulation-inhibiting gonadotropin-releasing hormone analogue (21). Although circulating concentrations of estrogen and progesterone do not discriminate women with PMDD from controls, women with PMDD appear to be more sensitive to the effects of fluctuations in these hormones (22). This idea has been examined by studying the effect of administering exogenous estrogen or progesterone to 1) women with a history of PMDD who were symptom-free while treated with ovulation inhibitors (23) and 2) menopausal women with a former history of PMDD (22). In both groups, the women with a history of PMDD were more likely to experience PMDD-like symptoms when exogenous female sex steroids were administered. In an elegant investigation, leuprolide (a gonadotropin-releasing hormone agonist) was administered monthly for 3 months to women with PMS, as well as to controls; after the 3-month treatment with either leuprolide or placebo, participants in this study received hormone therapy (transdermal 17β-estradiol and progesterone vaginal suppositories). Women with a history of PMDD reported fewer symptoms during leuprolide treatment and more symptoms during the hormone therapy phase, confirming that a subgroup of women is more susceptible to mood fluctuations in response to gonadal steroids.

The overlap in the clinical symptoms of PMDD and major depression has prompted many investigations.

For example, loss of appetite and decreased sleep are common symptoms of major depression. In contrast, food craving (24) and increased sleep are common symptoms in women with PMDD. Treatment response also differs; women with PMDD preferentially respond to selective serotonin reuptake inhibitors (SSRIs) and often do so more quickly and at lower doses (25) than women with a major depression. In fact, women with PMDD may respond to an SSRI in a few days, whereas treatment response for major depressive disorder requires 4–6 weeks on average (25). Clinically effective antidepressants that do not alter serotonin uptake have failed to effectively treat women with PMDD. Similar to major depression treatment studies in community samples, a review of the PMDD treatment studies with the most rigorous enrollment criteria demonstrates a placebo response rate of more than 40% (25, 26).

The treatment options for PMS and PMDD are discussed in the American College of Obstetricians and Gynecologists' Practice Bulletin No. 15. They include 1) calcium, 1,200 mg/d; 2) magnesium, 200– 400 mg/d; 3) supportive psychotherapy and SSRIs; 4) gonadotropin-releasing hormone agonists; and 5) drospironone-containing or extended-cycle oral contraceptives. Most investigations concur that women with premenstrual mood symptoms benefit from a regular exercise program.

Disorders During Pregnancy

Pregnancy historically has been perceived as a time of emotional well-being, but there is little evidence that pregnancy provides protection against psychiatric illness. A total of 10–14% of women experience a major depressive episode during pregnancy, and 25% of pregnant women experience elevated levels of depressive symptomatology (27). A recent study found that more than 25% of pregnant women with psychiatric illness experienced suicidal ideation during pregnancy (28). Depression during pregnancy is easily overlooked, because there is a notable overlap between normal sequelae of pregnancy and symptoms of major depressive disorder. The American College of Obstetricians and Gynecologists noted substantial evidence for the adverse effect of inadequately treated or untreated maternal mental illness (29).

The balancing of the risks and benefits of treatment during pregnancy has undergone extensive review (29). It suffices to summarize that treatment decisions should remain on a case-by-case basis. Prospective studies demonstrated a remarkably high rate of relapse (68–74%) during pregnancy for women discontinuing antidepressant therapy (30, 31).

The last decade has seen a dramatic increase in the available data on antidepressant medication use during pregnancy. An analysis of seven health care databases found that more than 6% of pregnant women receive a prescription for antidepressants at some point in pregnancy (32). The risks of antidepressant use in pregnancy can be broadly categorized as birth defects, obstetric complications, neonatal outcome, and long-term-developmental effects.

There is limited evidence that antidepressant exposure in pregnancy is associated with birth defects. The data on obstetric complications remain discordant. One report on persistent pulmonary hypertension of the newborn garnered considerable attention, although it lacks replication (33). The presence of neonatal symptoms, such as rapid respiration and tremor, after antidepressant exposure has been reviewed. Despite the widespread attention, most authors fail to point out that neonatal symptoms associated with medication exposure in pregnancy are not uncommon and fail to mention that the initial report of neonatal symptoms associated with antidepressant exposure was in 1973. To date, there is no conclusive evidence that such symptoms have long-term consequences, but infants should be observed in the neonatal period. The long-term follow-up data have failed to identify any adverse effects of antidepressant exposure (34).

Depression during pregnancy should be treated because of the risk of potential adverse consequences. The type of treatment—psychosocial, psychotherapeutic, or pharmacologic—remains a case-by-case decision. Given that more than 50% of pregnancies are unplanned, most cases of exposure, at least early in pregnancy, will have already occurred. Treatment history and prior fetal exposure to medication should be incorporated in the clinical decision. The amount of reproductive safety information is typically proportional to the duration of use (eg, "new and improved = less data"). Thus, in the absence of treatment history, prior fetal exposure, or both, older medications would be preferable choices.

Postpartum Disorders

Although most attention paid to mental illness that has an onset after delivery follows a tragic event involving a child, these events seldom represent illness whose onset was exclusively postpartum. The continuum of postpartum mood disturbances includes the relatively common postpartum blues; a major depressive episode termed *postpartum depression*; and the most severe, *postpartum psychosis*.

Postpartum Blues

The postpartum blues has such a high frequency (greater than 60%) that it is considered a normal sequela of childbirth. It is noteworthy that this purportedly normal condition appears to have many of the same risk factors as are seen for depression. Although clinical intervention is not typical, women experiencing the blues appear to be at greater risk for later depression. The role of the blues as a trigger for depression or

as a brief episode of mood disorder in a vulnerable population warrants further attention.

Postpartum Depression

The reported rate of major depression in the postpartum period is highly variable, with investigations citing 8–22% (35). There is evidence that teenaged women and women living in poverty have a higher rate of postpartum depression—26% and 27%, respectively (36). The onset of postpartum depression is typically within the first month postpartum (37). The symptoms of postpartum depression closely resemble the symptoms of depression at other times (38). Like depression during pregnancy, in postpartum depression there is considerable overlap between depressive symptoms (alterations in sleep, libido decline, fatigue, and appetite changes) and the normal sequelae of childbirth and the early postpartum period. To aid in the diagnosis, rating scales, such as the Edinburgh Postnatal Depression Rating Scale and the Postpartum Depression Checklist, have been developed, validated, and translated into several languages to help clinicians screen for depression in this population (39, 40). These scales minimize reliance on the presence of the overlapping symptoms but rather emphasize the quality of the symptoms. The treatment of postpartum depression is covered in the current edition of *Precis: Obstetrics*.

Postpartum Psychosis

Postpartum psychosis represents a severe mental illness. It is one of the few true psychiatric emergencies that require aggressive treatment, always in the inpatient setting. Postpartum psychosis affects 0.2% of women, with the onset most commonly within the first week after delivery but, by definition, within the first 4–6 weeks postpartum (41). Although 80% of women with postpartum psychosis have an onset after the birth of their first child (42), it is a highly recurrent illness for women choosing to have another child (43). Follow-up data indicate that most cases of postpartum psychosis are related to a mood disorder (eg, bipolar depression or major depression). This disorder is characterized by intense mood lability, obsessive ruminations about the baby, hallucinations, sleep disturbances, and paranoia (41). The strongest risk factors for postpartum psychosis are a history of bipolar disorder or a previous episode of postpartum psychosis (42, 44). One study of 486 women with postpartum psychosis who were admitted to an inpatient facility found that more than one third of patients had prior diagnoses of bipolar disorder; in comparison, less than 5% of patients had a diagnosis of schizophrenia (45).

Disorders During Menopause

The effect of the transition to menopause on mood disorders has provided an interesting set of data that clinicians often overlook. However, the effect of this transition is receiving increased attention. Several studies indicate higher rates of depression in the perimenopausal years relative to other periods in the reproductive life cycle, most notably among women with a history of mood disorder. For example, a 1996 cross-national study demonstrated an increase in the onset of depression in women aged 45–49 years (9). Moreover, women aged 45–64 years have the highest rate of completed suicide among women (46).

The transition to menopause (the climacteric period) can be of varying duration and of varying etiology (natural, surgical, chemical, or pharmacologic). Several studies have compared rates of depression in menopausal women with rates of depression at other points in a woman's life. Although no increase in depressive symptoms has been noted in post-menopausal women, more depressive symptoms have been reported in the climacteric period (47–50). One study of 3,302 women reported the rate of persistent depressive symptoms to be 14.9–18.4% for perimenopausal women as compared with 8–12% for premenopausal women (49). However, diagnosing depression in the perimenopausal woman can be challenging, because the symptoms of depression and the normal symptoms of menopause overlap (51). For example, irritability, insomnia, libido changes, loss of energy, and concentration difficulties have been described as common symptoms of menopause (51).

Sorting out the clinical diagnosis requires additional questions regarding the symptoms that are specific to menopause (eg, vaginal dryness), that are unique to psychiatric illness (eg, low self-esteem and thoughts of death and dying), or both. The clinician should be aware that both conditions can occur simultaneously; they are not mutually exclusive.

Another confounding factor in looking at the relationship between depression and menopause is the association between a history of major depression and an early age of onset of menopause. One study found that undergoing a natural menopause at a younger-than-average age (younger than 47 years) compared with an average age (50–55 years) was associated with a twofold to threefold increase in the likelihood of a history of depression (52).

The best predictor of perimenopausal depression is a past history of mood disorder; a past history significantly outweighs the effect of social circumstances or psychosocial stressors at this time (53). The presence and severity of vasomotor symptoms, a history of PMS, lack of employment, and possibly being African American appear to increase the risk of depression at this time (54).

Although estrogen has consistently been shown to enhance cognitive function in women (55), the effect of estrogen therapy on mood has been less clear. Several studies report that hormone therapy is effective in treating depression in menopausal women (56, 57); however, another investigation indicates that the women whose depression improves with estrogen therapy are the women who experience comorbid vasomotor symptoms (58). The decision of whether or not to treat perimenopausal and menopausal women with hormone therapy specifically for depression is not well supported. Several double-blind placebo-controlled studies do demonstrate the effectiveness of antidepressants (venlafaxine, fluoxetine, and paroxetine) in reducing the severity of hot flushes (59–62). Mood disorders and the reproductive life cycle are summarized in Box 42.

Dementia and Cognitive Decline

According to the *Diagnostic and Statistical Manual of Mental Disorders*, Fourth Edition, *dementia* is defined as a clinical syndrome characterized by acquired loss of memory and cognitive capacity severe enough to interfere with daily functioning and the quality of life. Alzheimer disease is the main cause of dementia, accounting for 50–70% of the cases, followed by vascular dementia (30–40% of cases) and mixed dementia (15–20% of cases). A variety of risk factors, many of which are more common in women than men, have been identified.

Box 42

Summary of Mood Disorders and the Reproductive Life Cycle

- Early onset puberty increases risk for depression.
- Mood symptoms may vary across the menstrual cycle.
- The luteal phase appears to be the highest risk period for symptoms and worsening of preexisting psychiatric illness.
- Maternal depression during pregnancy warrants identification and treatment.
- The use of antidepressant medication in pregnancy and lactation has not consistently been associated with adverse effects—obstetric, neonatal, or developmental.
- Pregnancy and lactation may complicate treatment decisions, but they do not preclude pharmacologic intervention, if appropriate.
- Postpartum mental illness is common and most cases can be identified by 6 weeks postpartum.
- The relationship between depression and the transition to the menopause remains obscure.
- The use of estrogen for the treatment of depressive symptoms in menopausal women warrants further investigation.

The strongest predictor for dementia is age. The prevalence of dementia increases sharply in individuals older than 80 years and is higher among old women than among their male counterparts. In men and women between the ages of 65 years and 80 years, the incidence of Alzheimer disease doubles every 4 years, reaching a prevalence of 30% by age 80 years (63).

Patients who have a first-degree relative with dementia have a 10–30% increased risk of developing Alzheimer disease (64). Approximately 7% of early-onset cases are familial, with an autosomal-dominant pattern of inheritance and penetrance (65).

Although there have been discordant results (66), women have higher rates of factors associated with vulnerability to the development of dementia, such as depression; a higher rate of silent cerebral ischemia and white matter changes associated with hypertension and diabetes mellitus (67); and a worse clinical outcome with a higher level of disability after stroke compared with men (68).

The use of pharmacologic intervention has expanded (69). Newer investigations have examined the role of pharmacogenetics in predicting treatment response in individuals with Alzheimer disease (70).

An association between estrogen and cognitive impairment or dementia has undergone extensive debate. Three meta-analyses showed a 20–40% reduction in risk of Alzheimer disease for women who underwent estrogen treatment after menopause (71–73). These data conflict with findings from the Women's Health Initiative clinical trials that showed an increased, rather than decreased, risk of dementia or mild cognitive impairment in women treated with estrogen alone or estrogen plus progestin when they were aged at least 65 years (74–76). Several investigators have proposed that these conflicting findings may be explained by an age-dependent effect of estrogen on the brain. Specifically, estrogen may have a protective effect on the brain if given to women early in the menopausal transition (eg, after oophorectomy and in the perimenopausal and early postmenopausal years). In contrast, estrogen may have deleterious effects on the brain if its administration begins many years after the onset of natural menopause. It has been posited that there may be a critical age window for the potential neuroprotective effects of estrogen.

References

1. King MB. Eating disorders in a general practice population. Prevalence, characteristics and follow-up at 12 to 18 months. Psychol Med Monogr Suppl 1989;14:1–34.

2. Patton GC, Carlin JB, Shao Q, Hibbert ME, Rosier M, Selzer R, et al. Adolescent dieting: healthy weight control or borderline eating disorder? J Child Psychol Psychiatry 1997;38:299–306.

3. Serdula MK, Collins ME, Williamson DF, Anda RF, Pamuk E, Byers TE. Weight control practices of U.S. adolescents and adults. Ann Intern Med 1993;119:667–71.

4. Krowchuk DP, Kreiter SR, Woods CR, Sinal SH, DuRant RH. Problem dieting behaviors among young adolescents. Arch Pediatr Adolesc Med 1998;152:884–8.

5. Field AE, Camargo CA, Jr, Taylor CB, Berkey CS, Frazier AL, Gillman MW, et al. Overweight, weight concerns, and bulimic behaviors among girls and boys. J Am Acad Child Adolesc Psychiatry 1999;38:754–60.

6. Morgan JF, Lacey JH, Sedgwick PM. Impact of pregnancy on bulimia nervosa [published erratum appears in Br J Psychiatry 1999;174:278]. Br J Psychiatry 1999;174:135–40.

7. Abraham S. Sexuality and reproduction in bulimia nervosa patients over 10 years. J Psychosom Res 1998;44:491–502.

8. Kessler RC, Berglund P, Demler O, Jin R, Koretz D, Merikangas KR, et al. The epidemiology of major depressive disorder: results from the National Comorbidity Survey Replication (NCS-R). National Comorbidity Survey Replication. JAMA 2003;289:3095–105.

9. Weissman MM, Bland RC, Canino GJ, Faravelli C, Greenwald S, Hwu HG, et al. Cross-national epidemiology of major depression and bipolar disorder. JAMA 1996;276:293–9.

10. Angold A, Costello EJ, Worthman CM. Puberty and depression: the roles of age, pubertal status and pubertal timing. Psychol Med 1998;28:51–61.

11. Stowe ZN, Newport DJ. Depression in women: recognition and treatment: myriad forms of depression occur throughout women's lives. Womens Health Prim Care 1998;1(suppl):29–39.

12. Cyranowski JM, Frank E, Young E, Shear MK. Adolescent onset of the gender difference in lifetime rates of major depression: a theoretical model. Arch Gen Psychiatry 2000;57:21–7.

13. Kessler RC, Walters EE. Epidemiology of DSM-III-R major depression and minor depression among adolescents and young adults in the National Comorbidity Survey. Depress Anxiety 1998;7:3–14.

14. Blyth DA, Hill JP, Smyth CK. The influence of older adolescents on younger adolescents: do grade-level arrangements make a difference in behaviors, attitudes, and experiences? J Early Adoles 1981;1:85–110.

15. Hayward C, Killen JD, Wilson DM, Hammer LD, Litt IF, Kraemer HC, et al. Psychiatric risk associated with early puberty in adolescent girls. J Am Acad Child Adolesc Psychiatry 1997;36:255–62.

16. Lewinsohn PM, Rohde P, Seeley JR. Major depressive disorder in older adolescents: prevalence, risk factors, and clinical implications. Clin Psychol Rev 1998;18:765–94.

17. Rivera-Tovar AD, Frank E. Late luteal phase dysphoric disorder in young women. Am J Psychiatry 1990;147:1634–6.

18. Bailey JW, Cohen LS. Prevalence of mood and anxiety disorders in women who seek treatment for premenstrual syndrome. J Womens Health Gend Based Med 1999;8:1181–4.

19. Cohen LS, Soares CN, Otto MW, Sweeney BH, Liberman RF, Harlow BL. Prevalence and predictors of premenstrual dysphoric disorder (PMDD) in older premenopausal women. The Harvard Study of Moods and Cycles. J Affect Disord 2002;70:125–32.

20. Girdler SS, Pedersen CA, Straneva PA, Leserman J, Stanwyck CL, Benjamin S, et al. Dysregulation of cardiovascular and neuroendocrine responses to stress in premenstrual dysphoric disorder. Psychiatry Res 1998;81: 163–78.

21. Sundstrom I, Nyberg S, Bixo M, Hammarback S, Backstrom T. Treatment of premenstrual syndrome with gonadotropin-releasing hormone agonist in a low dose regimen. Acta Obstet Gynecol Scand 1999;78:891–9.

22. Eriksson E, Andersch B, Ho HP, Landen M, Sundblad C. Diagnosis and treatment of premenstrual dysphoria. J Clin Psychiatry 2002;63 Suppl 7:16–23.

23. Leather AT, Studd JW, Watson NR, Holland EF. The treatment of severe premenstrual syndrome with goserelin with and without 'add-back' estrogen therapy: a placebo-controlled study. Gynecol Endocrinol 1999;13:48–55.

24. Bancroft J, Cook A, Williamson L. Food craving, mood and the menstrual cycle. Psychol Med 1988;18:855–60.

25. Steiner M, Steinberg S, Stewart D, Carter D, Berger C, Reid R, et al. Fluoxetine in the treatment of premenstrual dysphoria. Canadian Fluoxetine/Premenstrual Dysphoria Collaborative Study Group. N Engl J Med 1995;332: 1529–34.

26. Yonkers KA, Halbreich U, Freeman E, Brown C, Pearlstein T. Sertraline in the treatment of premenstrual dysphoric disorder. Psychopharmacol Bull 1996;32:41–6.

27. Evans J, Heron J, Francomb H, Oke S, Golding J. Cohort study of depressed mood during pregnancy and after childbirth. BMJ 2001;323:257–60.

28. Newport DJ, Levey LC, Pennell PB, Ragan K, Stowe ZN. Suicidal ideation in pregnancy: assessment and clinical implications. Arch Womens Ment Health 2007;10:181–7.

29. Use of Psychiatric Medications During Pregnancy and Lactation. ACOG Practice Bulletin No. 92. American College of Obstetricians and Gynecologists. Obstet Gynecol 2008;111:1001–20.

30. Cohen LS, Altshuler LL, Stowe ZN, Faraone SV. Reintroduction of antidepressant therapy across pregnancy in women who previously discontinued treatment. A preliminary retrospective study. Psychother Psychosom 2004;73:255–8.

31. Viguera AC, Whitfield T, Baldessarini RJ, Newport DJ, Stowe Z, Reminick A, et al. Risk of recurrence in women with bipolar disorder during pregnancy: prospective study of mood stabilizer discontinuation. Am J Psychiatry 2007; 164:1817–24; quiz 1923.

32. Andrade SE, Raebel MA, Brown J, Lane K, Livingston J, Boudreau D, et al. Use of antidepressant medications during pregnancy: a multisite study. Am J Obstet Gynecol 2008;198:194.e1–5.

33. Chambers CD, Hernandez-Diaz S, Van Marter LJ, Werler MM, Louik C, Jones KL, et al. Selective serotonin-reuptake inhibitors and risk of persistent pulmonary hypertension of the newborn. N Engl J Med 2006;354:579–87.

34. Nulman I, Rovet J, Stewart DE, Wolpin J, Pace-Asciak P, Shuhaiber S, et al. Child development following exposure to tricyclic antidepressants or fluoxetine throughout fetal life: a prospective, controlled study. Am J Psychiatry 2002; 159:1889–95.

35. O'Hara MW, Zekoski EM, Philipps LH, Wright EJ. Controlled prospective study of postpartum mood disorders: comparison of childbearing and nonchildbearing women. J Abnorm Psychol 1990;99:3–15.

36. Hobfoll SE, Ritter C, Lavin J, Hulsizer MR, Cameron RP. Depression prevalence and incidence among inner-city pregnant and postpartum women. J Consult Clin Psychol 1995;63:445–53.

37. Stowe ZN, Hostetter AL, Newport DJ. The onset of postpartum depression: implications for clinical screening in obstetrical and primary care. Am J Obstet Gynecol 2005; 192:522–6.

38. Suri R, Burt VK. The assessment and treatment of postpartum psychiatric disorders. J Pract Psychiatry Behav Health 1997;3:67–77.

39. Beck CT. Screening methods for postpartum depression. J Obstet Gynecol Neonatal Nurs 1995;24:308–12.

40. Cox JL, Holden JM, Sagovsky R. Detection of postnatal depression. Development of the 10-item Edinburgh Postnatal Depression Scale. Br J Psychiatry 1987; 150: 782–6.

41. Muller C. On the nosology of post-partum psychoses. Psychopathology 1985;18:181–4.

42. McNeil TF. A prospective study of postpartum psychoses in a high-risk group. 2. Relationships to demographic and psychiatric history characteristics. Acta Psychiatr Scand 1987;75:35–43.

43. Davidson J, Robertson E. A follow-up study of post partum illness, 1946–1978. Acta Psychiatr Scand 1985;71:451–7.

44. Marks MN, Wieck A, Checkley SA, Kumar R. Life stress and post-partum psychosis: a preliminary report. Br J Psychiatry Suppl 1991;(10):45–9.

45. Kendell RE, Chalmers JC, Platz C. Epidemiology of puerperal psychoses [published erratum appears in Br J Psychiatry 1987;151:135]. Br J Psychiatry 1987;150:662–73.

46. Kung HC, Hoyert DL, Xu J,Murphy SL. Deaths: final data for 2005. Natl Vital Stat Rep 2008;56(10):1–120. Available at: http://www.cdc.gov/nchs/data/nvsr/nvsr56/nvsr56_10.pdf. Retrieved November 12, 2008.

47. Avis NE, Brambilla D, McKinlay SM, Vass K. A longitudinal analysis of the association between menopause and depression. Results from the Massachusetts Women's Health Study. Ann Epidemiol 1994;4:214–20.

48. Ballinger CB. Psychiatric morbidity and the menopause; screening of general population sample. Br Med J 1975;3:344–6.

49. Bromberger JT, Assmann SF, Avis NE, Schocken M, Kravitz HM, Cordal A. Persistent mood symptoms in a multiethnic community cohort of pre- and perimenopausal women. Am J Epidemiol 2003;158:347–56.

50. Bungay GT, Vessey MP, McPherson CK. Study of symptoms in middle life with special reference to the menopause. Br Med J 1980;281:181–3.

51. Prior JC. Perimenopause: the complex endocrinology of the menopausal transition. Endocr Rev 1998;19:397–428.

52. Harlow BL, Wise LA, Otto MW, Soares CN, Cohen LS. Depression and its influence on reproductive endocrine and menstrual cycle markers associated with perimenopause: the Harvard Study of Moods and Cycles. Arch Gen Psychiatry 2003;60:29–36.

53. Schmidt PJ, Roca CA, Bloch M, Rubinow DR. The perimenopause and affective disorders. Semin Reprod Endocrinol 1997;15:91–100.

54. Freeman EW, Sammel MD, Liu L, Gracia CR, Nelson DB, Hollander L. Hormones and menopausal status as predictors of depression in women in transition to menopause. Arch Gen Psychiatry 2004;61:62–70.

55. Sherwin BB. Estrogen effects on cognition in menopausal women. Neurology 1997;48:S21–6.

56. Carranza-Lira S, Valentino-Figueroa ML. Estrogen therapy for depression in postmenopausal women. Int J Gynaecol Obstet 1999;65:35–8.

57. Zweifel JE, O'Brien WH. A meta-analysis of the effect of hormone replacement therapy upon depressed mood [published erratum appears in Psychoneuroendocrinology 1997;22:655]. Psychoneuroendocrinology 1997;22:189–212.

58. Hlatky MA, Boothroyd D, Vittinghoff E, Sharp P, Whooley MA. Quality-of-life and depressive symptoms in postmenopausal women after receiving hormone therapy: results from the Heart and Estrogen/Progestin Replacement Study (HERS) trial. Heart and Estrogen/ Progestin Replacement Study (HERS) Research Group. JAMA 2002; 287:591–7.

59. Barton D, La VB, Loprinzi C, Novotny P, Wilwerding MB, Sloan J. Venlafaxine for the control of hot flashes: results of a longitudinal continuation study. Oncol Nurs Forum 2002;29:33–40.

60. Loprinzi CL, Sloan JA, Perez EA, Quella SK, Stella PJ, Mailliard JA, et al. Phase III evaluation of fluoxetine for treatment of hot flashes. J Clin Oncol 2002;20:1578–83.

61. Treatment of menopause-associated vasomotor symptoms: position statement of The North American Menopause Society. North American Menopause Society. Menopause 2004;11:11–33.

62. Yonkers KA. Paroxetine treatment of mood disorders in women: premenstrual dysphoric disorder and hot flashes. Psychopharmacol Bull 2003;37(suppl 1):135–47.

63. Hebert LE, Scherr PA, Beckett LA, Albert MS, Pilgrim DM, Chown MJ, et al. Age-specific incidence of Alzheimer's disease in a community population. JAMA 1995;273: 1354–9.

64. van Duijn CM, Clayton D, Chandra V, Fratiglioni L, Graves AB, Heyman A, et al. Familial aggregation of Alzheimer's disease and related disorders: a collaborative re-analysis of case-control studies. EURODEM Risk Factors Research Group. Int J Epidemiol 1991;20 Suppl 2:S13–20.

65. Nussbaum RL, Ellis CE. Alzheimer's disease and Parkinson's disease [published erratum appears in N Engl J Med 2003;348:2588]. N Engl J Med 2003;348:1356–64.

66. Gao S, Hendrie HC, Hall KS, Hui S. The relationships between age, sex, and the incidence of dementia and Alzheimer disease: a meta-analysis. Arch Gen Psychiatry 1998;55:809–15.

67. Morin-Martin M, Gonzalez-Santiago R, Gil-Nunez AC, Vivancos-Mora J. Women and strokes. Hospital epidemiology in Spain [Spanish]. Rev Neurol 2003;37:701–5.

68. Di Carlo A, Lamassa M, Baldereschi M, Pracucci G, Basile AM, Wolfe CD, et al. Sex differences in the clinical presentation, resource use, and 3-month outcome of acute stroke in Europe: data from a multicenter multinational hospital–based registry. European BIOMED Study of Stroke Care Group. Stroke 2003;34:1114–9.

69. Cacabelos R, Alvarez A, Lombardi V, Fernandez-Novoa L, Corzo L, Perez P, et al. Pharmacological treatment of Alzheimer disease: from psychotropic drugs and cholinesterase inhibitors to pharmacogenomics. Drugs Today (Barc) 2000;36:415–99.

70. Cacabelos R. Pharmacogenomics and therapeutic prospects in dementia. Eur Arch Psychiatry Clin Neurosci 2008;258(suppl 1):28–47.

71. Yaffe K, Sawaya G, Lieberburg I, Grady D. Estrogen therapy in postmenopausal women: effects on cognitive function and dementia. JAMA 1998;279:688–95.

72. LeBlanc ES, Janowsky J, Chan BK, Nelson HD. Hormone replacement therapy and cognition: systematic review and meta-analysis. JAMA 2001;285:1489–99.

73. Hogervorst E, Williams J, Budge M, Riedel W, Jolles J. The nature of the effect of female gonadal hormone replacement therapy on cognitive function in post-menopausal women: a mate-analysis. Neuroscience 2000;101:485–512.

74. Shumaker SA, Legault C, Rapp SR, Thal L, Wallace RB, Ockene JK, et al. Estrogen plus progestin and the incidence of dementia and mild cognitive impairment in postmenopausal women: the Women's Health Initiative Memory Study: a randomized controlled trial. WHIMS Investigators. JAMA 2003;289:2651–62.

75. Rapp SR, Espeland MA, Shumaker SA, Henderson VW, Brunner RL, Manson JE, et al. Effect of estrogen plus progestin on global cognitive function in postmenopausal women: the Women's Health Initiative Memory Study: a randomized controlled trial. WHIMS Investigators. JAMA 2003;289:2663–72.

76. Shumaker SA, Legault C, Kuller L, Rapp SR, Thal L, Lane DS, et al. Conjugated equine estrogens and incidence of probable dementia and mild cognitive impairment in postmenopausal women: Women's Health Initiative Memory Study. Women's Health Initiative Memory Study. JAMA 2004;291:2947–58.

Sleep Disorders

Thomas E. Nolan

Sleep is a natural state of bodily rest. It appears to have restorative benefit and is essential for survival. Any sleep deprivation, but especially chronic sleep deprivation, may decrease job performance; adversely affect immunocompetence and inflammatory response; and increase accident rates, mood disturbances, and all-cause mortality (1). Sleep-related problems affect 50 million to 70 million Americans across the age spectrum and have a major impact on society. The most common disorders described in the literature are insomnia, sleep apnea, restless leg syndrome, and narcolepsy–cataplexy. The risk for women is comparable or higher than the risk for men. The prevalence of insomnia is higher in women than in men at all ages. The prevalence of sleep apnea increases in women during and after menopause. Sex-specific rates for restless leg syndrome have not been characterized well, but they appear to be higher in women than in men, particularly during pregnancy. Narcolepsy–cataplexy occurs in women at the same frequency as in men (2).

Sleep disorders, such as insomnia and sleep apnea, diabetes mellitus, and related cardiac disorders are a continuum in the aging process and are interrelated. These disorders in part are related to weight gain, which usually accompanies aging; affects the anatomy of the upper airway; and is associated with diabetes mellitus, hypertension, and cardiovascular disease. A linear relationship exists between weight or body mass index and sleep-related disorders. In women, sleep also be may affected by hormonal changes from menarche to menopause, followed by specific problems related to the menopause.

Sleep disorders among women have become more common with the increased stresses of employment outside the home and family needs. Risk factors for sleep deprivation are found in Box 43. Chronic sleep deprivation may have associated health problems, including depression-related tendencies, fibromyalgia, and chronic fatigue syndrome. New data suggest that sleep restrictions may lead to increased appetite and caloric intake (primarily of high-fat and salty foods), resulting in obesity and associated medical problems.

An interesting observation is the linkage of sleep disorders, primarily insomnia, with associated medical conditions of depression, chronic fatigue syndrome, and fibromyalgia. Abnormal levels of corticotropin-releasing factor have been considered by some researchers as a potential etiology and may lead to future contributions that can help physicians deal with these disorders more effectively (3).

Insomnia

Insomnia is defined as difficulty with the initiation, maintenance, duration, or quality of sleep that results in the impairment of daytime functioning, despite adequate opportunity and circumstances for sleep (4). Sleep maintenance problems involve waking after initiating sleep but before a defined wake time. A common definition of *delay of sleep* is an inability to fall asleep for 30 minutes after retiring. Insomnia is characterized as transient (less than 1 week's duration), short-term (duration of 1–4 weeks) and chronic (duration longer than 1 month). Individuals most affected by chronic insomnia are women, older adults, and patients with chronic medical and psychiatric diseases.

A working concept of insomnia is found in Box 44 (secondary insomnia is more common than primary

---

Resources

Sleep Disorders

American Academy of Sleep Medicine
http://www.aasmnet.org

American Sleep Apnea Association
http://www.sleepapnea.org

National Sleep Foundation
http://www.sleepfoundation.org

Restless Leg Syndrome Foundation
http://www.rls.org

Box 43

Risk Factors for Sleep Deprivation

- Employment and other lifestyle factors that lead to sleep deprivation
- Alcohol and substance use
- Smoking
- Depression
- Chronic medical conditions
- Stressful life events
- Pregnancy and postpartum period
- Menopause
- Aging

Hunt CE. Sleep problems and sleep disorders. Clin Update Womens Health Care 2004;III(2):1–108.

Box 44

Classification of Insomnia

Primary Insomnia

- *Idiopathic:* beginning in childhood and persistent and unremitting
- *Psychophysiologic:* maladaptive responsive to the bed environment where the individual has a heightened arousal state. Associated with an event that caused acute insomnia that did not resolve.
- *Paradoxical:* mismatch between individual's descriptions of sleep not supported by polysomnographic findings

Secondary Insomnia

- *Adjustment:* associated with secondary psychosocial stressors
- *Poor sleep hygiene:* lifestyle habits that interfere with sleep
- *Psychiatric:* active psychiatric disorder, such as depression or anxiety disorders
- *Medical:* chronic pain, cough, dyspnea, hot flushes, and restless leg syndrome
- *Drug or substance related:* consumption or discontinuation of medication, illicit drugs, caffeine, and alcohol

---

insomnia). A more extensive history of the sleep disorder should focus on the nature and length of the disorder. Acute insomnia may be the result of a recent stressor in the individual's life, such as work, financial, or family conditions. This stressor may lead to excessive worrying in bed. If the condition becomes chronic, it may lead to additional problems, including poor interpersonal relationships, occupational problems, and poor quality of life.

A physician who has recognized an insomnia disorder in a patient should interview a patient's bed partner or initiate keeping of a sleep diary. The patient should keep the diary for 2–4 weeks and include the time she goes to bed, the number of awakenings during the night, the time of waking, and the subjective quality of sleep. The diary also should note food intake and time, medication dosing, caffeine intake, and alcohol use. Once the diary is done, a strategy may be formalized. The most common interventions are primarily cognitive or behavioral therapy and pharmacologic therapies.

Unique to women is hormonal status and how it may affect sleep. Progesterone has a profound effect on sleep. Intravenously administered progesterone directly stimulates benzodiazepine receptors and γ-aminobutyric acid receptors. As progesterone levels begin to drop at the end of a normal menstrual cycle, the number of arousals increases. Estrogen decreases sleep latency, decreases the number of awakenings after sleep occurs, increases total sleep time, increases rapid eye movement sleep, and decreases the number of cyclic spontaneous arousals (5). Sleep-related breathing disorders associated with weight gain and hot flushes increase during menopause. Vasomotor instability is the most common reason for sleep disturbance in menopause because it leads to more frequent arousals and changed sleep architecture (6).

Therapy for insomnia usually begins with cognitive behavioral therapy (Box 45), primarily addressing lifestyle problems. Up to 50% of patients will respond to cognitive behavioral therapy. Combined therapy has been found to be more effective than individual components. In most cases, this therapy can be accomplished by primary care physicians or psychologists in three to six sessions. Other sources of therapy that may be used at the patient's convenience are videotapes and written manuals.

Box 45

Cognitive Behavioral Therapeutic Interventions

Stimulus Control Therapy*

- Use bedroom only for sleeping and sex
- Go to bed only when sleepy
- If unable to fall asleep in 20 minutes, leave bed and engage in quite activity or reading
- Avoid daytime napping
- Have a regular wake time, regardless of duration of sleep

Sleep Restrictive Therapy†

- Reduce time in bed to estimated total sleep time (5 hour minimum)
- Increase time in bed by 15 minutes per week when estimated sleep efficiency ratio is at least 90% (ratio of time asleep to time in bed)

Sleep-Hygiene Education‡

- Correction of extrinsic factors affecting sleep
  - Environmental factors, such as pets or snoring bed partner
  - Bedroom temperature
  - Fixation on bedside clock
  - Substance use (caffeine, alcohol, and nicotine)
  - Lack of exercise or exercise too close to bedtime

*Bootzin RR, Epstein D, Wood JM. Stimulus control instructions. In: Haurie PJ, editor. Case studies in insomnia. New York (NY): Plenum Medical Books; 1991. p. 19–28.

†Spielman AJ, Saskin P, Thorpy MJ. Treatment of chronic insomnia by restriction of time in bed. Sleep 1987; 10:45–56.

‡Haurie PJ. Sleep hygiene, relation therapy, and cognitive interventions. In: Case studies in insomnia. New York (NY): Plenum Medical Books; 1991. p. 65–84.

Pharmacologic interventions are used for short-term therapy or in more resistant cases of insomnia. Medications most commonly used that were approved by the U.S. Food and Drug Administration (FDA) are the benzodiazepines, the benzodiazepine-receptor agonists (γ-aminobutyric acid A receptors), and melatonin-receptor agonists. Commonly used formulations are listed in Table 17. Most of these agents have been shown to relieve short-term insomnia, but studies are lacking for use longer than 6 months. Short-acting agents work best for decreasing sleep latency, whereas the intermediate and long-term agents work best for increasing total sleep time. Benzodiazepines are FDA pregnancy category X. They are contraindicated in pregnancy because the risks involved with their use by pregnant women clearly outweigh the potential benefits. Benzodiazepine-receptor agonists are FDA pregnancy category C. Despite the lack of well-controlled human data, potential benefits of these agents may outweigh potential risks and warrant their use by pregnant women. Reduced dosages should be taken by elderly or debilitated patients and individuals with hepatic insufficiency. The use of over-the-counter medications, primarily sedating histamine derivatives, is not supported by data as being effective. The melatonin-receptor agonist ramelteon, although approved by the FDA, also has shown conflicting data concerning efficacy (7). Withdrawal symptoms and rebound insomnia are rare after discontinuation of the benzodiazepines, except triazolam, which may last 1–3 days.

Sleep Apnea

Obstructive sleep apnea is a clinical syndrome defined primarily as the intermittent cessation of airflow at the nose and mouth during sleep. Although the syndrome is most commonly found in men (incidence, 4%), the incidence is 2% in women aged 30–60 years (8). The disease may be underdiagnosed in women because of a lack of recognition among health care providers. Sleep apnea may stem from a central nervous system cause, but it primarily occurs when the soft tissues of the posterior pharynx relax and obstruct airflow to various degrees. When airflow ceases, the individual briefly awakens but often is not conscious that awakening has occurred.

Because the patient awakens anywhere from 400 to 500 times a night, restorative sleep does not take place. Lacking restorative sleep, patients fall asleep during routine work and activities. Because sleep can occur during operation of heavy machinery and automobiles, sleep apnea has the potential for very serious consequences (9).

The definitive event in an obstructive sleep apnea cycle is occlusion of the upper airway at the level of the oral pharynx. This apnea spell leads to progressive asphyxia until the patient briefly arouses from sleep, which then changes the tone of the airway and reverses the apnea. The upper airway is thought to collapse because of degeneration of critical subatmospheric pressure during inspiration, which exceeds the ability of

Table 17. Medications for Insomnia Approved by the U.S. Food and Drug Administration

Medication	Duration of Action, Half Life (Hours)	Dose	Indications	Side Effects
Benzodiazepines				
Temazepam	Intermediate, 8–15	7.5–30 mg	Sleep-maintenance insomnia	Drowsiness, dizziness, and incoordination
Estazolam	Intermediate, 10–24	0.5–2 mg	Sleep-maintenance insomnia	Drowsiness, dizziness, and incoordination
Triazolam	Short, 2–5	0.125–0.25 mg	Sleep-onset insomnia	Amnesia, drowsiness, dizziness, and incoordination
Benzodiazepine-Receptor Agonists				
Eszopiclone	Intermediate, 5–7	1–3 mg	Sleep-maintenance insomnia	Unpleasant taste, dry mouth, dizziness, and incoordination
Zolpidem	Short, 3	5–10 mg	Sleep-onset insomnia	Drowsiness, dizziness, and occasional amnesia
Zaleplon	Ultrashort, 1	5–20 mg	Sleep onset and sleep maintenance insomnia	Drowsiness

the airway dilator and abductor muscles to maintain stability and hence patency. Activity of the muscles in the upper airway is greater during the day, when the patient is awake and able to compensate for airway narrowing. Sleep reduces the activity of these muscles; therefore, the protective reflex response to subatmospheric airway pressure is overcome, resulting in transient obstruction.

A prominent observation in most patients with sleep apnea is that they snore excessively. Snoring is the result of relaxation of the upper airways, which sets up a vibratory response. Commonly found covariables in sleep apnea syndrome are alcohol use (which indirectly decreases muscular tone) and anatomic disturbances, such as adenotonsillar hypertrophy, retrognathia, and macroglossia. These anatomic variations result in narrowing of the upper airways, adding to the obstruction of flow. Many affected individuals have phenotypical characteristics, such as enlarged necks or small chins. These anatomic changes result in what is clinically described as "pharyngeal crowding" and may be demonstrated by imaging and acoustic reflection techniques. However, the primary problem in these individuals is increased fat deposition in the soft tissues of the pharynx that collapse during sleep, causing the obstruction.

A cyclic disorder occurs and leads to the overt clinical manifestation of sleep apnea. Sleep begins, followed by an episode of apnea that causes hypoxia and hypercapnia, which results in respiratory acidosis. These physiologic changes result in a brief arousal from sleep that may last anywhere from 10 seconds (the usual minimal interval that is classified as apnea) to 2–3 minutes. Airflow resumes on arousal, and the patient continues to sleep until the next episode of apnea. The major physiologic consequences of these episodes of apnea include vagal bradycardia with ectopic cardiac beats, pulmonary vasoconstriction, and systemic vasoconstriction with acute carbon dioxide retention. These events may lead to left-sided heart failure, unexplained death, systemic hypertension, and chronic hyperventilation. Arousal from sleep initiates a mechanism that results in cerebral dysfunction with a loss of deep sleep and manifests as excessive daytime sleepiness.

Screening and Diagnosis

Obstructive sleep apnea should be suspected among individuals who experience hypersomnolence and are obese, have hypertension, or are habitual snorers. In the primary care setting, patients at high risk meet two of the following three criteria: 1) they snore, 2) they experience persistent daytime sleepiness or drowsiness while driving, and (3) they have obesity or hypertension (10).

The following simple office test has been devised to predict which individuals are at high risk (11). The neck circumference is measured in centimeters. This mea-

surement is adjusted by adding centimeters for the patient who:

- Has hypertension—4 cm is added.
- Is a habitual snorer—3 cm is added.
- Is reported to choke or gasp most nights—3 cm is added.

Patients who have an adjusted neck circumference of less than 43 cm have a low probability of sleep apnea unless daytime symptoms are noticeable. Observation is recommended for this group. Patients with an intermediate neck measurement (43–48 cm) or a large adjusted circumference (greater than 48 cm) should be considered for polysomnography if this technique is readily available. Polysomnography consists of electroencephalography, electroculography, submental electromyography, and measurement of arterial oxygenation saturation by ear or finger oximetry, as well as heart rate and ventilatory variables that permit the identification of apneas and their classification as central or obstructive (12). The key diagnostic finding is episodes of airflow cessation at the nose and mouth despite continuing respiratory effort.

Because of the expense of polysomnography and its relative lack of availability, the use of overnight oximetry has been advocated (13). Essentially, oxygen desaturation is measured during sleep. By testing individuals with the clinical syndrome (eg, sleepiness, obesity, and high neck circumference), combined with at least 10–15 oxygen desaturation events per hour, one third of tested patients will have the diagnosis of obstructive sleep apnea either confirmed or excluded. The remaining subjects fall into the intermediate category, for which further studies are needed.

Management

Obstructive sleep apnea may be treated in several ways. A patient who has been ingesting alcohol and sedatives should avoid these drugs to increase upper airway muscle tone during sleep. Because most of these patients are obese, weight reduction and the avoidance of supine posture are helpful. Occasionally, patients can be fitted with an oral prosthesis that may improve nasal patency.

In most cases, nasal continuous positive airway pressure may be applied. Essentially, this technique mechanically increases the amount of airway pressure to avoid collapse of the upper airways. Devices to increase airway pressure are portable and are successful in up to 80% of patients with mild to moderate disorders (14).

The use of continuous positive airway pressure devices helps with sleep and reduces the daytime sleepiness in patients with mild to moderate obstruction. Patients who are compliant with these devices have increased maintenance of wakefulness and better daily functioning. However, compliance is a problem with the use of these devices; more than 50% of patients discontinue their use after weeks of therapy. Bilevel positive airway pressure is a variation of continuous positive airway pressure, but little difference in outcomes is seen (15, 16).

In severe cases of upper airway obstruction, an uvulopalatopharyngoplasty may be performed. Although palatopharyngoplasty has been successful in some cases, its success declines over time (17). Recently, surgeons have used laser surgery on the palate with various degrees of success. Finally, tracheostomy has been performed to bypass the upper airways in severe cases (8).

Medical implications of sleep apnea may reflect the overall etiology of obesity. Weight gain leads to type 2 diabetes mellitus, dyslipidemia, and pulmonary and systemic hypertension. Eventually, these factors may lead to right-sided congestive heart failure secondary to primary obstruction to pulmonary blood flow. Electrocardiographic evidence of *cor pulmonale* (right-sided heart failure) is a late finding. Individuals with sleep apnea have increased hypertension, pulmonary hypertension, right- and left-sided heart failure, coronary artery disease with myocardial infarction, and stroke (18).

Restless Leg Syndrome

Restless leg syndrome is estimated to affect approximately 7–10% of Americans; it disproportionately affects women more than men, reportedly at a 2:1 ratio. Affected participants perceive a disagreeable sensation typically in their legs, typically more often when they are inactive, and especially at night when they are asleep. The sensations decrease with activity, and patients have a strong urge to move. This syndrome interrupts normal sleep patterns.

Restless leg syndrome has a strong genetic component, with a positive family history reported in 63–92% of cases. Restless leg syndrome also is associated with iron deficiency (with or without anemia), pregnancy (with an incidence high as 19%), renal failure, periodic limb movements, and neuropathies, including essential tremor and some hereditary ataxias.

Asking patients with sleep disorders whether they perceive creeping, crawling, or uncomfortable, difficult-to-describe feelings; whether these feelings correlate with time of day, activity, or inactivity; and whether the feelings interfere with sleep may may yield the diagnosis of restless leg syndrome. Restless leg syndrome is a clinical diagnosis based on history. The International Restless Legs Syndrome Study Group has recommended clinical criteria for diagnosis (Box 46). Polysomnography is not routinely indicated. Evaluation for iron deficiency with ferritin level determination, for diabetes mellitus, and for renal failure should be considered.

Recent advances suggest that restless leg syndrome is associated with a dopaminergic dysfunction and brain iron deficiency. Patients with mild symptoms may not need medication therapy. The current first-line medication therapy, shown to be effective in decreasing symptoms of restless leg syndrome, is the use of dopaminergic agents (levodopa, carbidopa, pergolide, pramipexole, and ropinirole) (Table 18). Pramipexole has been approved by the FDA for the treatment of restless leg syndrome. Because of side effects and the potential for augmentation (continued therapy results in worse symptoms), therapy often should be individualized.

Box 46

Clinical Criteria for the Diagnosis of Restless Leg Syndrome

Minimal Criteria

- A compelling urge to move the limbs usually associated with paresthesias and dysesthesias
- Motor restlessness as seen in activities, such as floor pacing, tossing and turning in bed, and rubbing the legs
- Worsening of symptoms or symptoms exclusively present at rest (ie, lying and sitting) with variable and temporary relief by activity
- Worsening of symptoms in the evening and at night

Associated Features

- Sleep disturbance and daytime fatigue
- Normal neurologic examination (in patients with primary restless leg syndrome)
- Involuntary, repetitive, periodic, and jerking limb movements, either in sleep or while awake or at rest

Walters AS. Toward a better definition of the restless leg syndrome. The International Restless Legs Syndrome Study Group. Mov Disord 1995;10:634–42.x. © 1995 John Wiley & Sons, Inc. Reproduced with permission of John Wiley & Sons, Inc.

References

1. Dinges DF. Stress, fatigue, and behavioral energy. Nutr Rev 2001;59:S30–2.

2. Hunt CE. Sleep problems and sleep disorders. Clin Update Womens Health Care 2004;III(2):1–108.

3. Roth T, Roehrs T, Pies R. Insomnia: pathophysiology and implications for treatment. Sleep Med Rev 2007;11:71–9.

4. Costa e Silva JA, Chase M, Sartorius N, Roth T. Special report from a symposium held by the World Health Organization and the World Federation of Sleep Research Societies: an overview of insomnias and related disorders—recognition, epidemiology, and rational management. Sleep 1996;19:412–6.

5. Manber R, Armitage R. Sex, steroids, and sleep: a review. Sleep 1999;22:540–55.

6. Shaver JL, Giblin E, Paulsen V. Sleep quality subtypes in midlife women. Sleep 1991;14:18–23.

7. Rogers NL, Dinges DF, Kennaway DJ, Dawson D. Potential action of melatonin in insomnia. Sleep 2003;26:1058–9.

8. Bresnitz EA, Goldberg R, Kosinski RM. Epidemiology of obstructive sleep apnea. Epidemiol Rev 1994;16:210–27.

9. Sleep apnea, sleepiness, and driving risk. American Thoracic Society. Am J Respir Crit Care Med 1994;150: 1463–73.

10. Netzer NC, Stoohs RA, Netzer CM, Clark K, Strohl KP. Using the Berlin Questionnaire to identify patients at risk for the sleep apnea syndrome. Ann Intern Med 1999;131: 485–91.

11. Flemons WW, Whitelaw WA, Brant R, Remmers JE. Likelihood ratios for a sleep apnea clinical prediction rule. Am J Respir Crit Care Med 1994;150:1279–85.

12. Practice parameters for the indications for polysomnography and related procedures. Polysomnography Task Force, American Sleep Disorders Association Standards of Practice Committee. Sleep 1997;20:406–22.

13. Flemons WW. Clinical practice. Obstructive sleep apnea. N Engl J Med 2002;347:498–504.

14. McArdle N, Devereux G, Heidarnejad H, Engleman HM, Mackay TW, Douglas NJ. Long-term use of CPAP therapy for sleep apnea/hypopnea syndrome. Am J Respir Crit Care Med 1999;159:1108–14.

15. Marshall NS, Barnes M, Travier N, Campbell AJ, Pierce RJ, McEvoy RD, et al. Continuous positive airway pressure reduces daytime sleepiness in mild to moderate obstructive sleep apnoea: a meta-analysis. Thorax 2006;61:430–4.

16. Series F. Evaluation of treatment efficacy in sleep apnea hypopnea syndrome. Sleep 1996;19:S71–6.

17. Janson C, Gislason T, Bengtsson H, Eriksson G, Lindberg E, Lindholm CE, et al. Long-term follow-up of patients with obstructive sleep apnea treated with uvulopalatopharyngoplasty. Arch Otolaryngol Head Neck Surg 1997;123: 257–62.

18. Poirier P, Giles TD, Bray GA, Hong Y, Stern JS, Pi-Sunyer FX, et al. Obesity and cardiovascular disease: pathophysiology, evaluation, and effect of weight loss: an update of the 1997 American Heart Association Scientific Statement on Obesity and Heart Disease from the Obesity Committee of the Council on Nutrition, Physical Activity, and Metabolism. American Heart Association; Obesity Committee of the Council on Nutrition, Physical Activity, and Metabolism. Circulation 2006;113:898–918.

Table 18. Pharmacologic Treatment for Patients With Restless Leg Syndrome

Agent	Advantage	Disadvantage
Dopaminergic agents; eg, carbidopa and levodopa	Can be used on a one-time basis or as circumstances require, useful for control of intermittent RLS because dopamine antagonists take longer to be effective	Up to 80% of patients develop augmentation (symptoms worse with treatment)
Dopaminergic agents; eg, pergolide, pramipexole (FDA approved for RLS), and ropinirole	Useful in moderate to severe RLS, reports indicate high efficacy but role of their long-term use is unknown	Can cause severe sleepiness, limiting use in daytime; agonists can cause nausea
Opioids; eg, codeine, hydrocodone, oxycodone, propoxyphene, and tramadol	Can be used on a intermittent basis but also on a daily basis	Tolerance and dependence possible, can cause constipation, urinary retention, sleepiness, or cognitive changes
Benzodiazepines; eg, clonazepam and temazepam	Helpful in some patients when other medications not tolerated and may improve sleep	Can cause daytime sleepiness and cognitive impairment
Anticonvulsants; eg, carbamazepine and gabapentin	Consider when dopaminergic agents fail, may be useful when RLS coexists with peripheral neuropathy or when RLS sensations are described as pain	Side effects vary depending on agent, but include gastrointestinal disturbance, such as nausea, sedation, and dizziness.
Iron (ferrous sulfate)	Use in patient with ferritin levels less than 50 ng/mL	Ideal means of administration not established; oral route may take months and is poorly tolerated
Clonidine	May be useful in hypertensive patients	Potential to cause hypotension, dermatitis, and sleepiness

Abbreviations: FDA indicates U.S. Food and Drug Administration; RLS, restless leg syndrome.

Diabetes Mellitus

Siri L. Kjos and Thomas Buchanan

Diabetes mellitus is a chronic disorder of metabolism characterized by an absolute or relative lack of insulin that results in metabolic derangements ranging from asymptomatic hyperglycemia that imparts a risk of chronic complications to severe decompensation manifested as ketoacidosis, a hyperosmolar state, or both. The long-term complications of diabetes mellitus (retinopathy, nephropathy, neuropathy, and accelerated atherosclerosis) account for most of the morbidity and mortality that result from this condition.

Classification and Related Conditions

Diabetes

Diabetes results from the failure of pancreatic β-cells to secrete sufficient insulin to meet the needs of liver and skeletal muscle, the primary insulin-responsive tissues in the body (1). The β-cell failure can have a variety of causes. Autoimmune destruction of the β-cells (type 1 diabetes mellitus) occurs chiefly in young individuals and leads to absolute insulin deficiency. Type 1 diabetes mellitus accounts for less than 10% of all cases of diabetes, whereas β-cell failure (usually progressive) that occurs on a background of insulin resistance (type 2 diabetes mellitus) accounts for most cases (more than 90%). Obesity is the most common cause of insulin resistance that leads to type 2 diabetes mellitus in developed countries. Other causes of insulin resistance (eg, insulin receptor mutations, acromegaly, and Cushing syndrome) are less common. Specific genetic abnormalities that alter β-cell function can lead to a relatively mild form of diabetes mellitus with autosomal-dominant inheritance (maturity-onset diabetes of youth). At least six separate genes have been identified as causes of distinct types of maturity-onset diabetes of youth

Diabetes that occurs without an obvious precipitating disease, such as acromegaly or Cushing disease, is sometimes referred to as *primary diabetes mellitus*, whereas diabetes mellitus without an obvious cause may be called *secondary diabetes mellitus*. This arbitrary distinction loses relevance as distinct causes of "primary" diabetes mellitus are defined. Nonpregnant individuals whose glucose levels are outside the reference range but below the diabetic range have impaired fasting glucose or impaired glucose tolerance (Table 19), also called *prediabetes*. Those individuals are at increased risk of developing diabetes mellitus compared with people with normal glucose tolerance (1–4).

Gestational Diabetes Mellitus

Gestational diabetes mellitus is defined as glucose intolerance with an onset or first recognition during pregnancy (5). Criteria for gestational diabetes mellitus identify women without a known history of diabetes mellitus whose glucose levels are in the upper portion of the population distribution. These women impart to their babies an increased risk of perinatal complications and, possibly, a long-term risk of obesity and diabetes mellitus. Women with gestational diabetes mellitus also are at increased risk for developing diabetes mellitus when they are not pregnant, as are people with other forms of abnormal glucose tolerance. Because of these increased risks, mothers with prior gestational diabetes mellitus and their offspring should be educated to avoid obesity and should be tested periodically for the development of diabetes. After delivery, women should undergo glucose tolerance testing (75-g, 2-hour test) to reclassify their status as having diabetes mellitus, impaired fasting glucose or glucose tolerance, or normoglycemia. Thereafter, if they do not have diabetes, they should undergo testing for this disease 1 year after delivery and subsequently at a minimum of every 3 years.

Metabolic Syndrome

Of increasing interest and prevalence is the metabolic syndrome, also known as insulin resistance syndrome or syndrome X. Different authoritative bodies recommend different definitions of metabolic syndrome; all include obesity, lipid abnormalities, and elevated blood pressure (6–9). One approach to the diagnosis is listed in Table 20. Most individuals with *metabolic syndrome* have insulin resistance, and metabolic syndrome is a risk factor for type 2 diabetes mellitus. In addition to diabetes mellitus, individuals with metabolic syndrome are at increased risk for conditions, such as polycystic ovary syndrome (PCOS), fatty liver, cholesterol gallstones, asthma, and sleep apnea.

Resources

Diabetes Mellitus

American Diabetes Association
http://www.diabetes.org

National Diabetes Education Program
http://www.ndep.nih.gov

National Institute of Diabetes and Digestive and
Kidney Diseases
http://www2.niddk.nih.gov

Table 19. Diagnosis of Diabetes Mellitus in Nonpregnant Adults

Classification	Normal Levels (mg/dL)	Impaired levels (mg/dL)	Diabetes[‡] (mg/dL)
Random glucose levels with symptoms of overt hyperglycemia (fatigue, weight loss, thirst, and polyuria)	–	–	200 or greater[‡]
Fasting plasma glucose levels*	Less than 100	100–125	126 or greater[‡]
Two-hour glucose levels[†]	Less than 140	140–199	200 or greater[‡]

*Measured on plasma in a certified clinical laboratory, fasting is defined as no caloric intake for a least 8 hours.

[†] 75-g, 2 hour oral glucose tolerance test

[‡]Confirm diagnosis on a subsequent day by any one of the three methods listed, eg, fasting plasma glucose levels of 126 mg/dL or greater.

Data from Diagnosis and classification of diabetes mellitus. American Diabetes Association. Diabetes Care 2008;31(suppl 1):S55-60.

Table 20. Clinical Features of the Metabolic Syndrome*

Risk Factor	Defining Level
Abdominal obesity (waist circumference)	Greater than 102 cm (40 in) for men Greater than 88 cm (35 in) for women
High-density lipoprotein cholesterol	Less than 40 mg/dL for men Less than 50 mg/dL for women
Triglycerides	Greater than or equal to 150 mg/dL
Fasting glucose	Greater than or equal to 110 mg/dL
Blood pressure	Greater than or equal to 130 mm Hg systolic Greater than or equal to 85 mm Hg diastolic

*Metabolic syndrome is present if three of the five risk factors are abnormal.

Modified from Third Report of the National Cholesterol Education Program (NCEP) Expert Panel on Detection, Evaluation, and Treatment of High Blood Cholesterol in Adults (Adult Treatment Panel III) final report. National Cholesterol Education Program (NCEP) Expert Panel on Detection, Evaluation, and Treatment of High Blood Cholesterol in Adults (Adult Treatment Panel III). Circulation 2002;106:3143–421.

The National Cholesterol Education Program recommends intervention to reverse the underlying risk factors for metabolic syndrome, namely, overweight (having a body mass index of 25–29.9 [expressed as weight in kilograms divided by height in meters squared]) and obesity (body mass index of 30 or greater), physical inactivity, and atherogenic diet. Lifestyle modifications, targeting weight loss, and exercise are the first line of therapy (6). Weight loss decreases the levels of serum low-density lipoprotein cholesterol (LDL-C) and triglycerides; increases the levels of high-density lipoprotein cholesterol (HDL-C); decreases blood pressure, glucose levels, and insulin resistance; and decreases the levels of C-reactive protein and plasminogen activator inhibitor-1.

The most effective and healthful strategies for long-term weight loss are reduced-energy diets with a modest reduction in intake of 500–1,000 kcal/d and a weight loss target of approximately 7–10% per 6–12 months. Healthful eating habits need to be incorporated; eg, setting goals, eating regular and planned meals, reading labels, reducing portion sizes, and avoiding eating binges. For detailed recommendations for healthy eating and weight reduction, see "Role of Exercise, Diet, and Medical Intervention in Weight Management." Nutritional recommendations include avoiding extreme intake of either carbohydrates or fats; maintaining a low intake of saturated fats, trans fats, and cholesterol; limiting intake of simple sugars; and increasing intake of vegetables, fruit, and whole grains.

Behavioral and medical therapy to stop or reduce cigarette smoking should not be neglected. A minimum of 30 minutes daily of moderate-intensity exercise is recommended for all adults. Initiating daily exercise in sedentary individuals involves changes in behavior (reducing television and computer use), starting with short (10- to 15-minute) bouts of exercise, adding exercise into daily routines (taking stairs or walking at lunchtime), and self-monitoring (10). Several clinical trials have demonstrated that combining daily exercise with weight reduction can reduce the progression of impaired glucose tolerance to type 2 diabetes mellitus by one half, but the effect of lifestyle on reducing cardiovascular (CV) disease risk has yet to be demonstrated.

Medical therapy may be needed for atherogenic dyslipidemia. The administration of statins in combination with fibrates has been shown to improve atherogenic dyslipidemia and possible CV disease end points (11). Similarly, recommendations from the *Seventh Report of the Joint National Committee on Prevention, Detection, Evaluation, and Treatment of High Blood Pressure* on medical therapy for the treatment of hypertension should be followed (12). The report recognized "prehypertension" (120–139/80–89 mm Hg) as a risk category for CV disease. Categorical hypertension (140 or greater/90 or greater mm Hg) should be treated medically. The selection of antihypertensive agent appears to be less important than achieving normal-range blood pressure and should take into account comorbidities, such as diabetes mellitus and dyslipidemia. Daily aspirin therapy should be considered for patients whose 10-year risk of coronary artery disease is 10% or greater (13).

Polycystic Ovary Syndrome

Polycystic ovary syndrome may be associated with metabolic syndrome. A not uncommon condition in women of reproductive age, PCOS was originally described as an association of amenorrhea, hirsutism, obesity, and enlarged, cystic ovaries (14). Some of the softer surrogate markers of coronary artery disease, such as intimal medial thickness, carotid plaque index, coronary artery calcification, endothelin-1, and homocysteine, have been shown to be present or increased in patients with PCOS. However, no outcomes studies have established a relationship between these markers and levels of CV risk associated with PCOS (14).

Obesity in patients with PCOS is centripetal and characterized by a pattern of fat distribution that is a predictor of diabetes mellitus and dyslipidemia. The association of hypertension and PCOS appears to be variable (15). The importance of hypertension as a CV risk factor, as well as the end-organ complications of the disease, warrant close and consistent monitoring of blood pressure in patients with PCOS. Insulin resistance, glucose intolerance, and the development of diabetes mellitus also are associated with PCOS (15). Diabetes mellitus elevates the level of CV risk of the PCOS patient, because diabetes mellitus is a CV risk equivalent to the presence of coronary artery disease (16). Polycystic ovary syndrome is consistently associated with dyslipidemia. Lipid profile abnormalities include elevated levels of triglycerides and LDL-C, with lower levels of HDL-C. Although none of these abnormalities is profound, the abnormalities are nevertheless associated with increased CV risk (7).

In summary, although specific outcomes data regarding PCOS patients and their associated CV factors are not available, it is prudent to assess PCOS patents for all relevant CV risk factors (a so-called global CV risk assessment), irrespective of age. Where appropriate,

aggressive treatment of any abnormalities according to the guidelines is recommended (7, 12, 16–22).

Pathophysiology

Type 1 diabetes mellitus occurs most often when an autoimmune destruction of the pancreatic β-cells leads to a complete lack of insulin production. Without exogenous insulin, patients with type 1 diabetes mellitus experience ketoacidosis. Generally, type 1 diabetes mellitus has an acute onset before age 30 years.

Type 2 diabetes mellitus includes the remaining forms of chronic hyperglycemia severe enough to meet the diagnostic criteria for diabetes mellitus (1). The wide variation in the degree of decreased insulin production relative to the increased insulin demand or peripheral insulin resistance in these patients supports a heterogeneous etiology of type 2 diabetes mellitus. Type 2 diabetes mellitus results from resistance of the muscle, adipose tissue, and liver to insulin action and the failure of β-cells to secrete sufficient insulin, coupled with excess glucose production by the liver in response to circulating glucose and insulin levels (23). Patients with type 2 diabetes mellitus rarely have ketoacidosis. Although some may require insulin for adequate glycemic control, they are not dependent on insulin for survival. Onset of type 2 diabetes mellitus generally is insidious, progressing over years from normal to impaired glucose tolerance, then to asymptomatic diabetes mellitus, and finally to symptomatic hyperglycemia. Based on large surveys, it is estimated that in one third of patients with actual type 2 diabetes mellitus, the disease is undiagnosed and untreated; and the diagnosis often is made after permanent diabetic sequelae have developed (24).

Diagnosis

The diagnosis of diabetes mellitus is based on persistent hyperglycemia, detected in the absence of acute illness that is sufficiently elevated to impart a risk of long-term diabetic complications, such as retinopathy. The current diagnostic criteria used in the United States require one of the three criteria listed in Table 19 (1). The diagnosis of diabetes mellitus can be made based on a certified clinical laboratory identifying one of these criteria by measuring venous serum or plasma glucose levels. Reflectance meters and glycosylated hemoglobin levels should not be used for diagnosis. Determining the fasting plasma glucose level is the preferred method for diagnosing diabetes mellitus in children and nonpregnant adults.

Screening

Type 2 diabetes mellitus accounts for 90% of diabetes mellitus cases. The prevalence of diagnosed diabetes mellitus has increased. According to the National

Health and Nutrition Examination Survey in 2003–2004, the prevalence was 7.8%, with the greatest increases in women, patients aged 40–59 years, non-Hispanic whites, and obese people (24). Screening studies from the United States suggest that an additional 2–3% of the population has undiagnosed type 2 diabetes mellitus. These individuals may have subtle or no symptoms of diabetes mellitus, but they are at risk for long-term diabetic complications (25). Detection of these individuals is the goal of screening programs. No screening program is recommended for type 1 diabetes mellitus, because symptoms of acute hyperglycemia (weight loss, weakness, polydipsia, polyuria, and ketoacidosis) merit immediate testing. Recommendations for screening that apply primarily to type 2 diabetes mellitus are presented in Box 47 (1).

Screening for diabetes mellitus is preferable after 8-hour overnight fasting, but a random serum or plasma glucose level also may be measured in a nonfasting individual (see Table 19). A fasting plasma glucose level of 126 mg/dL or greater defines diabetes mellitus (1). The diagnosis must be confirmed by a subsequent repeated elevated glucose level in the fasting state. Diabetes also can be diagnosed by a 2-hour glucose level of 200 mg/dL or greater after a 75-g, 2-hour oral glucose tolerance test. This method generally is not recommended for the routine diagnosis of diabetes mellitus except after a pregnancy complicated by gestational diabetes mellitus.

Individuals with impaired glucose tolerance or impaired fasting glucose are at increased risk for diabetes mellitus and CV disease compared with individuals with normal glucose levels. Studies have shown that weight loss and regular physical activity, as well as treatment with certain medications that improve insulin resistance or lower glucose levels, can delay or prevent type 2 diabetes mellitus in people with impaired glucose tolerance (2–4). Thus, patients with impaired fasting glucose or impaired glucose tolerance should be advised to implement lifestyle changes, such as weight loss and exercise to reduce their risk of diabetes mellitus and CV disease (3).

Among individuals with gestational diabetes mellitus, risk factors for diabetes mellitus include fasting hyperglycemia requiring insulin during pregnancy, impaired glucose tolerance at postpartum testing, or marked weight gain after delivery (5). All women with prior gestational diabetes mellitus should be considered at risk for diabetes mellitus and be counseled regarding that risk; effective ways to reduce their risk by diet, weight loss, and exercise; and the need to be tested for diabetes mellitus at regular intervals and before any future pregnancies. Identifying women in whom type 2 diabetes mellitus (which may be asymptomatic) has developed before another pregnancy should be a priority. Within 10–20 years after delivery, type 2 diabetes mellitus will have developed in more than one half of women with previous gestational diabetes mellitus (26);

in certain ethnic groups the rate is even higher (up to 50% in 5 years in Hispanic women) (27).

Women with type 1 and type 2 diabetes mellitus in poor glycemic control during embryogenesis impart an increased risk of major congenital anomalies to their babies. The increased teratogenic risk appears to be related to increasing hyperglycemia rather than oral antidiabetic therapy (28). Women with prior gestational diabetes mellitus and women with established type 1 and type 2 diabetes mellitus should practice effective family planning so they can participate in preconception assessment of glucose and hemoglobin (Hb) A_{1c} levels and, for those with diabetes mellitus, preconception diabetes mellitus care. The goal of care is to achieve low-risk glucose levels

---

Box 47

Screening for Prediabetes and Diabetes in Asymptomatic Adult Individuals

1. Testing should be considered in all adults who are overweight (body mass index 25 or greater; expressed as weight in kilograms divided by height in meters squared) and have these additional risk factors:

   - Physical inactivity
   - Family history of diabetes in parents or siblings
   - High-risk ethnicity group for diabetes (Native American, Hispanic, African American, Pacific Islander, and Asian American)
   - History of gestational diabetes or giving birth to a baby weighing more than 9 lb at birth
   - History of impaired fasting glucose or impaired glucose tolerance
   - Hypertension (blood pressure of greater than or equal to 140/90 mmHg) or undergoing therapy for hypertension
   - Total triglyceride level greater than 250 mg/dL, or high-density lipoprotein cholesterol level less than 35 mg/dL
   - History of cardiovascular disease
   - Polycystic ovary syndrome
   - Conditions associated with insulin resistance (severe obesity and *acanthosis nigricans*)

2. In absence of above criteria, testing should begin at age 45 years

3. If results are normal, testing should be repeated at least every 3 years with consideration for more frequent testing depending on initial results and risk status

during embryogenesis. Patients should continue effective contraception until the lowest possible Hb A_{1c} level is achieved without undue risk of hypoglycemia (preferably less than 7%) (1). At each medical visit, pregnancy planning and contraceptive use should be reviewed.

Management

Initial Evaluation

Initial medical evaluation in type 2 diabetes mellitus is similar to that in type 1 diabetes mellitus. Because patients with newly diagnosed type 2 diabetes mellitus could have had unrecognized diabetes mellitus for several years, the physician should perform a thorough examination to detect signs and symptoms of atherosclerosis, neuropathy, retinopathy, and nephropathy, all of which may be present already (25, 29). The initial evaluation should include detailed questions regarding the patient's history; a complete physical examination targeting organs affected by diabetes mellitus; and laboratory screening for glycemia, renal function, hyperlipidemia, and CV disease (Box 48).

Initial Diabetic Education and Medical Management

Although type 1 and type 2 diabetes mellitus differ, they share similar complications, and both require monitoring and management of hyperglycemia. Thus, the two conditions will be considered together here, and differences in management will be described where applicable.

Patients with diabetic complications (retinopathy, neuropathy, nephropathy, and atherosclerosis) and those with type 1 diabetes mellitus should be cared for by a physician with expertise in diabetes mellitus. Similarly, patients who require insulin therapy should have a physician who is experienced in diabetes mellitus management and should have access to a diabetes support team, including a certified diabetic educator and a nutritionist. Obstetrician–gynecologists who assume the role of diabetologist should be familiar with intensive diabetes mellitus management using a team approach (28). When diabetes mellitus care is provided by a diabetes mellitus specialist, the obstetrician–gynecologist should ensure that appropriate management of reproductive issues is in place. Specific issues include effective contraception and the importance of attaining low-risk glycemia during embryogenesis to reduce the risk of malformations. The preconception evaluation should assess and attempt to reduce maternal and fetal risk.

Routine care should be directed toward the prevention of diabetic complications and maintenance of a good quality of life. The risk of developing diabetic retinopathy, nephropathy, and neuropathy increases with the severity and duration of hyperglycemia. For each percentage point of decrease in Hb A_{1c} level, there is an asso-

---

Box 48

Initial Evaluation of Type 2 Diabetes Mellitus

History

- Any symptoms of hyperglycemia (polyuria, polydipsia, blurred vision, weight loss, ketoacidosis, or coma)
- Any symptoms of hypoglycemia (diaphoresis, tachycardia, tremor, confusion, nightmares, and current or previous glucose self-monitoring skills or insulin or oral antihyperglycemic medication use)
- Current or previous evaluation and treatment of diabetic complications (retinopathy, nephropathy, neuropathy, or atherosclerosis)
- Current dietary habits and nutritional education
- Daily exercise and activity habits
- Other cardiovascular risk factors (smoking, hypertension, obesity, hyperlipidemia, menopause, and family history)
- Reproductive status and, if fertile, contraceptive methods and fertility desires
- Current medications use, prescribed and over-the-counter
- Smoking, alcohol consumption, and illicit drug use
- Social support structure and level of education

Physical Examination

- Evaluation of body habitus (height, weight, waist circumference, and calculation of body mass index and percentile of ideal body weight)
- Blood pressure
- Fundiscopic examination with referral to an ophthalmologist for a baseline evaluation
- Periodontal examination with referral, if periodontal disease present
- Cardiovascular examination (including peripheral pulses and bruits)
- Foot and skin examination, including screening for fungal infections (tinea cruris, tinea pedis with onycomycosis, and candidal vaginitis)
- Neurologic examination for peripheral sensation and autonomic dysfunction (lack of sweating or tachycardia)

Laboratory Evaluation

- Fasting plasma glucose
- Hemoglobin A_{1c}
- Fasting lipid profile (total, low-density lipoprotein and high-density lipoprotein cholesterol, and total triglycerides)
- Serum creatinine (+/− 24-hour urine collection for creatinine clearance)
- Random spot urine for albumin/creatinine ratio
- Electrocardiogram

Data from Standards of medical care in diabetes-2008. American Diabetes Association. Diabetes Care 2008;31 (suppl 1): S12-54.

ciated 20–30% reduction in risk of developing sequelae (29, 30). Thus, normalization of Hb A_{1c} levels should be a primary goal of diabetic therapy. Atherosclerosis, a macrovascular complication, leads to coronary artery disease and stroke, and it has been less closely correlated with glycemic control (25). Nonetheless, reductions in glycemia have generally reduced the risk of clinical events, such as heart attack and stroke. Diabetes care also should minimize these risks by aggressively treating hyperlipidemia and hypertension through a medical diet, regular exercise, and appropriate medications.

The Diabetes Control and Complications Trial (31) and the United Kingdom Prospective Diabetes Study (32) showed conclusively that decreasing blood glucose levels in patients with type 1 diabetes mellitus and type 2 diabetes mellitus greatly reduces the risk of microvascular complications and, at least in patients with type 2 diabetes mellitus, reduces the risk of CV events. Thus, attaining low-risk glycemia (Hb A_{1c} less than 7%) is a primary therapeutic goal (29).

Treatment

GENERAL APPROACH

Early in the course of type 2 diabetes mellitus, glycemic control often can be achieved by weight loss, a diabetic diet, and daily exercise. Lifestyle interventions to decrease weight and increase activity, when successful, can decrease Hb A_{1c} levels by 1–2%. Patients with diabetes mellitus may find it easier to understand estimated average glucose values than Hb A_{1c} values. The Hb A_{1c} level can be translated into an estimated average glucose value by a simple equation:

$$\text{Average glucose (mg/dL)} = 28.7 \times \text{Hb } A_{1c} (\%) - 46.7$$

For example, an Hb A_{1c} of 6% translates into an estimated average glucose value of 126 mg/dL, and an Hb A_{1c} of 8% translates to an estimated average glucose value of 183 mg/dL (33). If hyperglycemia persists above low-risk targets, oral antidiabetic therapy is required. Specific agents will be discussed in detail later.

Sulfonylurea drugs, metformin, thiazolidinediones, and acarbose all lower glucose levels through different mechanisms, so they can be used in combination in a stepped-care approach to achieve a target glycemia. The first three classes generally decrease Hb A_{1c} levels by 1–1.5%, whereas acarbose generally is approximately one half as effective (30, 32, 34, 35). There is no standard approach to therapy, so factors, such as adverse effects, cost, and frequency of dosing should be used to select initial and add-on therapies for individual patients. Exogenous insulin may be administered if control is suboptimal, or it may be required as the patient's β-cell function severely deteriorates. The primary treatment goal in patients with type 1 and type 2 diabetes mellitus is an Hb A_{1c} level below 7% (29).

GLUCOSE SELF-MONITORING

The ability to self-monitor blood glucose levels, along with improved medications and insulin delivery systems, has made it possible for many patients to achieve the low-risk glycemic targets defined earlier. Self-monitoring is essential for all patients with type 1 diabetes mellitus to achieve low-risk glycemia with the minimum of hypoglycemia. These patients require multiple (four to seven) daily measurements to adjust the appropriate basal and preprandial insulin doses or insulin infusion rates. In patients with type 2 diabetes mellitus, the optimal frequency and timing of glucose monitoring has not been established, and less frequent self-monitoring may suffice. Glycemic goals and monitoring plans should be established and adjusted according to the individual patient's needs and frequency of hypoglycemic and hyperglycemic episodes.

MEDICAL NUTRITIONAL THERAPY

Medical nutritional therapy is directed at achieving target glucose levels. It should take into account body weight and possible coexisting hypertension, renal insufficiency, and hyperlipidemia (36). Dietary planning should be individualized and involve the patient in order to address her lifestyle, work, family schedule, and cultural habits if it is to be successful. The caloric intake should be set to achieve and maintain a healthy body weight (Box 49). Most patients with type 2 diabetes mellitus are obese, and a moderate caloric restriction that achieves a 5–10% weight loss will contribute to improved glycemic control.

EXERCISE THERAPY

Diet therapy is most effective when accompanied by an exercise program that targets the CV system. Exercise additionally has been shown to reduce CV risk, hypertension, and hypercholesterolemia. The American Diabetes Association guidelines recommend aerobic exercise at least three times a week at 50–70% of an individual's maximum target heart rate, lasting 20–45 minutes with appropriate warm-up and cool-down periods (29). The prescription should be appropriate for the patient's general health and fitness. A preexercise evaluation should assess the patient's general physical condition and uncover any serious contraindications, such as underlying heart disease.

PHARMACOLOGIC THERAPY

Oral medications should be added when diet and exercise are insufficient to control glucose levels in patients with type 2 diabetes mellitus. These agents have no role in the treatment of type 1 diabetes mellitus. Various classes of oral medications are available, several of which have been marketed only within the past decade. The oldest and best-studied of these medications in clinical outcome trials are the sulfonylureas, biguanides, and thiazolidinediones.

Box 49

Medical Nutritional Management

Goal

Individualized medical nutritional therapy to meet target glucose levels and to address body weight, coexisting medical conditions, lifestyle and culture

Guidelines

- Prescribe caloric intake to achieve and maintain healthy body weight:
  - In overweight and obese individuals a modest weight loss (5–10%) improves insulin resistance.
  - Low-carbohydrate or low fat calorie restricted diets may be effective short term (up to 1 year). High-protein diets are not recommended.
- Monitor carbohydrate (carbohydrate counting and exchanges) intake:
  - Carbohydrates should include fruit, vegetables, nuts, whole grains, high-fiber foods, legumes, and low-fat milk.
  - Glycemic index and load may be used.
  - Sucrose containing foods can be substituted for other carbohydrates.
  - Sugar alcohols and nonnutritive sweeteners are safe when consumed within the recommendations of the U.S. Food and Drug Administration.
- Limit intake of saturated fat to 7% or less and intake of trans fat to a minimum.
  - Encourage two or more servings of fish per week to provide n-3 polyunsaturated fatty acids.
  - Decrease dietary cholesterol intake to less than 200 mg per day.
- Protein intake should be approximately 15–20% of total calories.
  - Limit protein intake to 0.8–1.0 g per kilogram of body weight per day with chronic kidney disease.
- Reduce sodium intake to less than 2,300 mg per day in normotensive and hypertensive individuals.
- Limit alcohol intake.
  - Consume less than one drink per day.
  - To reduce nocturnal hypoglycemia (with insulin or insulin secretagogues) consume alcohol with food. Coingestion of carbohydrate may raise blood glucose levels.
- Hypoglycemia should be treated with ingestion of 15–20 g of glucose (or a carbohydrate containing glucose can be used).

Bantle JP, Wylie-Rosett J, Albright AL, Apovian CM, Clark NG, Franz MJ, et al. Nutrition recommendations and interventions for diabetes: a position statement of the American Diabetes Association. American Diabetes Association. Diabetes Care 2008;31(suppl 1):S61–78.

Insulin Secretogogues (Including Sulfonylureas). Sulfonylureas stimulate endogenous insulin release from the pancreas, thus lowering blood glucose levels. The newer sulfonylurea compounds—glimepiride, gliclazide, glipizide, and glipizide GITS—have fewer hypoglycemic adverse effects than does glyburide. The major side effects are weight gain and hypoglycemia. New short-acting insulin secretogogues—the glinides, repaglinide, and nagletinide—are not sulfonylureas; they have a similar, but shorter, mechanism of action and cause less hypoglycemia. The dosage of glinides and sulfonylureas should be gradually increased and adjusted to attain glycemic targets. As the course of type 2 diabetes mellitus progresses, endogenous insulin secretion generally declines and the use of a secretagogue alone becomes insufficient to control hyperglycemia.

Biguanides (Metformin). Biguanides enhance the liver's response to insulin, reducing fasting hepatic glucose production. Also they increase peripheral insulin sensitivity. Metformin is the only biguanide currently available for clinical use. It does not increase pancreatic secretion of insulin and, therefore, generally does not produce hypoglycemia. Metformin has been shown to decrease serum triglycerides and increase HDL-C levels in diabetic patients, most likely the result of decreasing of glucose levels. In general, weight either does not increase or decreases with metformin use. Also, the United Kingdom Prospective Diabetes Study found that risk reduction for CV events was significant for patients taking metformin. Therefore, metformin is an attractive first-line therapy in obese patients. The medication should be taken with meals and the dose gradually increased during the first 3–4 weeks of therapy to minimize gastrointestinal upset. Metformin can cause lactic acidosis in people with congestive heart failure or renal functional impairment.

Thiazolidinediones (Pioglitazone, Rosiglitazone). Thiazolidinediones work by uncoupling obesity from insulin resistance. There appear to be two mechanisms: 1) redistribution of fatty acids out of liver and muscle, where they cause insulin resistance, and back into adipose tissue, and 2) changes in adipocyte hormones that cause insulin resistance in liver and muscle. The net effect is enhanced insulin action to suppress glucose production from the liver (lowering fasting glucose levels) and to stimulate glucose uptake by skeletal muscle (lowering postprandial glucose levels).

As a result, the drugs reduce endogenous and exogenous insulin needs. Their major side effect is fluid retention. These drugs should not be taken by people with congestive heart failure and should be administered cautiously in patients with risk factors for heart failure (hypertension, advanced age, and long-lasting diabetes mellitus) (37). Recent studies have suggested a link between thiazolidinedione use and increased risk of myocardial infarction.

α-Glucosidase Inhibitors (Acarbose). The α-glucosidase inhibitors slow the digestion and absorption of carbohydrates from the gut, thus lowering postprandial glucose levels. They are less effective in reducing glucose levels than either sulfonylureas or biguanides. They are most useful as adjuncts, especially in patients with significant postprandial hyperglycemia. Gastrointestinal upset and flatulence may limit their use. Dosing should start small and increase slowly to minimize side effects. As predicted from the mechanism of action, doses must be taken with meals to be effective.

Other Drugs. Three additional categories of drugs have recently become available: 1) amylin analogues; eg, pramlintide; 2) agonists of glucagon-like peptide 1 (GLP-1) receptor (GLP-1 analogues); eg, exenatide and liraglutide; and 3) dipeptidyl-peptidase 4 inhibitors, eg, sitagliptin and vildagliptin. The GLP-1 agonists and dipeptidyl-peptidase 4 inhibitors appear to preserve β-cell mass, and all these drugs have been shown to improve glycemic control with less hypoglycemia. Adequate studies demonstrating a reduction in diabetic sequelae, morbidity, or mortality remain to be done.

Combination Therapy in Type 2 Diabetes. Over time, monotherapy is rarely sufficient to control hyperglycemia. The availability of medications with different sites and mechanisms of action has permitted the stepwise addition of additional agents when monotherapy is insufficient to control hyperglycemia (Fig. 16). At this point, referral is most appropriate.

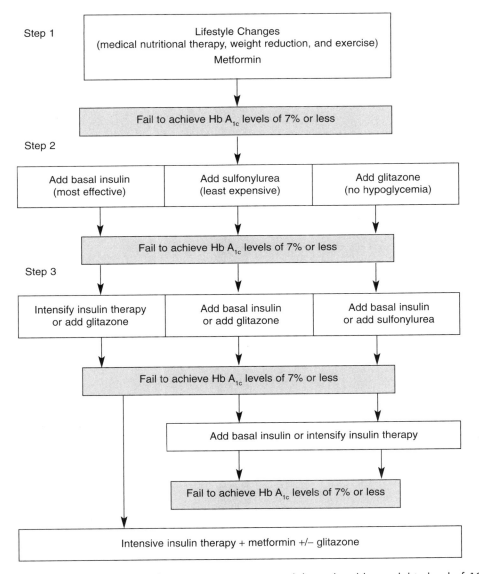

Figure 16. Outpatient treatment interventions for asymptomatic patients (glycosylated hemoglobin level of 10% or less) with newly diagnosed type 2 diabetes who do not have diabetic ketoacidosis or hyperosmolar coma. Abbreviation: Hb A$_{1c}$ indicates glycosylated hemoglobin. (Data from Nathan DM, Buse JB, Davidson MB, Ferrannini E, Holman RR, Sherwin R, et al. Management of hyperglycemia in type 2 diabetes: a consensus algorithm for the initiation and adjustment of therapy [published erratum appears in Diabetes Care 2008;31:522]. Diabetes Care 2008;31:173–5.)

PRIMARY INSULIN THERAPY

Initial insulin therapy for patients newly diagnosed with type 1 diabetes mellitus often takes place in the hospital setting because the diagnosis frequently is accompanied by ketoacidosis or severe hyperglycemia. Patients with newly diagnosed type 2 diabetes mellitus who have symptoms—eg, the presence of catabolism, diuresis, or severe hyperglycemia (Hb A_{1c} level greater than 10%)—initially should begin taking insulin. Generally, they can be educated in an outpatient setting.

CONTINUING CARE

Until glycemic care has become stabilized and patients have become skilled at assessing their own glycemic status and managing their therapy regimens, they require frequent visits and ready access to the diabetic team. Initially, their visits could be daily to weekly. Once blood glucose is stabilized, patients should be monitored at quarterly intervals with blood pressure and glycosylated hemoglobin measurements to assess overall control (Table 21).

References

1. Diagnosis and classification of diabetes mellitus. American Diabetes Association. Diabetes Care 2008;31(suppl 1):S55-60.

2. Knowler WC, Barrett-Connor E, Fowler SE, Hamman RF, Lachin JM, Walker EA, et al. Reduction in the incidence of type 2 diabetes with lifestyle intervention or metformin. Diabetes Prevention Program Research Group. N Engl J Med 2002;346:393-403.

3. Pan XR, Li GW, Hu YH, Wang JX, Yang WY, An ZX, et al. Effects of diet and exercise in preventing NIDDM in people with impaired glucose tolerance. The Da Qing IGT and Diabetes Study. Diabetes Care 1997;20:537-44.

4. Tuomilehto J, Lindstrom J, Eriksson JG, Valle TT, Hamalainen H, Ilanne-Parikka P, et al. Prevention of type 2 diabetes mellitus by changes in lifestyle among subjects with impaired glucose tolerance. Finnish Diabetes Prevention Study Group. N Engl J Med 2001;344:1343-50.

5. Metzger BE, Buchanan TA, Coustan DR, de Leiva A, Dunger DB, Hadden DR, et al. Summary and recommendations of the Fifth International Workshop-Conference on Gestational Diabetes Mellitus [published erratum appears in Diabetes Care 2007;30:3154]. Diabetes Care 2007;30 (suppl 2):S251-60.

6. Grundy SM, Hansen B, Smith SCJ, Cleeman JI, Kahn RA. Clinical management of metabolic syndrome: report of the American Heart Association/National Heart, Lung, and Blood Institute/American Diabetes Association conference on scientific issues related to management. American Heart Association; National Heart, Lung, and Blood Institute; American Diabetes Association. Circulation 2004; 109:551-6.

Table 21. Summary of Recommendations for Glycemic, Blood Pressure, and Lipid Control for Patients With Diabetes

Evaluation	Frequency	Target for Intervention
Preprandial glucose	3–4 times per day	70–130 mg/dL
Postprandial glucose	1–3 times per day	Less than 180 mg/dL
Blood pressure	Quarterly	Less than 130/80 mm Hg
Hb A_{1c}	Semi-annually to quarterly	Less than 7%
LDL-C	Annually	Without CV disease: less than 100 mg/dL
		With CV disease: less than 70 mg/dL
Random spot urine microalbumin/creatinine ratio	Annually	Microalbuminuria: 30–299 mcg/mg of creatinine
		Macroalbuminuria: 300 mcg/mg or more of creatinine
Serum creatinine	Annually	Less than 1.5 mg/dL
Glomerular filtration rate	Annually	Mild decrease: 60–89 mL/min
		Moderate decrease: 30–59 mL/min
		Severe decrease: 12–29 mL/min
		Kidney failure: less than 15 mL/min or dialysis
Dilated retinal examination	Annually	Macular edema, severe nonproliferative retinopathy, or any proliferative retinopathy

Abbreviations: CV indicates cardiovascular; Hb A_{1c}, glycosylated hemoglobin; LDL-C, low-density lipoprotein cholesterol.
Data from Standards of medical care in diabetes–2008. American Diabetes Association. Diabetes Care 2008;31(suppl 1):S12-54.

7. Third Report of the National Cholesterol Education Program (NCEP) Expert Panel on Detection, Evaluation, and Treatment of High Blood Cholesterol in Adults (Adult Treatment Panel III) final report. National Cholesterol Education Program (NCEP) Expert Panel on Detection, Evaluation, and Treatment of High Blood Cholesterol in Adults (Adult Treatment Panel III). Circulation 2002;106: 3143–421.

8. World Health Organization. Definition, diagnosis and classification of diabetes mellitus and its complications: report of a WHO Consultation. Geneva: WHO; 1999. Available at: http://whqlibdoc.who.int/hq/1999/WHO_NCD_NCS_99.2.pdf. Retrieved November 12, 2008.

9. Alberti KG, Zimmet P, Shaw J. Metabolic syndrome-a new world-wide definition. A Consensus Statement from the International Diabetes Federation. Diabet Med 2006;23: 469–80.

10. Thompson PD, Buchner D, Pina IL, Balady GJ, Williams MA, Marcus BH, et al. Exercise and physical activity in the prevention and treatment of atherosclerotic cardiovascular disease: a statement from the Council on Clinical Cardiology (Subcommittee on Exercise, Rehabilitation, and Prevention) and the Council on Nutrition, Physical Activity, and Metabolism (Subcommittee on Physical Activity). American Heart Association Council on Clinical Cardiology Subcommittee on Exercise, Rehabilitation, and Prevention; American Heart Association Council on Nutrition, Physical Activity, and Metabolism Subcommittee on Physical Activity. Circulation 2003;107:3109–16.

11. Rubins HB. Triglycerides and coronary heart disease: implications of recent clinical trials. J Cardiovasc Risk 2000;7:339–45.

12. Chobanian AV, Bakris GL, Black HR, Cushman WC, Green LA, Izzo JL Jr, et al. The Seventh Report of the Joint National Committee on Prevention, Detection, Evaluation, and Treatment of High Blood Pressure: the JNC 7 report. National Heart, Lung, and Blood Institute Joint National Committee on Prevention, Detection, Evaluation, and Treatment of High Blood Pressure; National High Blood Pressure Education Program Coordinating Committee [published erratum appears in JAMA 2003;290:197]. JAMA 2003;289:2560–72.

13. Pearson TA, Blair SN, Daniels SR, Eckel RH, Fair JM, Fortmann SP, et al. AHA Guidelines for Primary Prevention of Cardiovascular Disease and Stroke: 2002 Update: Consensus Panel Guide to Comprehensive Risk Reduction for Adult Patients Without Coronary or Other Atherosclerotic Vascular Diseases. American Heart Association Science Advisory and Coordinating Committee. Circulation 2002;106:388–91.

14. Lakhani K, Prelevic GM, Seifalian AM, Atiomo WU, Hardiman P. Polycystic ovary syndrome, diabetes and cardiovascular disease: risks and risk factors. J Obstet Gynaecol 2004;24:613–21.

15. Wild RA. Polycystic ovary syndrome: a risk for coronary artery disease? Am J Obstet Gynecol 2002;186:35–43.

16. Nixon JV. Lower is better—the contemporary concept of low-density lipoprotein lowering in the preventive management of cardiovascular risk: does this apply to all patients? Prev Cardiol 2006;9:219–25; quiz 226–7.

17. Smith SC Jr, Allen J, Blair SN, Bonow RO, Brass LM, Fonarow GC, et al. AHA/ACC guidelines for secondary prevention for patients with coronary and other atherosclerotic vascular disease: 2006 update endorsed by the National Heart, Lung, and Blood Institute. American Heart Association. American College of Cardiology. National Heart, Lung, and Blood Institute. J Am Coll Cardiol 2006; 47:2130–9.

18. Mosca L, Appel LJ, Benjamin EJ, Berra K, Chandra-Strobos N, Fabunmi RP, et al. Evidence-based guidelines for cardiovascular disease prevention in women. American Heart Association. Circulation 2004;109:672–93.

19. Goldstein LB, Adams R, Alberts MJ, Appel LJ, Brass LM, Bushnell CD, et al. Primary prevention of ischemic stroke: a guideline from the American Heart Association/ American Stroke Association Stroke Council: cosponsored by the Atherosclerotic Peripheral Vascular Disease Interdisciplinary Working Group; Cardiovascular Nursing Council; Clinical Cardiology Council; Nutrition, Physical Activity, and Metabolism Council; and the Quality of Care and Outcomes Research Interdisciplinary Working Group: the American Academy of Neurology affirms the value of this guideline. American Heart Association/ American Stroke Association Stroke Council; Atherosclerotic Peripheral Vascular Disease Interdisciplinary Working Group; Cardiovascular Nursing Council; Clinical Cardiology Council; Nutrition, Physical Activity, and Metabolism Council; Quality of Care and Outcomes Research Interdisciplinary Working Group; American Academy of Neurology [published erratum appears in Stroke 2007;38: 207]. Stroke 2006;37:1583–633.

20. Krauss RM, Eckel RH, Howard B, Appel LJ, Daniels SR, Deckelbaum RJ, et al. AHA Dietary Guidelines: revision 2000: a statement for healthcare professionals from the Nutrition Committee of the American Heart Association. Circulation 2000;102:2284–99.

21. Grundy SM, Cleeman JI, Daniels SR, Donato KA, Eckel RH, Franklin BA, et al. Diagnosis and management of the metabolic syndrome: an American Heart Association/ National Heart, Lung, and Blood Institute Scientific Statement. American Heart Association; National Heart, Lung, and Blood Institute [published erratum appears in Circulation 2005;112:e297]. Circulation 2005;112:2735–52.

22. Grundy SM, Cleeman JI, Merz CN, Brewer HB Jr, Clark LT, Hunninghake DB, et al. Implications of recent clinical trials for the National Cholesterol Education Program Adult Treatment Panel III guidelines. National Heart, Lung, and Blood Institute; American College of Cardiology Foundation; American Heart Association [published erratum appears in Circulation 2004;110:763]. Circulation 2004;110:227–39.

23. Reaven GM. Banting lecture 1988. Role of insulin resistance in human disease. Diabetes 1988;37:1595–607.

24. Ong KL, Cheung BM, Wong LY, Wat NM, Tan KC, Lam KS. Prevalence, treatment, and control of diagnosed diabetes in the U.S. National Health and Nutrition Examination Survey 1999–2004. Ann Epidemiol 2008;18:222–9.

25. Donahue RP, Orchard TJ. Diabetes mellitus and macrovascular complications. An epidemiological perspective. Diabetes Care 1992;15:1141–55.

26. O'Sullivan JB. The Boston gestational diabetes studies: review and perspectives. In: Sutherland HW, Stowers JM, Pearson DW, editors. Carbohydrate metabolism in pregnancy and the newborn. London: Springer-Verlag; 1989. p. 287–94.

27. Kjos SL, Peters RK, Xiang A, Henry OA, Montoro M, Buchanan TA. Predicting future diabetes in Latino women with gestational diabetes. Utility of early postpartum glucose tolerance testing. Diabetes 1995;44:586–91.

28. Preconception care of women with diabetes. American Diabetes Association. Diabetes Care 2004;27(suppl 1):S76–8.

29. Standards of medical care in diabetes—2008. American Diabetes Association. Diabetes Care 2008;31(suppl 1):S12–54.

30. Implications of the United Kingdom Prospective Diabetes Study. American Diabetes Association. Diabetes Care 1998;21:2180-4.

31. The effect of intensive treatment of diabetes on the development and progression of long-term complications in insulin-dependent diabetes mellitus. The Diabetes Control and Complications Trial Research Group. N Engl J Med 1993;329:977–86.

32. United Kingdom Prospective Diabetes Study 24: a 6-year, randomized, controlled trial comparing sulfonylurea, insulin, and metformin therapy in patients with newly diagnosed type 2 diabetes that could not be controlled with diet therapy. United Kingdom Prospective Diabetes Study Group. Ann Intern Med 1998;128:165-75.

33. Nathan DM, Kuenen J, Borg R, Zheng H, Schoenfeld D, Heine RJ. Translating the A1C assay into estimated average glucose values. A1c-Derived Average Glucose Study Group. Diabetes Care 2008;31:1473–8.

34. Intensive blood-glucose control with sulphonylureas or insulin compared with conventional treatment and risk of complications in patients with type 2 diabetes (UKPDS 33). UK Prospective Diabetes Study (UKPDS) Group. Lancet 1998;352:837–53.

35. Effect of intensive blood-glucose control with metformin on complications in overweight patients with type 2 diabetes (UKPDS 34). UK Prospective Diabetes Study (UKPDS) Group. Lancet 1998;352:854-65.

36. Bantle JP, Wylie-Rosett J, Albright AL, Apovian CM, Clark NG, Franz MJ, et al. Nutrition recommendations and interventions for diabetes: a position statement of the American Diabetes Association. American Diabetes Association. Diabetes Care 2008;31(suppl 1):S61–78.

37. Nesto RW, Bell D, Bonow RO, Fonseca V, Grundy SM, Horton ES, et al. Thiazolidinedione use, fluid retention, and congestive heart failure: a consensus statement from the American Heart Association and American Diabetes Association. Diabetes Care 2004;27:256–63.

Gastrointestinal Disorders

Jeanne M. Schilder

Gastrointestinal and gynecologic disorders can have similar symptoms. As a woman's primary health care provider, the obstetrician–gynecologist must be comfortable in differentiating gastrointestinal disorders from gynecologic disorders, as well as be familiar with the available diagnostic and therapeutic tools. One such tool, the Rome criteria, is a set of diagnostic criteria for diagnosing functional gastrointestinal disorders. It was first issued in 1990 (now referred to as the Rome I criteria) by the Rome committee and was most recently revised in 2006 (Rome III criteria). One objective of the Rome III criteria is to provide diagnostic standards for clinical trials and clinical care (Box 50).

Dyspepsia

Dyspepsia is commonly referred to as *indigestion* by the lay population. The term *dyspepsia*, however, pertains to a multitude of symptoms—ranging from abdominal pain or pressure to heartburn—that can vary significantly among individuals. It is, therefore, important for the clinician to obtain a precise description of the reported symptoms from the patient to elucidate the etiology.

Studies on the prevalence of dyspepsia report that it varies from 14% to 44%, depending on the definition of dyspepsia used (1). One method of categorizing dyspepsia is to define it as structural (when organic disease is identified) or functional (when no organic disease is identified by endoscopy) (1). Patients treated in primary care settings generally have uninvestigated dyspepsia. Their symptoms may have an underlying structural cause (eg, peptic ulcer disease, reflux esophagitis, or endoscopic-negative gastroesophageal reflux disease [GERD]). However, a substantial number of these patients have functional dyspepsia in which there is no definite structural or biochemical explanation for their symptoms, even after appropriate investigation.

Resources

Gastrointestinal Disorders

American Cancer Society
http://www.cancer.org

American College of Gastroenterology
http://www.acg.gi.org

American Gastroenterological Association
http://www.gastro.org

National Institute of Diabetes and Digestive and Kidney Diseases
http://www2.niddk.nih.gov

Peptic Ulcer Disease

Duodenal and gastric ulcers are types of peptic ulcer disease. They are a common cause of morbidity, affecting approximately 7 million people annually in the United States and up to 10% of the population at some point during their lifetime. Gastric ulcer disease occurs on average one decade later than duodenal ulcers, and its incidence continues to increase in individuals, especially women, older than 65 years (2).

Symptoms

Dyspepsia is the cardinal symptom of peptic ulcer disease (1). Duodenal ulcers classically result in pain that is gnawing and burning, is localized to the epigastrium, and may radiate to the back. Pain often is episodic and nocturnal. Duodenal ulcer pain usually occurs 2–4 hours after a meal, whereas gastric ulcer pain is more likely to occur while eating; however, the relationship of the pain to meals is highly variable. The pain usually is relieved by antacids, and food intake sometimes relieves the pain from duodenal, but not gastric, ulcers. Complications from peptic ulcer disease include hemorrhage, perforation, penetration (into the liver, colon, or biliary tract), and gastric outlet obstruction.

Etiology

Peptic ulcers occur as the result of an imbalance between gastric acid and the mucosal defenses that protect cells from acid-induced injury (1). Since the identification of *Helicobacter pylori*, this organism has been associated with 90–100% of duodenal ulcers and 60–75% of gastric ulcers (1). Recognition of *H pylori* as a causative agent has changed the clinical view of peptic ulcer from being a surgically managed condition to that of a potentially medically curable disease.

The presence of gastric ulcers should raise the suspicion of malignancy. Strong evidence exists that *H pylori* is a major etiologic factor in the development of gastric carcinoma as well as peptic ulcer disease. A recent consensus report recommending treatment strategies and management of *H pylori* infections concludes that eradication of *H pylori* can reduce the prevalence of gastric carcinoma (3). This gram-negative rod thrives within a narrow acidic pH range and produces large amounts of urease, two properties that are used to diagnose and suppress infection. Approximately 15–30% of *H pylori*-infected individuals develop ulcer disease (1). Acute dyspepsia occurs within 1–2 weeks of acute infection

---

Box 50

Rome III Criteria of Functional Gastrointestinal Disorders

A. Functional Esophageal Disorders
A1. Functional heartburn
A2. Functional chest pain of presumed esophageal origin
A3. Functional dysphagia
A4. Globus

B. Functional Gastrointestinal Disorders
B1. Functional dyspepsia
   B1a. Postprandial distress syndrome
   B1b. Epigastric pain syndrome
B2. Belching disorders
   B2a. Aerophagia
   B2b. Unspecified excessive belching
B3. Nausea and vomiting disorders
   B3a. Chronic idiopathic nausea
   B3b. Functional vomiting
   B3c. Cyclic vomiting syndrome
B4. Rumination syndrome in adults

C. Functional Bowel Disorders
C1. Irritable bowel syndrome
C2. Functional bloating
C3. Functional constipation
C4. Functional diarrhea
C5. Unspecified functional bowel disorder

D. Functional Abdominal Pain Syndrome

E. Functional Gallbladder and Sphincter of Oddi Disorders
E1. Functional gallbladder disorder
E2. Functional biliary sphincter of Oddi disorder
E3. Functional pancreatic sphincter of Oddi disorder

F. Functional Anorectal Disorders
F1. Functional fecal incontinence
F2. Functional anorectal pain
   F2a. Chronic proctalgia
      F2a1. Levator ani syndrome
      F2a2. Unspecified functional anorectal pain
   F2b. Proctalgia fugax
F3. Functional defecation disorders
   F3a. Dyssynergic defecation
   F3b. Inadequate defecatory propulsion

---

and is followed by gastritis. Asymptomatic infected persons are noted to have a 25% rate of ulceration. Recurrence of dyspepsia symptoms, which is common with acid-suppressive therapy alone, is decreased with eradication of H $pylori$.

After H $pylori$, nonsteroidal anti-inflammatory drugs (NSAIDs) are the second most common cause of peptic ulcer disease, especially in elderly women. The prevalence of peptic ulcer disease is increased approximately fourfold in long-term NSAID users. For women with NSAID-associated peptic ulcer disease who cannot discontinue the use of NSAIDs, risk reduction can be achieved with adjuvant treatment with prostaglandins (misoprostol) or histamine$_2$ (H$_2$)-receptor antagonists. Of patients with NSAID-associated peptic ulcer disease, 50% also have H $pylori$ infection (1). Definitive treatment requires therapy directed at H $pylori$.

Detection of *Helicobacter Pylori* Infection

The detection of H $pylori$ infection includes invasive modalities (eg, endoscopy with biopsy) and noninvasive modalities (eg, serology and urea breath tests) (4). Serology with commercial tests performed in the clinical laboratory yields sensitivity and specificity generally greater than 90%. Confirmation of cure (ie, eradication of H $pylori$) with noninvasive tests is best done with the urea breath test rather than serology. Endoscopy, though expensive and invasive, offers the advantage of defining the pathology and extent of disease.

Evaluation

Individuals older than 55 years who have dyspepsia accompanied by "alarm symptoms" (hemorrhage, anemia, dysphagia, odynophagia, and weight loss) should undergo esophagogastroduodenoscopy. Other patients may be managed either with H $pylori$ testing or a 4–8-week empiric course of a proton-pump inhibitor (5). Lack of an appropriate response or recurrent symptoms should prompt further evaluation, including endoscopy.

Therapy

Initial therapy is to remove any associated factor, especially NSAIDs but also cigarette smoking and alcohol use. Treatment depends on whether H $pylori$ is present. For managing peptic ulcer disease without H $pylori$ infection, H$_2$-receptor antagonists are widely used and are potent inhibitors of gastric acid secretion. Antacids (aluminum–magnesium preparations, not calcium-containing antacids, which stimulate gastrin release), sucralfate, and misoprostol (which inhibits acid secretion) are as effective as the H$_2$-receptor antagonists. Use of misoprostol in pregnancy is contraindicated because it is uterotonic and may promote contractions, bleeding, and abortion. Proton blockers are effective and are associated with more rapid healing of ulcers, especially gastric ulcers, than are H_2-receptor antagonists. Proton blockers inhibit the H^+-K^+ adenosine triphosphatase pump, the final step in luminal acid secretion. These agents require acid activation and, therefore, should not be taken concomitantly with antacids, sucralfate, or H_2-receptor antagonists.

The H_2-receptor antagonists are currently available over-the-counter in lower doses than prescription doses. Although published data are scarce, these agents appear to be effective in the treatment and prevention of heartburn, with few adverse effects. However, the lower doses would not be sufficient to manage an unsuspected peptic ulcer and could delay the diagnosis of gastric carcinoma. Persistence of symptoms necessitates a more extensive evaluation.

When *H pylori* infection is documented in association with peptic ulcer disease or gastritis, treatment is recommended (4). The best treatment of *H pylori* infection is based on consensus and consists of combination therapy, including a proton pump inhibitor and antibiotic therapy. Omeprazole or bismuth and two types of antibiotics—usually amoxicillin, clarithromycin, or metronidazole—is the standard treatment (3) Taking amoxicillin alone yields a 20% eradication rate, which increases to 60–80% when amoxicillin is combined with omeprazole. The reduction in gastric acid produced by omeprazole appears to promote greater antibiotic effectiveness. Reinfection is uncommon, occurring in less than 1% of patients.

Gastroesophageal Reflux Disease

Gastroesophageal reflux disease is estimated to affect 4–7% of the population. However, only a small percentage of affected individuals seek medical attention (6).

Symptoms

The most common presenting symptoms of GERD are heartburn and acid regurgitation. The diagnosis is further secured if symptoms are positional (ie, are increased when the patient is supine or stooping), occur postprandially and at night, and are transiently relieved with antacids. Gastroesophageal reflux disease, however, can present with atypical symptoms, such as chest pain (present in 40–50% of patients with unexplained noncardiac chest pain), water brash (heartburn with regurgitation of fluid into the mouth), globus sensation (the sensation of having a ball in the throat), dysphagia, odynophagia, hoarseness, gastrointestinal bleeding, and asthma (6). Long-term complications from GERD and reflux esophagitis include stricture, anemia, and Barrett esophagus. The latter complication, characterized by specialized columnar epithelium of greater than 2–3 cm above the gastroesophageal junction, occurs in approximately 10% of longstanding cases of GERD and is asso-

ciated with an approximately 10% risk of esophageal adenocarcinoma (6).

Etiology

The pathogenic mechanism of GERD is related to the loss of pressure in the lower esophageal sphincter, reduction in esophageal motility, and esophageal mucosal resistance. The integrity of the lower esophageal sphincter is affected by hiatal hernia, cigarette smoking, alcohol use, obesity, pregnancy, medications (eg, anticholinergics, calcium channel blockers, and nitrates), and certain food products (eg, fatty foods, coffee, and chocolate). Acid is the mediator of mucosal injury that leads to esophagitis and long-term complications.

Evaluation

Patients with typical or mild symptoms compatible with GERD can be treated empirically, without further evaluation. Patients with atypical symptoms, such as chest pain or evidence of tissue injury (eg, anemia, dysphagia, or odynophagia) require a more extensive evaluation. Such an evaluation may include ambulatory esophageal pH level monitoring and endoscopy. In ambulatory pH level monitoring, a pH electrode is placed within the esophagus just above the lower esophageal sphincter. This test is especially useful in documenting acid reflux in patients who have typical or atypical symptoms that are not associated with endoscopic evidence of esophagitis and who fail to respond to conventional antacid therapy.

Therapy

Initial therapy for mild symptomatic GERD has traditionally consisted of modifying lifestyle and avoiding factors (eg, medications) that exacerbate the reflux. Weight loss is useful for obese women. Simple measures, such as elevating the head of the bed, eating small meals, avoiding cigarettes and alcohol, and avoiding the supine position immediately after eating, may be all that is needed for most patients. The next traditional line of therapy consists of antacids and sucralfate, followed by H_2-receptor antagonists (cimetidine, ranitidine, famotidine, or nizatidine), prokinetic agents (metoclopramide or cisapride), or both, followed finally by proton pump inhibitors (omeprazole or lansoprazole) (6).

The logic of such a stepwise approach is questionable, given the superior and prompt response of GERD to proton pump inhibitor therapy (7). The stepwise therapies just described are less likely to provide prompt relief of symptoms and confirmation of the diagnosis. Therefore, initial, short-term treatment with proton pump inhibitors is reasonable. If this treatment is unsuccessful, either the diagnosis is incorrect or the chosen treatment has not been sufficiently effective. If it is determined on review that GERD remains the most likely diagnosis, therapy can be intensified with the use of a proton pump inhibitor twice daily or possibly with the addition of an H_2-receptor antagonist (7). The exact role of prokinetic agents in primary or adjuvant therapy remains undefined.

Because GERD is thought to be a chronic, relapsing disorder, strategies are needed for long-term care after the initial control of reflux symptoms. The choice for long-term therapy should be determined by individual patient characteristics. Options include continuation of initial therapy, withdrawal of initial therapy, taking steps down in therapy, or even antireflux surgery. Patients with persistent symptomatic GERD that is unresponsive to medical therapy are candidates for surgery, but fundoplication outcomes vary substantially even among centers of excellence (7).

Follow-up

Although endoscopy has been used frequently for follow-up of reflux disease, data on how this modality helps in patient management are lacking. The use of endoscopy for patients with progressive disease or long-standing problems might be reasonable, but a subsequent, well-performed endoscopy should define risks and guide management for many years (7). Patients with Barrett esophagus (scarring of the lower esophagus caused by chronic reflux) represent a special category. Endoscopic evaluation of 150 consecutive individuals with proven GERD noted that 25 patients (16.7%) had evidence of Barrett esophagus. All these individuals had evidence of a structurally defective sphincter, whereas those with a structurally normal sphincter had a 0% incidence of Barrett esophagus (8). No definitive reports suggest screening intervals for Barrett esophagus, but one acceptable method is to screen patients with no or low-grade dysplasia every 2 or 3 years by upper endoscopy and biopsy (6).

There is little evidence-based consensus regarding the treatment of patients with GERD who have Barrett esophagus. Options include medical and surgical management. In a study evaluating 554 patients with GERD, 60 patients were found to have Barrett esophagus. Of these patients, 32 were randomized to receive laparoscopic antireflux surgery, and 28 were randomized to receive 20–40 mg of esomeprazole daily. Three-year follow-up demonstrated similar outcomes in both groups, with few treatment failures in either arm. Thus, well-controlled surgical management can match the success of optimized medical management in these patients (9).

Irritable Bowel Syndrome

Irritable bowel syndrome (IBS) is defined as a functional bowel disorder characterized by symptoms of abdominal pain or discomfort that are associated with disturbed defecation (10). In North America, the prevalence of IBS is approximately 10–15% (11). Patients with IBS are typically aged 30–50 years and are predominantly female (2:1).

Symptoms

The symptoms of IBS can occur frequently, waxing and waning over years. Patients present with long-term (of 3 months' duration) abdominal pain and altered bowel habits. Flares may be associated with stress, travel, medications, menstrual cycles, or eating certain foods. The pain is typically described as lower midabdominal, crampy pain. Altered bowel habits may consist of diarrhea, constipation, or diarrhea alternating with constipation. Irritable bowel syndrome can present in variations, such as abdominal pain only, chronic pelvic pain, or painless diarrhea. Patients with IBS also have a higher prevalence of other functional disorders of the gastrointestinal tract, such as chest pain of unexplained origin (GERD or esophageal spasm), nonulcer dyspepsia, and biliary dyskinesia (12).

Etiology

The etiology of IBS is unknown, and the mechanisms responsible for abdominal pain and altered bowel habits occur in both healthy control subjects and in patients with the disorder. Symptoms can occur in response to a disruption of functioning of the gastrointestinal tract from an infection; medications (eg, antacids and antibiotics); dietary indiscretions (eg, increased fat or alcohol intake); lifestyle changes (eg, traveling or exercise); depression; anxiety disorders; physical, sexual, or substance abuse; and psychologic stress (12). The differences between patients with IBS and healthy control subjects are quantitative rather than qualitative. Findings of motility observations in the stomach, small intestine, colon, and rectum are qualitatively similar, but patients with IBS show an exaggerated response to a variety of provocative stimuli. In addition, enhanced perception of visceral events is documented throughout the gastrointestinal tract (12). There is no consensus on the patterns of motility that are responsible for diarrhea and constipation, although accelerated transit is seen in patients with diarrhea, and slowed transit is seen in patients with constipation.

Diagnosis

The diagnosis of IBS is based on identifying positive symptoms (using Rome III criteria) that are consistent with the syndrome while excluding other, similar clinical presentations in a cost-effective manner. The differential diagnosis includes organic and functional disorders, as well as the multiple causes of chronic pelvic pain. Alarm features, such as weight loss, refractory diarrhea, and family history of colon cancer, should be considered and used to help guide the workup. If alarm features are absent, the risk of missing organic disease is low, because the specificity of the symptom-based Rome criteria for IBS is greater than 98% (12). Irritable bowel syndrome is considered a diagnosis of exclusion. Symptoms of nocturnal abdominal pain or diarrhea, weight loss, hematochezia, or fever are incompatible with a diagnosis of IBS and suggest an organic cause.

Evaluation

Evaluation for IBS should include assessing underlying etiologies. Results of a complete physical examination, including special attention to the abdominal examination (to rule out hepatomegaly, masses, and signs of bowel obstruction), pelvic examination (eg, to rule out pelvic floor abnormality), and rectal examination, usually are normal. The screening studies to consider, if they have not already been performed, are complete blood count and a three-card fecal occult blood test. If their use is supported by clinical features, the following studies may be performed: sedimentation rate; ova and parasite; thyroid-stimulating hormone; serum chemistries; and colonoscopy, flexible sigmoidoscopy, or both (12). In many cases, a therapeutic trial can be undertaken before further diagnostic studies are done.

Therapy

Irritable bowel syndrome is a benign syndrome, and although a cure is not expected, its symptoms can be modified. The most important element in the management of this chronic disorder is a reassuring, therapeutic patient–physician relationship. The health care provider must listen actively, provide a thorough explanation, respond to the patient's concerns and expectations, set realistic and consistent limits, involve the patient in the treatment, and establish a long-term relationship with a primary care provider. The treatment strategy should be based on the nature and severity of the symptoms, the correlation of symptoms with food intake or defecation, the degree of functional impairment, and the presence of psychosocial or psychiatric problems (12).

Most patients with IBS have mild symptoms. The usual first step in therapy includes avoiding foods associated with symptoms and increasing the daily dietary fiber intake. The type of food consumed does not usually contribute to symptoms, but patients are more likely to experience symptoms as a generalized effect of eating. However, some substances, such as caffeine, lactose (in lactose-intolerant individuals), and excessive fiber, may aggravate symptoms. Having the patient keep a symptom diary for 2–3 weeks is helpful to assess the timing and severity of symptoms, the presence of aggravating factors, and the emotional or cognitive effect on the patient.

For patients with continued symptoms or moderate to severe IBS, pharmacotherapy often targets specific symptoms. For pain and bloating, antispasmodic (anticholinergic) medicines, such as dicyclomine and hyoscyamine, are used in the United States, but their clinical effectiveness is not proved (11). These drugs are best used on an as-needed basis for acute attacks of pain or before meals when postprandial symptoms are a problem. Adverse events associated with these medications (dry mouth, visual disturbances, urinary retention, and constipation) can limit their dose range.

High-fiber diets (25 g/d) decrease colonic transit time and are recommended for the treatment of simple constipation, but their effectiveness in reducing pain in constipation-predominant IBS is unproved (12). In addition, the value of high-fiber diets for the relief of diarrhea is controversial. If fiber is not helpful, osmotic laxatives, such as milk of magnesia, sorbitol, and polyethylene glycol, may be used. For the treatment of diarrhea-predominant IBS, loperamide or diphenoxylate can reduce loose stools, urgency, and fecal soiling.

Tricyclic antidepressants are prescribed in patients with IBS with the rationale that these agents will manage psychiatric comorbidity, alter gastrointestinal physiology (visceral sensitivity, motility, and secretion), and reduce central pain perception. Low doses of tricyclic antidepressants are recommended for the treatment of pain and sleep disturbances associated with IBS (12). For the same reasons, selective serotonin reuptake inhibitors often are prescribed, but randomized controlled trials documenting their effectiveness have not been published.

Constipation

Constipation is estimated to affect 34% of the population. It is prevalent in young children, older individuals, and pregnant women (13).

Symptoms

In general, constipation is defined objectively as fewer than three bowel movements a week and subjectively as hard stools, excessive straining, and a feeling of incomplete evacuation and lower abdominal fullness. The differential diagnosis of constipation is broad. Acute onset of constipation in middle-aged or older women should prompt an evaluation (barium enema or colonoscopy) for possible colonic obstruction, specifically to exclude the possibility of carcinoma. Other etiologies that may lead to colonic obstruction include ischemia, diverticulosis, prior abdominal surgery, and inflammatory bowel disease.

Evaluation

The initial clinical evaluation for chronic constipation is directed toward detection of exacerbating factors, colonic disease, or systemic disease. Exacerbating factors include medications, inactivity, immobility, and lack of adequate dietary fiber and water intake. Medications associated with constipation include anticholinergic agents, antidepressants, antipsychotics, codeine and other analgesics, calcium- and aluminum-containing antacids, iron supplements, sucralfate, and calcium antagonists. Systemic illnesses associated with constipation include neurologic illnesses, such as multiple sclerosis, stroke, Parkinson disease, and spinal cord injury; diabetes mellitus; hyperparathyroidism; and hypothyroidism. Other conditions associated with constipation include hemorrhoids, rectal fissure, rectal prolapse, and rectocele (14). However, most chronic constipation is of unknown origin.

Severe constipation, which is seen mostly in young and middle-aged women, is associated with infrequent defecation and excessive straining and is unresponsive to increased dietary fiber intake and mild laxatives. Colonic studies demonstrate slow colonic transit in 70% of patients. In the remaining 30%, colonic transit time is normal, but patients demonstrate abnormal anorectal sensory and motor function (ie, outlet obstruction and anismus).

Therapy

For the typical patient with mild to moderate symptoms, reassurance, adjustment of medications, correction of insufficient fiber and water intake, and counseling may be all that is needed. An initial 20- to 30-g increase in daily dietary fiber intake often is successful. Fiber supplements can be increased gradually to minimize side effects (eg, bloating) and encourage compliance. Fiber therapy requires 3–4 weeks to exert its effects. Laxatives generally are used as second-line therapy. Patients with severe constipation and abnormal anorectal sensory function may be helped with biofeedback therapy (15). Often they require specialist care and specialized studies.

Available laxatives include emollients, osmotic agents, and stimulants. Emollients, such as docusate sodium and mineral oil, improve the penetration of water and fats into feces. Osmotic agents are generally nonabsorbable salts or carbohydrates that increase fecal water retention. They include milk of magnesia, magnesium citrate solutions, lactulose, and lavage solutions. Lactulose is used primarily in patients with hepatic disorders because it facilitates the clearance of elevated-serum ammonia. Stimulants include phenolphthalein, castor oil, bisacodyl, and extracts of cascara and senna. Phenolphthaleins stimulate the secretion of fluids and electrolytes into the bowel lumen, effectively softening feces. Castor oil and bisacodyl stimulate peristalsis and generally effect evacuation within the hour. Extracts of cascara and senna also promote bowel motility, but their effect generally is not seen for 6–10 hours. The latter two agents are not recommended for long-term use

because they are associated with colonic denervation and atony. Definitive studies to show which laxative is the most clinically effective do not exist. In general, the safest are the bulk fiber laxatives. The use of stimulant laxatives should be limited to once or twice weekly to reduce adverse effects and dependence.

Constipation is a particular problem in the elderly, possibly because of inadequate fluid and food intake, blunted rectal sensation, inactivity, and lack of regular bowel habits (14). Untreated constipation may lead to fecal impaction, overflow incontinence, and bowel obstruction. Therapy consists of correcting the factors previously noted, encouraging patients to sit on the toilet twice a day, and recommending the judicious use of osmotic and bulk stool softeners and stimulants.

Diverticulitis and Diverticulosis

Acute diverticulitis affects men more often than women. In an older patient it generally manifests as abdominal pain and is accompanied by signs of peritoneal irritation, guarding, fever, and leukocytosis. Constipation is commonly reported. The inflamed diverticula may progress to free perforation into the peritoneal space, resulting in peritonitis, sepsis, and shock.

Treatment of mild cases of diverticulosis and diverticulitis consists of bed rest, stool softeners, and broad-spectrum antibiotics. Recently, the traditionally prescribed liquid diets have been found to be of marginal benefit. More acutely ill patients may require hospitalization, intravenous antibiotics, and possible surgical intervention (16).

Colorectal Cancer

Colorectal cancer is the second most common cancer in the United States. In women, it is the third most common form of cancer, after lung and breast cancer. Colorectal cancer accounts for approximately 26,000 deaths in women each year. Incidence and mortality rates for colorectal cancer have declined for men and women since the mid-1980s (17). Survival is linked to the extent of disseminated disease. The 5-year survival rate is 91% with localized disease, 61% with regional spread, and 7% with distant metastases (18). Approximately 60% of patients have regional or distant metastases at the time of diagnosis.

Etiology

It is generally accepted that colorectal cancer evolves from adenomatous polyps in a process that takes 7–12 years. Adenomatous polyps occur in 30% of older individuals, and approximately 5–10% of these polyps become malignant. When colorectal cancer is detected at the stage of adenomatous polyps or localized cancer, it is potentially curable by surgery.

Risk factors for colorectal cancer are listed in Box 51. Patients with familial syndromes (eg, hereditary polyposis, hereditary nonpolyposis, or colorectal cancer) and long-standing ulcerative colitis are at greatest risk but account for only 6% of all cases of colorectal cancer. In a postmenopausal woman, iron deficiency anemia should be considered a sign of gastrointestinal lesion or cancer until proved otherwise.

Screening

Colorectal cancer is rare before age of 50 years. Most patients with colorectal cancer have few, if any, identified risk factors. Therefore, screening is recommended at age 50 years. In 1999, however, fewer than 30% of eligible individuals had a screening test for colorectal cancer (18). Evaluation of Behavioral Risk Factor Surveillance System surveys demonstrates that overall screening increased between 2002 and 2004, indicating improved awareness and compliance (19). The digital rectal examination is limited in its ability to detect polyps or colorectal cancer, because only 10% of all types of colorectal cancer are within reach of the examining finger. Testing of a single fecal sample for occult blood is common in the United States after a rectal examination, but this approach has not been studied in randomized clinical trials. Rectal examination with fecal occult blood testing may be associated with higher rates of false-positive and false-negative results. Occult blood testing of three serially obtained samples of stool at home has been studied with randomized controlled trials and is preferred (20). If any of the three samples has a positive test result, a workup of the entire colon is recommended because the probability of finding cancer or a large adenoma is 17–46%.

When using fecal occult blood testing for asymptomatic patients, the physician must keep in mind that most positive tests are falsely positive. False-positive results may be caused by nonspecific bleeding (eg, angiodysplasia), diet, or rehydration of samples. Health care providers may want to recommend that patients avoid consuming red meat, horseradish, or aspirin before a test to reduce false-positive results. Rehydrating the samples increases sensitivity but causes a loss of specificity and an increase in false-positive results. In general, with fecal occult blood testing, 1–10% of patients will have a positive result. Of these patients, 5–12% will have cancer, and 20–50% will have polyps; there will be no explanation for the positive results of the other patients (18).

Sigmoidoscopy, performed without sedation in a patient who has received a laxative or an enema, is highly sensitive and specific for lesions within reach of the instrument. Sigmoidoscopy will miss roughly 50% of neoplasms that are proximal or right sided (20). Unlike fecal occult blood testing, sigmoidoscopic screening has not been assessed in any randomized controlled trial.

The U.S. Preventive Services Task Force has recommended screening of the average-risk individual with three sample fecal occult blood tests, sigmoidoscopy, or both (21). The American College of Obstetricians and Gynecologists recommends screening patients who are at average risk starting at age 50 years with one of five options, including fecal occult blood tests, flexible sigmoidoscopy, double-contrast barium enema, colonoscopy, and combinations at various intervals (22). Guidelines for screening and surveillance of women at increased risk are listed in Table 22. Although the best screening method is still unclear, it is evident that screening can reduce the rate of death from colorectal cancer. Diagnosis and management of colorectal cancer go beyond the scope of this overview; details can be found in the current edition of *Precis: Oncology*.

Fecal Incontinence

Estimates of the prevalence of fecal incontinence in the adult female population range between 1% and 17% (12). This disorder, defined as involuntary passage of gas, liquid, or solid stool, is even more stigmatized than urinary incontinence. Approximately one in five women with urinary incontinence also have some form of anal incontinence. Obstetric trauma is usually the cause of involuntary fecal loss in most women seeking care for this symptom. Symptoms of fecal urgency, fecal incontinence, or both may be present in up to 50% of patients with a history of third- or fourth-degree perineal lacerations, despite primary repair. Generally, an initial approach to evaluating fecal loss follows the routine for evaluating urinary incontinence; ie, understanding the specific symptoms and inquiring about normal bowel habits and prior treatments.

Box 51

Risk Factors for Colorectal Cancer

- History of colorectal, endometrial, ovarian, or breast cancer
- History of adenomatous polyps
- Family history of colorectal cancer (two or more first-degree relatives)
- Ulcerative colitis or Crohn colitis
- Previous radiation exposure to the bowel
- Familial adenomatous polyposis
- Cancer familial syndrome (Lynch syndrome II)
- Possibly, diets high in fat and low in fiber

Data from Ferrante JM. Colorectal cancer screening. Med Clin North Am 1996;80:27–43.

Table 22. American Cancer Society Guidelines for Screening and Surveillance for the Early Detection of Colorectal Adenomas and Cancer in Individuals at Increased and High Risk

Risk Category	Age to Begin	Recommendation	Comment
Increased Risk—Patients With History of Polyps Before Colonoscopy			
Patients with small rectal hyperplastic polyps*	—	Colonoscopy or other screening options at intervals recommended for average-risk individuals	An exception are patients with a hyperplastic polyposis syndrome. They are at increased risk for adenomas and colorectal cancer and need to be identified for more intensive follow-up.
Patients with one or two small tubular adenomas with low-grade dysplasia*	5–10 years after the initial polypectomy	Colonoscopy	The precise timing within this interval should be based on other clinical factors (such as prior colonoscopy findings, family history, and the preferences of the patient and judgment of the physician).
Patients with three to 10 adenomas, or one adenoma greater than 1 cm, or any adenoma with villous features, or high-grade dysplasia*	3 years after the initial polypectomy	Colonoscopy	Adenomas must have been completely removed. If the follow-up colonoscopy is normal or shows only one or two small, tubular adenomas with low-grade dysplasia, then the interval for the subsequent examination should be 5 years.
Patients with more than 10 adenomas on a single examination*	Less than 3 years after the initial polypectomy	Colonoscopy	Consider the possibility of an underlying familial syndrome.
Patients with sessile adenomas that are removed piecemeal*	2–6 months to verify complete removal	Colonoscopy	Once complete removal has been established, subsequent surveillance needs to be individualized based on the endoscopist's judgment. Completeness of removal should be based on both endoscopic and pathologic assessments.
Increased Risk—Patients With Colorectal Cancer			
Patients with colon and rectal cancer should undergo high-quality perioperative clearing.†	3–6 months after cancer resection, if no unresectable metastases are found during surgery; alternatively, colonoscopy can be performed intraoperatively	Colonoscopy	In the case of nonobstructing tumors, this can be done by preoperative colonoscopy. In the case of obstructing colon cancers, CTC with intravenous contrast or DCBE can be used to detect neoplasms in the proximal colon.

(continued)

Table 22. American Cancer Society Guidelines for Screening and Surveillance for the Early Detection of Colorectal Adenomas and Cancer in Individuals at Increased and High Risk (*continued*)

Risk Category	Age to Begin	Recommendation	Comment
Increased Risk—Patients With Colorectal Cancer (continued)			
Patients undergoing curative resection for colon or rectal cancer[‡]	1 year after the resection (or 1 year after the performance of the colonoscopy that was performed to clear the colon of synchronous disease)	Colonoscopy	This colonoscopy at 1 year is in addition to the perioperative colonoscopy for synchronous tumors. If the examination performed at 1 year is normal, then the interval before the next subsequent examination should be 3 years. If that colonoscopy is normal, then the interval before the next subsequent examination should be 5 years. Following the examination at 1 year, the intervals before subsequent examinations may be shortened if there is evidence of HNPCC or if adenoma findings warrant earlier colonoscopy. Periodic examination of the rectum for the purpose of identifying local recurrence, usually performed at 3- to 6-month intervals for the first 2 or 3 years, may be considered after low-anterior resection of rectal cancer.
Increased Risk—Patients With a Family History			
Either colorectal cancer or adenomatous polyps in a first-degree relative before age 60 years or in two or more first-degree relatives at any age[§]	Age 40 years or 10 years before the youngest affected relative in the immediate family	Colonoscopy	Every 5 years
Either colorectal cancer or adenomatous polyps in a first-degree relative aged 60 years or older or in two second-degree relatives with colorectal cancer	Age 40 years	Screening options at intervals recommended for average-risk individuals	Screening should begin at an earlier age, but individuals may choose to be screened with any recommended form of testing.
High Risk			
Genetic diagnosis of FAP without genetic testing evidence[§]	Age 10–12 years	Annual FSIG to determine if the individual is expressing the genetic abnormality and counseling to consider genetic testing	If the genetic test is positive, colectomy should be considered.

(continued)

Table 22. American Cancer Society Guidelines for Screening and Surveillance for the Early Detection of Colorectal Adenomas and Cancer in Individuals at Increased and High Risk (*continued*)

Risk Category	Age to Begin	Recommendation	Comment
	High Risk (continued)		
Genetic or clinical diagnosis of HNPCC or individuals at increased risk of HNPCC[§]	Age 20 to 25 years or 10 years before the youngest affected relative in the immediate family	Colonoscopy every 1–2 years and counseling to consider genetic testing	Genetic testing for HNPCC should be offered to first-degree relatives of persons with a known inherited MMR gene mutation. It also should be offered when the family mutation is not already known, but one of the first three of the modified Bethesda criteria is present.
Inflammatory bowel disease[§], chronic ulcerative colitis, and Crohn colitis	Cancer risk begins to be significant 8 years after the onset of pancolitis or 12 to 15 years after the onset of left-sided colitis	Colonoscopy with biopsy for dysplasia	Every 1 to 2 years; these patients are best referred to a center with experience in the surveillance and management of inflammatory bowel disease.

*Winawer SJ, Zauber AG, Fletcher RH, Stillman JS, O'brien MJ, Levin B, et al. Guidelines for colonoscopy surveillance after polypectomy: a consensus update by the US Multi-Society Task Force on Colorectal Cancer and the American Cancer Society. CA Cancer J Clin 2006;56:143–59; quiz 184–5.

[†]Rex DK, Kahi CJ, Levin B, Smith RA, Bond JH, Brooks D, et al. Guidelines for colonoscopy surveillance after cancer resection: a consensus update by the American Cancer Society and the US Multi-Society Task Force on Colorectal Cancer. American Cancer Society; US Multi-Society Task Force on Colorectal Cancer. Gastroenterology 2006;130:1865–71.

[‡]Ries LA, Melbert D, Krapcho M, Stinchcomb DG, Howlader N, Horner MJ, et al. SEER cancer statistics review, 1975–2005. Bethesda (MD): National Cancer Institute; 2007. Available at: http://seer.cancer.gov/csr/1975_2005. Retrieved November 14, 2008.

[§]Winawer S, Fletcher R, Rex D, Bond J, Burt R, Ferrucci J, et al. Colorectal cancer screening and surveillance: clinical guidelines and rationale–Update based on new evidence. Gastrointestinal Consortium Panel. Gastroenterology 2003;124:544–60.

Abbreviations: CTC indicates computed tomographic colonography; DCBE, double-contrast barium enema; FAP, familial adenomatous polyposis; FSIG, flexible sigmoidoscopy; HNPCC, hereditary nonpolyposis colon cancer; MMR, mismatch repair.

Levin B, Lieberman DA, McFarland B, Smith RA, Brooks D, Andrews KA, et al. Screening and surveillance for the early detection of colorectal cancer and adenomatous polyps, 2008: a joint guideline from the American Cancer Society, the US Multi-Society Task Force on Colorectal Cancer, and the American College of Radiology. CA Cancer J Clin 2008;58(3):130–60 and Reprinted from Gastroenterology, Vol 134, Levin B, Lieberman DA, McFarland B, Smith RA, Brooks D, Andrews KA, et al. Screening and surveillance for the early detection of colorectal cancer and adenomatous polyps, 2008: a joint guideline from the American Cancer Society, the US Multi-Society Task Force on Colorectal Cancer, and the American College of Radiology, Pages 1570–95, Copyright 2008, with permission from Elsevier.

Etiology

Anal incontinence has several causes. However, a growing body of literature documents the hazards of pregnancy and vaginal delivery for the anal sphincter. Studies in which anatomic and functional characteristics of the anus were compared before and after uncomplicated deliveries show a significant decrease in anal pressure and a high rate of anatomic disruption that is unrecognized and unrepaired. Injuries can have anatomic components, neuromuscular components, or both. Women whose sphincter injuries are recognized and repaired according to current techniques are still more likely to become symptomatic than are women with uninjured sphincters, possibly because of concomitant neuromuscular damage.

In general, the causes of fecal incontinence in women are divided into two groups: causes related to an abnormal sphincter mechanism and causes related to impaired storage in the rectal reservoir. Chiefly considered here are the events that contribute to the damage of the rectal sphincter. The entities that most commonly affect the storage function, or distensibility, of the rectum are radiation therapy to the pelvis, inflammatory bowel diseases, scleroderma, and diabetes mellitus. Like the problem of poor compliance, this limitation of rectal function diminishes the storage ability and reduces the rectum's ability to discern between gas, fluid, and solid waste.

Evaluation

The history must include the patient's bowel habits, the frequency of leakage, the characteristics of the substances passed (solid, liquid, or gas), the need for perineal pads or diapers, the timing of incontinence, the effect on lifestyle, and the dietary or medical therapies attempted. Physical examination includes a brief neurologic examination that includes checking the reflexes of the lower extremities and the cutaneous anal reflex, or anal wink, bilaterally. The vagina, perineal body, and anus should be examined visually for any deformity, including the appearance of descent, prolapse, or incontinence with the Valsalva maneuver. The digital examination should assess for masses, palpable defects, impacted stool, and sphincter tone at rest and with maximal squeeze. Contraction of the puborectalis muscle can be felt along the posterior rectal wall just above the external anal sphincter.

When the certainty of fecal incontinence is in doubt, a form of stress test can be performed by introducing tap water or saline into the rectum to assess the presence and severity of rectal incontinence. The same neurologic assessment recommended for urinary incontinence should be performed for fecal incontinence; the test should include pudendal nerve function assessment, which can pinpoint a cause for both conditions. Other forms of testing, although unavailable to many obstetrician–gynecologists, include the following:

- Endoscopic evaluation of the rectosigmoid colon or beyond
- Anal manometry for compliance testing
- Neurodiagnostic testing, electromyelography, and nerve testing
- Anal ultrasonography and magnetic resonance imaging

Several of these techniques are in the investigative phase, but they are revealing new information that has expanded the understanding of this troublesome disorder.

Therapy

Therapeutic considerations for patients with fecal incontinence depend on the diagnosis discovered by the evaluation. If no surgical defect is demonstrated, the goal of therapy is to help the patient maintain a state of formed stool and to make every effort to keep the rectum empty. Recommendations include dietary modifications (mostly to increase fiber) and muscle exercises much like those recommended for certain bladder conditions. Dietary modifications, such as appropriate fiber intake (25–30 g/d) result in improved symptoms in 50% of patients. Properly performed Kegel exercises result in reduced symptoms in more than 60% of users (see "Urinary Tract Disorders"). Biofeedback methods have been used with results similar to those achieved in patients with bladder dysfunction. If an anatomic disruption of the rectal sphincter or pudendal nerve dysfunction has been demonstrated, surgical intervention may be considered. However, the results are less rewarding in the latter condition.

Follow-up and Referral

The safest route of delivery for a woman who has had a prior anal sphincter repair or whose sphincter is minimally symptomatic is based on expert opinion. Proponents of subsequent cesarean delivery cite the known neuromuscular damage with vaginal delivery and the increased chance of symptoms in such patients. Proponents of repeated vaginal delivery suggest that the primary damage occurs with the first delivery and that the second delivery poses little additional risk. These important epidemiologic questions remain unanswered. Until scientific data are available, discussions with patients should include the uncertainty of current knowledge and the recognized risks of all routes of delivery.

Crohn Disease

Crohn disease comprises a spectrum of clinical and pathologic patterns manifested by focal, asymmetric, transmural, and occasionally granulomatous inflammation affecting the gastrointestinal tract. Occasionally, it can be systemic or extraintestinal (affecting the vulva, eyes, skin, and joints). The onset of the disease is most common in the second and third decades, and its prevalence in the United States is approximately 50 per 100,000 (23). Characteristic symptoms include chronic or nocturnal diarrhea and abdominal pain, weight loss, fever, and rectal bleeding. Clinical signs include pallor; cachexia; abdominal mass or tenderness; and perianal fissures, fistulae, or abscess.

The ileum and colon are the most commonly affected sites. The onset of Crohn disease is typically insidious, but it can present with a fulminant onset or toxic megacolon. The diagnosis is based on documentation of focal, asymmetric, transmural, or granulomatous features with endoscopic, radiographic, and pathologic studies. The differential diagnosis includes other inflammatory bowel diseases (infectious, ischemic, radiation-induced, and medication-induced disorders), idiopathic disease (eg, ulcerative colitis and celiac disease), and IBS.

The severity of Crohn disease is classified according to clinical parameters, systemic manifestations, and the effect of the disease on the patient's life. Therapy is determined by the severity of the disease, response to therapy, and tolerance of medical intervention (23). Mild to moderate disease frequently is managed with an oral aminosalicylate (mesalamine or sulfasalazine), high-dose metronidazole, or ciprofloxacin. Moderate to severe disease frequently is managed with prednisone until resolution of symptoms occurs. Infliximab, a human–mouse chimeric monoclonal immunoglobulin G1 antibody directed at tumor necrosis factor-α, is now used in the management of moderate to severe disease. Patients with severe–fulminant disease frequently are managed with hospitalization and parenteral steroids, with the possible addition of cyclosporine. Surgery is warranted in patients who have obstruction with a tender abdominal mass.

Because Crohn disease is not curable, the aim of treatment is disease remission. Azathioprine and 6-mercaptopurine have demonstrated benefits for use as maintenance therapy after initial therapy with corticosteroids (23).

References

1. Agreus L, Talley NJ. Dyspepsia: current understanding and management. Annu Rev Med 1998;49:475–93.

2. Ashley SW, Evoy D, Daly JM. Stomach. In Schwartz SI, Fisher JE, Spencer FC, Shires GT, Daly JM, editors. Principles of surgery. 7th ed. New York (NY): McGraw-Hill; 1999. p. 1181–216.

3. Malfertheiner P, Megraud F, O'Morain C, Bazzoli F, El-Omar E, Graham D, et al. Current concepts in the management of Helicobacter pylori infection: the Maastricht III Consensus Report. Gut 2007;56:772–81.

4. Soll AH. Consensus conference. Medical treatment of peptic ulcer disease. Practice guidelines. Practice Parameters Committee of the American College of Gastroenterology [published erratum appears in JAMA 1996;275:1314]. JAMA 1996;275:622–9.

5. Talley NJ, Vakil N. Guidelines for the management of dyspepsia. Practice Parameters Committee of the American College of Gastroenterology. Am J Gastroenterol 2005;100:2324–37.

6. Weinberg DS, Kadish SL. The diagnosis and management of gastroesophageal reflux disease. Med Clin North Am 1996;80:411–29.

7. Sexuality and Sexual Dysfunction. Dent J. Management of reflux disease. Gut 2002;50 Suppl 4:iv67–71.

8. Peters JH, DeMeester TR. Esophagus and diaphragmatic hernia. In Schwartz SI, Fisher JE, Spencer FC, Shires GT, Daly JM, editors. Principles of Surgery. 7th ed. New York (NY): McGraw-Hill; 1999. p. 1081–180.

9. Attwood SE, Lundell L, Hatlebakk JG, Eklund S, Junghard O, Galmiche JP, et al. Medical or surgical management of GERD patients with Barrett's esophagus: the LOTUS trial 3-year experience. J Gastrointest Surg 2008;12:1646–54; discussion 1654–5.

10. Drossman DA, Camilleri M, Mayer EA, Whitehead WE. AGA technical review on irritable bowel syndrome. Gastroenterology 2002;123:2108–31.

11. Brandt LJ, Bjorkman D, Fennerty MB, Locke GR, Olden K, Peterson W, et al. Systematic review on the management of irritable bowel syndrome in North America. Am J Gastroenterol 2002;97:S7–26.

12. Jackson SL, Hull TL. Fecal incontinence in women. Obstet Gynecol Surv 1998;53:741–7; quiz 748–51.

13. Velio P, Bassotti G. Chronic idiopathic constipation: pathophysiology and treatment. J Clin Gastroenterol 1996;22:190–6.

14. Read NW, Celik AF, Katsinelos P. Constipation and incontinence in the elderly. J Clin Gastroenterol 1995;20:61–70.

15. Weber J, Ducrotte P, Touchais JY, Roussignol C, Denis P. Biofeedback training for constipation in adults and children. Dis Colon Rectum 1987;30:844–6.

16. Jacobs DO. Clinical practice. Diverticulitis. N Engl J Med 2007;357:2057–66.

17. Jemal A, Siegel R, Ward E, Hao Y, Xu J, Murray T, et al. Cancer statistics, 2008. CA Cancer J Clin 2008;58:71–96.

18. Ferrante JM. Colorectal cancer screening. Med Clin North Am 1996;80:27–43.

19. Increased use of colorectal cancer tests--United States, 2002 and 2004. Centers for Disease Control and Prevention. MMWR Morb Mortal Wkly Rep 2006;55:308–11.

20. Ransohoff DF, Sandler RS. Clinical practice. Screening for colorectal cancer. N Engl J Med 2002;346:40–4.

21. Screening for Colorectal Cancer—United States, 1997. Centers for Disease Control and Prevention. MMWR Morb Mortal Wkly Rep 1999;48:116–21.

22. Colonoscopy and colorectal cancer screening and prevention. ACOG Committee Opinion No. 384. American College of Obstetricians and Gynecologists. Obstet Gynecol 2007;110:1199–202.

23. Hanauer SB, Sandborn W. Management of Crohn's disease in adults. Practice Parameters Committee of the American College of Gastroenterology. Am J Gastroenterol 2001;96:635–43.

Osteoporosis

Robert L. Barbieri

Osteoporosis is a disease of the bone that is characterized by a predisposition to low-trauma fractures caused by low bone mass and disordered microarchitecture. Approximately 1.5 million osteoporotic fractures occur annually in the United States, and approximately 50% of women older than 50 years will experience an osteoporotic fracture. Of patients with an osteoporotic hip fracture, 50% are unable to walk independently after their fracture heals.

Diagnosis and Screening

The measurement of bone mineral density (BMD) is central to the detection and treatment of osteoporosis (Box 52). Bone mineral density should be measured in all women older than 65 years and in all menopausal women with a clinical risk factor for osteoporosis (1). Clinical risk factors include early menopause, prolonged premenopausal amenorrhea, parental history of a hip fracture, current cigarette smoking, and a body weight of less than 57.7 kg (127 lb). The use of certain medications, such as corticosteroids and heparin, and some metabolic conditions, such as hyperthyroidism and malabsorption, are associated with osteoporosis. In general, men have higher BMD values than women. African-American women have higher BMD values than white women. White, Latina, and Asian women have similar BMDs when controlled for body mass index (BMI) (2). Most data on osteoporosis treatment are based on the study of white women.

The technologies available for measuring bone density include dual-energy X-ray absorptiometry (DXA), single-energy X-ray absorptiometry, ultrasonography, radiographic absorptiometry, and quantitative computed tomography. Dual- and single-energy X-ray absorptiometry and radiographic absorptiometry have radiation exposures in the range of 1–5 mrem—less than the radiation exposures of mammography. Quantitative computed tomography has a radiation exposure in the range of 50 mrem.

Measurements of BMD at the hip and spine are more predictive of hip and spine fractures than are measurement of BMD at the forearm or heel. Bone mineral density at the hip is the best predictor of hip fracture. Because the risk of hip fracture increases rapidly in women older than 65 years, it may be especially important to focus on hip BMD in women of this age (Table 23). Spine and hip BMD valueshave similar clinical efficacy in predicting spine fractures. In women aged 65 years and older, degenerative arthritis and calcifications near the vertebral bodies may limit the diagnostic and predictive value of spine BMD measurements. Because BMD in the spine changes rapidly in women taking oral corticosteroids, the spine might be the best site for monitoring osteoporosis in these women.

Resources

Osteoporosis

National Institute of Arthritis and Musculoskeletal and Skin Diseases
http://www.niams.nih.gov

National Osteoporosis Foundation
http://www.nof.org

North American Menopause Society
http://www.menopause.org

Women's Health Initiative
http://www.nhlbi.nih.gov/whi

Box 52

Bone Disease Terminology

Osteopenia: A term developed by the World Health Organization to refer to T scores between −1.0 and −2.5.

Osteoporosis: A term defined by the World Health Organization as a bone density T score at or below −2.5 standard deviations of normal peak bone density values for sex-matched young adults. A diagnosis of osteoporosis also can be made by proving the presence of a low-impact vertebral, hip, or wrist fracture.

T score: The difference in standard deviations between the value for a patient being tested and the mean value of a sex-matched group of adults aged 25–45 years. A T score of 0 indicates that the person being tested has a bone mineral density that is the mean for adults aged 25–45 years. For any measurement, the range from the 5th to the 95th percentile of a group covers approximately 4 standard deviations.

Z score: The difference in standard deviations between the mean bone mineral density of a patient being tested and a group of people of the same age and sex.

Cummings SR, Bates D, Black DM. Clinical use of bone densitometry: scientific review [published erratum appears in JAMA 2002;288:2825]. JAMA 2002;288:1889–97.

Table 23. Lifetime Risk (in %) of Hip Fracture for White Women Based on Femoral Neck Bone Mineral Density T Score*

Age (years)	T Score							
	-3.5	-3	-2.5	-2	-1.5	-1	-0.5	0
50	49	41	33	27	21	16	13	10
60	47	40	33	27	21	17	13	10
70	46	39	33	27	21	17	13	10
80	41	35	30	24	21	16	12	10

*These estimates are based on a stochastic model using a logistic model of the relationship between bone mineral density and risk of hip fracture derived from the Study of Osteoporotic Fractures (relative risk, 2.6/standard deviation decrease). T scores were based on bone mineral density results from Hologic QDR 1000 densitometers, with T scores derived from the National Helath and Nutrition Examination Survey III 1995 database. Overall mortality rates are based on US Vital Statistics. Statistical methods are published in part in Black DM, Cummings SR, Melton III LJ. Appendicular bone mineral and a woman's lifetime risk of hip fracture. J Bone Miner Res 1992;7:639-46.

Cummings SR, Bates D, Black DM. Clinical use of bone densitometry: scientific review [published erratum appears in JAMA 2002;288:2825]. JAMA 2002;288:1889-97. Copyright © 2002 American Medical Association. All right reserved.

Measurements of BMD at peripheral sites (eg, forearm and heel) are less expensive than measurements of hip and spine BMD, but they also are less predictive of hip fracture. Measurement of peripheral sites may be cost-effective to identify women who should be referred for DXA of the hip and spine.

The cost-effectiveness of monitoring BMD during treatment is not well studied. Small changes in BMD values may be caused by the random variability of the test. Bone mineral density should not be measured more frequently than every 1–2 years during treatment.

Biochemical markers of bone resorption (collagen cross-linked C-telopeptide, peptide-bound N-telopeptide cross-links, and free deoxypyridinoline) provide a single assessment of bone resorption at one point in time and are not clinically useful for diagnosing osteoporosis. After adjusting for age and BMD, these markers have limited usefulness in assessing initial response to therapies that reduce bone resorption.

The use of algorithms that combine BMD measurement with clinical factors, such as age and preexisting fractures, is a good way to identify women most likely to benefit from treatment (3). The purpose of combining BMD measurement and clinical risk factors in a single prediction algorithm is to better identify women who will most benefit from therapy and to try to avoid treating women with osteoporosis who are at lowest risk of fracture (4).

Secondary Causes

The chance of finding a secondary cause of osteoporosis in a primary care setting is unknown, and the cost-effectiveness of screening for secondary causes is not well characterized. Some diseases associated with secondary osteoporosis include intestinal malabsorption, hyperparathyroidism, hyperthyroidism, multiple myeloma, Cushing disease, and Paget disease. Box 53 lists laboratory tests commonly performed in the evaluation of secondary osteoporosis.

Intestinal malabsorption is a common cause of secondary osteoporosis. Celiac disease is associated with the chronic malabsorption of vitamin D and calcium. Population-based screening studies report that approximately 1% of white women have celiac disease; however, the disease is diagnosed in only one third of these women. In one study of more than 250 patients with osteoporosis, 4.5% had celiac disease, compared with 1% of patients without osteoporosis (5). Measurement of antiendomysial antibodies is a sensitive screening test for celiac disease.

Box 53

Laboratory Evaluation for Secondary Causes of Osteoporosis

Serum Chemistry for
- Calcium
- Phosphorus
- Albumin
- Alkaline phosphate

Endocrine Measurements of Circulating
- Parathyroid hormone
- Thyroid-stimulating hormone
- 25-hydroxyvitamin D

Data from Wagman RB, Marcus R. Beyond bone mineral density-navigating the laboratory assessment of patients with osteoporosis. J Clin Endocrinol Metab 2002;87: 4429-30 and Tannenbaum C, Clark J, Schwartzman K, Wallenstein S, Lapinski R, Meier D, et al. Yield of laboratory testing to identify secondary contributors to osteoporosis in otherwise healthy women. J Clin Endocrinol Metab 2002;87:4431-7.

The administration of corticosteroids is a common cause of osteoporosis. The cumulative dose of corticosteroids correlates with the magnitude of the decrease in BMD and the rate of fracture. A daily dose of less than 7.5 mg of prednisone or equivalent is associated with minimal bone loss in euestrogenic women. At higher doses, corticosteroids are associated with appreciable bone loss and a clinically important increase in fracture risk. Skeletal bones with a high proportion of trabecular bone, such as the spine and ribs, are most susceptible to bone loss during corticosteroid treatment. Measurement of BMD is useful in estimating the effect of corticosteroid treatment on bone density. Bisphosphonates and teriparatide (PTH 1-34) have been demonstrated to be effective treatments for patients with corticosteroid-induced osteoporosis.

Osteomalacia is the disordered mineralization of newly formed bone protein matrix. Causes of osteomalacia include vitamin D deficiency and hypophosphatemia. In osteomalacia, but not in primary osteoporosis, the serum phosphate level is reduced and the serum alkaline phosphatase level is elevated. The combination of hypophosphatemia and hypocalcemia is typical of severe vitamin D deficiency. Isolated hypophosphatemia often is seen in patients with renal tubular phosphate wasting syndrome.

Prevention and Treatment

Diet and Exercise

An optimal diet for the prevention and treatment of osteoporosis includes 1,000–1,500 mg of elemental calcium per day in divided doses with meals, 800 international units of vitamin D per day, and adequate calories to avoid malnutrition (6). Vitamin D intake of 400 international units daily does not appear to be sufficient to prevent fractures. Adequate protein in the diet helps to preserve bone density.

Many claims have been made for the possible benefits of specific nutrients on bone health. For example, isoflavones, which have mixed estrogen agonist–antagonist properties, have been advocated for the treatment of menopausal symptoms and osteoporosis. The clinical efficacy and safety of isoflavones have not been completely characterized. In one study of the isoflavone ipriflavone (200 mg, administered three times daily) compared with placebo, there was no difference in BMD or vertebral fractures in the two groups. In addition, ipriflavone treatment induced lymphocytopenia in 13% of the subjects (7). This study indicates that some herbs and "nutrients" advocated for the treatment of menopausal symptoms have no benefit and may cause appreciable clinical risks.

Physical activity reduces the risk of fracture by improving muscle strength and balance, which reduces the risk of falling, and by increasing BMD. Clinical trials have reported that hip bone density can be increased with weight-bearing exercise or resistance training. In a clinical trial, 40 postmenopausal women were randomly assigned to groups receiving either high-intensity strength training 2 days per week or standard activity. After 1 year, hip and spine BMD values increased by 0.9% and 1% in the strength-training group and decreased by 2.5% and 1.8% in the control group, respectively (8).

Recent studies have reported that even modest amounts of physical activity can reduce fracture risk. For example, 1 hour of walking at a moderate pace is equivalent to three metabolic equivalents; three metabolic equivalents of activity per week was associated with a 6% decrease in the risk of hip fracture, and 24 metabolic equivalents of activity per week was associated with a 55% decrease in hip fracture. Reduction in hip fracture risk was seen in low-risk (high-BMI) and high-risk (low-BMI) groups. For women who walked at an average pace for 4 hours per week and did no other exercise, the risk of hip fracture was reduced by 41% (relative risk, 0.59; 95% confidence interval, 0.37–0.94), as compared with a group who walked less than 1 hour per week. Women who walked at a brisk pace further reduced their risk of fracture. In addition, sedentary women who began walking for 4 hours per week reduced their risk of hip fracture as compared with sedentary women who remained sedentary. Paradoxically, "healthy" lifestyle changes that include decreased saturated fat and caloric intake and increased exercise may be associated with successful weight loss and increased loss of BMD at the hip (9).

Cessation of smoking is strongly recommended for all women. In a study of female twins who were discordant for smoking, a dosage of one pack of cigarettes per day during adult life was associated with a 5–10% reduction in bone density in the smoking twin compared with that of the nonsmoking twin (10).

Pharmacologic Prevention and Treatment

Pharmacologic treatment should be offered to women with known osteoporosis and women with a history of osteoporotic fracture (11). According to community-based studies, most women with documented osteoporotic fractures have had neither evaluation nor treatment for osteoporosis (12). Women without preexisting fractures and a T score of less than –2, as well as women with a T score of –1.5 and another clinical risk factor, should be offered treatment. Clinicians must diligently ensure that women with osteoporotic fractures are offered evaluation and treatment.

ORAL BISPHOSPHONATES

The bisphosphonates—alendronate (70 mg once per week or 10 mg daily), risedronate (5 mg daily, 35 mg once per week, 75 mg on each of 2 consecutive days each month, or one monthly dose of 150 mg), and ibandronate (150 mg once per month or 5 mg daily)—are approved by the U.S. Food and Drug Administration (FDA) for the prevention and treatment of osteoporosis. Clinical trials have demonstrated that alendronate and risedronate reduce vertebral, hip, and other fractures. Compliance is an important factor in predicting the effectiveness of bisphosphonate therapy. Once-weekly or once-monthly dosing is associated with better compliance than is daily dosing.

The use of the bisphosphonates can be associated with adverse gastrointestinal events, such as nausea, vomiting, epigastric pain, and diarrhea. Most studies demonstrate that when alendronate, risedronate, and ibandronate are properly administered, the rate of gastrointestinal adverse effects is low. For example, esophagitis occurs in approximately 1 person per 8,000 person–years of use of a bisphosphonate. To reduce gastrointestinal side effects and enhance bioavailability, it is recommended that bisphosphonates be administered with 240 mL (8 fl oz) of water with the patient in a fasting state, after which the patient is advised to remain upright for at least 30 minutes. No food or beverage should be consumed within the first 30 minutes after taking the medicine. The potential risks of bisphosphonate therapy, including osteonecrosis, must be weighed against the clear protective effect of continuing therapy for as long as possible over 10 years. The optimal duration of therapy with bisphosphonates is not known.

Bisphosphonate therapy may be associated with the development of osteonecrosis of the jaw. In one study of 368 cases of osteonecrosis of the jaw, 85% of the cases had prevalent multiple myeloma or breast cancer, and 94% of the cases had received bisphosphonates intravenously. Only 4% of the cases had been taking a bisphosphonate orally for the treatment of postmenopausal osteoporosis. A history of recent dental surgery was found in 60% of the cases (13). A recent review reported that the estimated risk of osteonecrosis was approximately 1 per 100,000 person–years for postmenopausal women taking an oral bisphosphonate and 1 per 100 person–years for cancer patients receiving bisphosphonates intravenously (14).

There are no clinical trials that guide recommendations for preventing bisphosphonate-associated osteonecrosis of the jaw. However, many dental surgeons recommend that patients receiving long-term bisphosphonate treatment stop therapy 3 months before a planned tooth extraction or tooth implant and not reinitiate therapy until the jaw is fully healed (15). Given the evidence that bisphosphonates have a long biologic half-life and that bone mineral changes occur over relatively long periods, a 6-month bisphosphonate holiday is unlikely to be associated with detrimental bone loss.

INTRAVENOUS BISPHOSPHONATES

Two intravenous bisphosphonate regimens are currently approved by the FDA: zoledronic acid, 5 mg intravenous bolus annually, and ibandronate, 3 mg intravenously every 3 months. Compared with oral regimens, intravenous bisphosphonate therapy increases the likelihood that patients will comply with treatment. In one trial of intravenous zoledronic acid, 2,127 patients who experienced a hip fracture within the previous 90 days were randomized to receive intravenous zoledronic acid or a placebo. After 1.9 years of therapy, there was a 35% decrease in new clinical fractures in the zoledronic acid group compared with the placebo group (16). According to data from a large trial (N=7,765) that focused on postmenopausal women with osteoporosis, 14 women would need to be treated with intravenous zoledronic acid to prevent one vertebral fracture, and 98 women would need to be treated to prevent one hip fracture (17).

To reduce the risk of renal toxicity, it is important that zoledronic acid be infused over 15–30 minutes and that it not be administered to women with renal insufficiency. Intravenous bisphosphonates are more expensive than generic alendronate.

RALOXIFENE

Raloxifene is a selective estrogen receptor modulator that is approved for the prevention and treatment of osteoporosis (18). In the Raloxifene Use for the Heart (RUTH) trial, 10,101 postmenopausal women with coronary heart disease or multiple risk factors for that disease were randomly assigned to receive raloxifene or placebo, with a median treatment interval of 5.6 years (19). Raloxifene therapy was associated with a 35% reduction in vertebral fractures. Raloxifene also was associated with a 44% reduction in invasive breast cancer. Raloxifene and placebo were associated with a similar risk of coronary events, but raloxifene was associated with more cases of deep venous thromboembolism and fatal stroke. In a separate trial of women at increased risk of developing breast cancer as determined by the Gail scoring system (5-year risk, 4%), raloxifene and tamoxifen therapy were associated with similar rates of breast cancer, but the raloxifene group had 30% fewer cases of deep vein thrombosis and 38% fewer cases of uterine cancer than the tamoxifen group (20).

ESTROGEN AND ESTROGEN–PROGESTIN TREATMENT

The Women's Health Initiative reported that in postmenopausal women, the combination of conjugated equine estrogen (0.625 mg) and medroxyprogesterone acetate (2.5 mg) daily, as well as conjugated equine estrogen as daily monotherapy, was associated with a reduced risk of hip fractures and total fractures (21). In a trial of combination estrogen–progestin treatment, the average age of the subjects on entry into the study was 63 years, and the mean follow-up was 5.2 years. Estrogen–progestin therapy was associated with 34% fewer hip fractures and 34% fewer vertebral fractures than was placebo. The reduction in fracture risk was most prominent in women with a BMI of less than 25 (measured as weight in kilograms divided by height in meters squared). Estrogen–progestin treatment was not associated with a statistically significant reduction in fracture risk in obese women (BMI greater than 30).

The effect of estrogen on BMD is dosage dependent. Dosages of estrogen as low as conjugated equine estrogen 0.3 mg daily or transdermal estradiol 14 micrograms daily have been reported to be associated with an increase in lumbar spine and hip BMD compared with placebo. However, these low-dose and ultralow-dose estrogen regimens have not definitively been demonstrated to reduce hip fracture in large clinical trials.

The relative benefits and risks of estrogen monotherapy and estrogen–progestin combination treatment suggest that other agents, such as the bisphosphonates, should be considered as first-line therapy for osteoporosis. Estrogen monotherapy and estrogen–progestin therapy may be indicated for the treatment of osteoporosis in women with vasomotor symptoms requiring hormone treatment. Additional indications for estrogen treatment in women with osteoporosis include not being able to tolerate other treatments, such as alendronate or risedronate. For menopausal women who are stopping estrogen treatment, bone loss is likely to increase in the 2 years after discontinuation of estrogen treatment. When women with a history of osteoporosis discontinue estrogen treatment, they should consider initiating bisphosphonate or raloxifene therapy.

In premenopausal women with osteoporosis and hypoestrogenism, estrogen remains a primary treatment option. In one clinical trial, 48 women with hypoestrogenism caused by anorexia were randomly assigned to receive estrogen or no estrogen. After 1.5 years of treatment, BMD increased 4% in the estrogen group and decreased 20% in the women not treated with estrogen (22).

CALCITONIN

The use of calcitonin nasal spray, 200 international units daily, increases BMD in the spine and hip, but not as much as treatment with alendronate (23). In women with acute osteoporotic fracture and appreciable musculoskeletal pain, calcitonin may have benefit as first-line therapy in the first month of treatment, because its use is associated with a decrease in pain.

TERIPARATIDE

Chronic hyperparathyroidism is associated with bone loss. Paradoxically, administration of teriparatide (PTH 1-

34) increases bone formation and BMD over the first 18 months of treatment. The FDA has approved the use of teriparatide for the treatment of osteoporosis at a dose of 20 micrograms by daily subcutaneous injection.

COMBINATION TREATMENT

The combination of estrogen plus a bisphosphonate increases BMD more than either agent alone (24). In addition, the combination of raloxifene plus a bisphosphonate increases BMD more than either agent independently. (25). The combination of teriparatide plus a bisphosphonate does not increase BMD compared with teriparatide monotherapy. In general, combination therapy has clinical limitations because of the lack of long-term studies demonstrating fracture reduction and safety. The use of two antiresorptive agents in combination may oversuppress bone turnover (26). In most cases, a woman with osteoporosis who continues to lose bone while taking one agent typically is given an alternative agent rather than combination therapy.

Once the treatment is established, the patient's response to therapy should be monitored. This follow-up should not be repeated more often than 1–2 years after initiation of therapy (Box 54).

Box 54

Monitoring Therapy for Osteoporosis in Postmenopausal Women

For monitoring the patient's response to therapy, dual-energy X-ray absorptiometry testing should be performed 1–2 years after the initiation of therapy. The continued management decision depends on the test result:

- If the result of the bone mineral density measurement is increased, stable, or has decreased less than 0.3 g/cm^2 from the baseline, the current therapy should be continued. Repeated dual-energy X-ray absorptiometry monitoring has not proved to be necessary, but may be repeated every 2 years, if desired.

- If the result of the bone mineral density measurement is decreased more than 0.3 g/cm^2 from the baseline, evaluation should be performed for secondary causes of osteoporosis. If workup results are normal, compliance issues should be discussed with the patient and consideration given to changing the regimen to one that is more acceptable to the patient.

References

1. Low bone mass (osteopenia) and fracture risk. ACOG Committee Opinion No. 407. American College of Obstetricians and Gynecologists. Obstet Gynecol 2008;111: 1259–61.

2. Finkelstein JS, Lee ML, Sowers M, Ettinger B, Neer RM, Kelsey JL, et al. Ethnic variation in bone density in pre-menopausal and early perimenopausal women: effects of anthropometric and lifestyle factors. J Clin Endocrinol Metab 2002;87:3057–67.

3. Dawson-Hughes B, Tosteson AN, Melton LJ 3rd, Baim S, Favus MJ, Khosla S, et al. Implications of absolute fracture risk assessment for osteoporosis practice guidelines in the USA. National Osteoporosis Foundation Guide Committee. Osteoporos Int 2008;19:449–58.

4. De Laet C, Oden A, Johansson H, Johnell O, Jonsson B, Kanis JA. The impact of the use of multiple risk indicators for fracture on case-finding strategies: a mathematical approach. Osteoporos Int 2005;16:313–8.

5. Stenson WF, Newberry R, Lorenz R, Baldus C, Civitelli R. Increased prevalence of celiac disease and need for routine screening among patients with osteoporosis. Arch Intern Med 2005;165:393–9.

6. Bischoff-Ferrari HA, Willett WC, Wong JB, Giovannucci E, Dietrich T, Dawson-Hughes B. Fracture prevention with vitamin D supplementation: a meta-analysis of random-ized controlled trials. JAMA 2005;293:2257–64.

7. Alexandersen P, Toussaint A, Christiansen C, Devogelaer JP, Roux C, Fechtenbaum J, et al. Ipriflavone in the treat-ment of postmenopausal osteoporosis: a randomized con-trolled trial. Ipriflavone Multicenter European Fracture Study. JAMA 2001;285:1482–8.

8. Nelson ME, Fiatarone MA, Morganti CM, Trice I, Greenberg RA, Evans WJ. Effects of high-intensity strength training on multiple risk factors for osteoporotic fractures. A randomized controlled trial. JAMA 1994;272:1909–14.

9. Park HA, Lee JS, Kuller LH, Cauley JA. Effects of weight control during the menopausal transition on bone mineral density. J Clin Endocrinol Metab 2007;92:3809–15.

10. Hopper JL, Seeman E. The bone density of female twins discordant for tobacco use. N Engl J Med 1994;330:387–92.

11. Qaseem A, Snow V, Shekelle P, Hopkins R Jr, Forciea MA, Owens DK. Pharmacologic treatment of low bone density or osteoporosis to prevent fractures: a clinical practice guideline from the American College of Physicians. Ann Int Med 2008;249:303–15.

12. Bellantonio S, Fortinsky R, Prestwood K. How well are community-living women treated for osteoporosis after hip fracture? J Am Geriatr Soc 2001;49:1197–204.

13. Woo SB, Hellstein JW, Kalmar JR. Narrative [corrected] review: bisphosphonates and osteonecrosis of the jaws [published erratum appears in Ann Intern Med 2006;145:235]. Ann Intern Med 2006;144:753–61.

14. Khosla S, Burr D, Cauley J, Dempster DW, Ebeling PR, Felsenberg D, et al. Bisphosphonate-associated osteonecro-sis of the jaw: report of a task force of the American Society for Bone and Mineral Research. American Society for Bone and Mineral Research. J Bone Miner Res 2007;22:1479–91.

15. Migliorati CA, Casiglia J, Epstein J, Jacobsen PL, Siegel MA, Woo SB. Managing the care of patients with bisphos-phonate–associated osteonecrosis: an American Academy of Oral Medicine position paper [published erratum appears in J Am Dent Assoc 2006;137:26]. J Am Dent Assoc 2005;136:1658–68.

16. Lyles KW, Colon-Emeric CS, Magaziner JS, Adachi JD, Pieper CF, Mautalen C, et al. Zoledronic acid and clinical fractures and mortality after hip fracture. HORIZON Recurrent Fracture Trial. N Engl J Med 2007;357:1799–809.

17. Black DM, Delmas PD, Eastell R, Reid IR, Boonen S, Cauley JA, et al. Once-yearly zoledronic acid for treatment of postmenopausal osteoporosis. HORIZON Pivotal Fracture Trial. N Engl J Med 2007;356:1809–22.

18. Selective estrogen receptor modulators. ACOG Practice Bulletin No. 39. American College of Obstetricians and Gynecologists. Obstet Gynecol 2002;100:835–43.

19. Barrett-Connor E, Mosca L, Collins P, Geiger MJ, Grady D, Kornitzer M, et al. Effects of raloxifene on cardiovascular events and breast cancer in postmenopausal women. Raloxifene Use for The Heart (RUTH) Trial Investigators. N Engl J Med 2006;355:125–37.

20. Vogel VG, Costantino JP, Wickerham DL, Cronin WM, Cecchini RS, Atkins JN, et al. Effects of tamoxifen vs ralox-ifene on the risk of developing invasive breast cancer and other disease outcomes: the NSABP Study of Tamoxifen and Raloxifene (STAR) P-2 trial. National Surgical Adjuvant Breast and Bowel Project (NSABP) [published errata appear in JAMA 2006;296:2926; JAMA 2007;298:973]. JAMA 2006;295:2727–41.

21. Anderson GL, Limacher M, Assaf AR, Bassford T, Beresford SA, Black H, et al. Effects of conjugated equine estrogen in postmenopausal women with hysterectomy: the Women's Health Initiative randomized controlled trial. Women's Health Initiative Steering Committee. JAMA 2004;291:1701–12.

22. Klibanski A, Biller BM, Schoenfeld DA, Herzog DB, Saxe VC. The effects of estrogen administration on trabecular bone loss in young women with anorexia nervosa. J Clin Endocrinol Metab 1995;80:898–904.

23. Downs RW Jr, Bell NH, Ettinger MP, Walsh BW, Favus MJ, Mako B, et al. Comparison of alendronate and intranasal calcitonin for treatment of osteoporosis in postmenopausal women. J Clin Endocrinol Metab 2000;85:1783–8.

24. Bone HG, Greenspan SL, McKeever C, Bell N, Davidson M, Downs RW, et al. Alendronate and estrogen effects in post-menopausal women with low bone mineral density. Alendronate/Estrogen Study Group. J Clin Endocrinol Metab 2000;85:720–6.

25. Johnell O, Scheele WH, Lu Y, Reginster JY, Need AG, Seeman E. Additive effects of raloxifene and alendronate on bone density and biochemical markers of bone remod-eling in postmenopausal women with osteoporosis. J Clin Endocrinol Metab 2002;87:985–92.

26. Pinkerton JV, Dalkin AC. Combination therapy for treat-ment of osteoporosis: a review. Am J Obstet Gynecol 2007;197:559–65.

Thyroid Diseases

Keith A. Hansen

Thyroid diseases are more common in women than in men, primarily because of an increased frequency of autoimmune thyroid dysfunction in females. The exact mechanism underlying increased thyroid autoimmunity in women is unknown. Recent studies suggest that the increased autoimmunity is due to persistent fetal cells from a previous pregnancy that reside in the thyroid gland and stimulate an immune response.

Hypothyroidism is common in women; an estimated 0.3–0.5% of women have overt hypothyroidism, whereas 2–3% have subclinical hypothyroidism during pregnancy. Approximately 7% of women have postpartum thyroiditis 6–12 months after delivery. Of women older than 65 years, 10–15% have evidence of hypothyroidism. Whereas autoimmune hypothyroidism is common in developed countries, iodine deficiency is a common cause of hypothyroidism worldwide and a significant cause of severe neurologic damage in the newborn.

Screening

Universal thyroid dysfunction screening of women, especially of women attempting pregnancy or those in the early stages of pregnancy, is controversial. Arguments for screening include the fact that thyroid diseases are common in women, overt hypothyroidism during pregnancy has been associated with preterm delivery and neurodevelopmental abnormalities in the newborn, screening tests are readily available and sensitive, and once the disease is diagnosed it can be treated effectively. The primary arguments against universal screening are the fact that treatment of subclinical hypothyroidism has not been proved to benefit the pregnancy and that the case finding is not cost-effective.

In regard to adult women who are not pregnant, the U.S. Preventive Services Task Force stated in 2004 that "the evidence is insufficient to recommend for or against routine screening for thyroid disease in adults"(1). However, physicians should have a high level of suspicion for thyroid disease in women and test those who are at high risk.

The highly sensitive (third-generation) thyroid-stimulating hormone (TSH) assay is recommended as a single test to screen for thyroid dysfunction. In patients with overt or subclinical hypothyroidism, the TSH level is elevated. Hypothyroidism caused by central (pituitary or hypothalamic) disease, however, can result in a normal or low TSH level. In the patient at risk for central hypothyroidism, free thyroxine (T_4) also must be measured to determine thyroid function. The TSH level will be suppressed in patients with overt or subclinical primary hyperthyroidism. One of the clear advantages of the highly sensitive TSH assay is that it allows discrimination between patients who are hyperthyroid and euthyroid. If central hyperthyroidism is suspected, a free T_4 level also should be measured (Table 24 and Figure 17).

Thyroid Function Tests

Thyroid function can be assessed by two methods: 1) measuring the level of thyroid hormones in the blood and 2) measuring the level of TSH in the blood as a reflection of the thyroid status of the patient. In many cases, both measurements are needed to ascertain the patient's true thyroid status.

THYROID-STIMULATING HORMONE

Thyroid-stimulating hormone levels are measured by assays. The third-generation assays have a lower detection limit of 0.01 milli-international units/mL and the usual reference range of 0.4–4.5 milli-international units/mL. This improvement in the lower detection limit of the assay allows discrimination between the euthyroid and mildly hyperthyroid state, which was not possible with earlier assays (2).

Heterophile antibodies can result in spuriously high TSH levels. Heterophile antibodies are antibodies in the test subject that are directed against the assay antibodies. These heterophile antibodies can form when the patient is inadvertently (eg, when the patient is an animal handler) or therapeutically (eg, when the patient is undergoing monoclonal antibody-directed cancer therapy) immunized with antigens from the animal in which the assay antibodies are developed. One should consider such assay interference when the test result does not correlate with the clinical findings.

Table 24. Guide to Thyroid Function Testing

Condition	Free Thyroxine	Triiodothyronine	Thyroid-stimulating Hormone	Comment
Primary hypothyroidism	↓	↓	↑	Caused by primary thyroid failure
Subclinical hypothyroidism	↔	↔	↑	Usually caused by auto-immune thyroid failure
Primary hyperthyroidism	↑	↑	↓	Graves disease is the main cause
Triiodothyronine thyrotoxicosis	↔	↑	↓	Seen in approximately 10% of hyperthyroidism cases caused by Graves disease or toxic multinodular goiter
Subclinical hyperthyroidism	↔	↔	↓	Usually seen in patients with underlying multinodular goiter
Nonthyroidal illness	↔ or ↓	↓	↔ or ↓	Thyroid-stimulating hormone levels may be increased in recovery phase

Abbreviations: ↑ indicates elevated; ↓, decreased; ↔, normal.

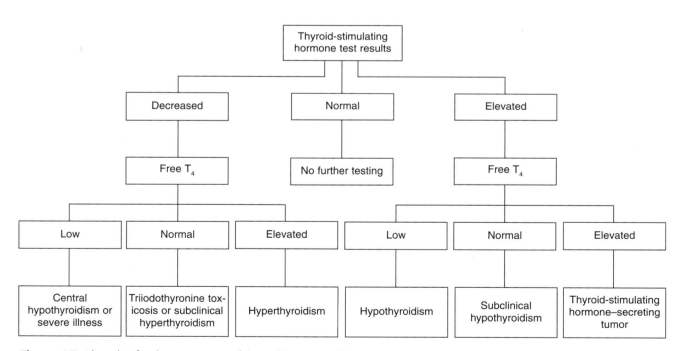

Figure 17. Algorithm for the assessment of thyroid function. Abbreviation: T_4 indicates thyroxine.

THYROXINE MEASUREMENT

The measurement of total T_4 is a good estimate of thyroid function. A number of conditions can alter total T_4 level but not change the biologically active free T_4 level. In females, pregnancy and taking oral estrogen will result in elevated levels of thyroid-binding protein. These elevations in thyroid-binding protein result in an increased total T_4 level but no change in free T_4 level. In the past, the free T_4 level was estimated (free T_4 index) by measuring total T_4 and multiplying it by the triiodothyronine (T_3) resin uptake (an estimate of unoccupied binding sites). The free T_4 index has been replaced by immunoassays for free T_4. The free T_4 assays better determine the biologically active T_4 level, but with limitations. In most assays for free T_4, the reference range is developed using samples from nonpregnant individuals. The suggestion of using laboratory-specific or trimester-specific free T_4 assays has been made but remains controversial (3).

TRIIODOTHYRONINE MEASUREMENT

Total T_3 measurement also is influenced by qualitative and quantitative changes in thyroid-binding proteins. Free T_3 levels can be determined by immunoassay and give a better idea of biologically active T_3 levels in patients with altered thyroid-binding proteins. In patients with a suppressed TSH level and a normal free T_4 level, the measurement of free T_3 can be helpful in the diagnosis of T_3 thyrotoxicosis.

MEASUREMENT OF THYROID ANTIBODIES

Autoimmune thyroid disease comprises a spectrum from hypothyroidism (Hashimoto thyroiditis) to hyperthyroidism (Graves disease). A patient with Hashimoto thyroiditis has antibodies directed against thyroglobulin, thyroid peroxidase, and the TSH receptor. The antibody profile for each patient is highly individualized—so much so that it can be used as an antibody fingerprint. Asymptomatic patients with thyroid antibodies are at increased risk of having postpartum thyroiditis.

Graves disease is characterized by an activating antibody against the TSH receptor, which results in unregulated thyroid hormone production. This TSH receptor antibody is known as *thyroid-stimulating immunoglobulin* or *thyroid-binding inhibitory immunoglobulin*. In pregnant patients with Graves disease, it is suggested that thyroid-stimulating immunoglobulin levels be measured. High maternal levels of thyroid-stimulating immunoglobulins can cross the placenta and increase the risk of fetal thyrotoxicosis.

Imaging

The radioactive isotopes iodine 123 and iodine 131 have biologic properties that are similar to those of native iodine. In thyroid scanning, radioactive iodine or technetium is administered to the patient and the fractional uptake by the thyroid gland determined. Patients with hyperthyroidism secondary to Graves disease, toxic uninodular goiter, or toxic multinodular goiter will have increased uptake of the radioactive isotope. Patients with primary hypothyroidism will have decreased uptake of the radioactive isotope. In the United States, the fractional uptake is 5–25%, but it can be significantly lower in iodine-replete areas. Radioactive isotopes of iodine should not be administered to pregnant or breast-feeding women.

The usual procedure for the clinical evaluation of thyroid nodules is history gathering, physical examination, and fine-needle aspiration. Thyroid ultrasonography may be helpful in confirmation and monitoring, as well as in directing fine-needle aspiration of thyroid nodules. Thyroid ultrasonography also may be helpful in monitoring a thyroid goiter.

Hyperthyroidism

Thyrotoxicosis is the constellation of physical manifestations caused by excess circulating thyroid hormone. *Hyperthyroidism* is the generic term for excess circulating free thyroid hormone. It affects approximately 2% of women throughout their lifetimes, including the reproductive years (4).

Causes

The most common cause of primary hyperthyroidism is Graves disease. The hyperthyroidism of Graves disease results from unregulated stimulation of the TSH receptor by immunoglobulins. Patients with Graves disease often have a spectrum of blocking and stimulating immunoglobulins directed against the TSH receptor. The relative predominance of one isoform over the other immunoglobulin determines the degree of hyperthyroidism. These immunoglobulins also are responsible for the characteristic ophthalmopathy and pretibial myxedema of Graves disease. Graves disease is considered multifactorial, with an underlying genetic predisposition triggered by unknown environmental stimuli. Environmental factors that increase the risk of Graves disease include smoking, stress, and the postpartum period.

Another cause of hyperthyroidism is an autonomously functioning thyroid adenoma, either a solitary nodule or a multinodular goiter. The clinical course of multinodular goiters usually is prolonged, with long periods of subclinical hyperthyroidism followed by the onset of overt hyperthyroidism. Because of the slow development of hyperthyroidism, patients with multinodular goiters usually present at older ages with cardiovascular and gastrointestinal symptoms.

Patients with subacute thyroiditis (which is painful) or postpartum thyroiditis (which is painless, silent, or lymphocytic) can present with transient thyrotoxicosis due to the uncontrolled release of thyroid hormone after injury to the thyroid follicles. Other rare forms of hyperthyroidism include choriocarcinoma with markedly elevated human chorionic gonadotropin levels, a TSH-producing pituitary adenoma, or an ovarian teratoma (struma ovarii). Exogenous ingestion of T_4 or T_3 also can result in hyperthyroidism. The rare forms of hyperthyroidism discussed in this paragraph are typified by low uptake on a radioactive iodine uptake scan. Patients with iatrogenic or factitious ingestion of thyroid hormone will have low thyroid uptake on a radioactive iodine scan but also will have low thyroglobulin levels.

Clinical Features

Most clinical findings of thyrotoxicosis can be explained as an increased sensitivity to adrenergic stimulation, but the exact molecular mechanism remains an enigma. The common, classic symptoms of thyrotoxicosis include heat intolerance, fatigue, palpitations, dyspnea, nervousness, and weight loss. Approximately one fourth of young women with thyrotoxicosis gain weight. Pregnant patients with thyrotoxicosis may present with *hyperemesis gravidarum*. Signs of thyrotoxicosis include tachycardia, lid lag, tremor, proximal muscle weakness, and warm, moist skin. Elderly patients may present with atypical symptoms, including unexplained weight loss, atrial fibrillation, osteoporosis, or angina pectoris. Most women with hyperthyroidism have regular menses, but they may have lighter flow. Anovulation and irregular menses can occur and depend on the severity of the hyperthyroidism.

Extrathyroidal manifestations of Graves disease include ophthalmopathy and pretibial myxedema. These findings can appear any time during the clinical course of the disease, including after the successful treatment of hyperthyroidism. The presence of extrathyroidal findings of Graves disease will help the clinician make the appropriate diagnosis, especially during pregnancy.

The goiter in patients with Graves disease is usually smooth, diffusely enlarged, and not tender, with a vascular bruit. Of patients with Graves disease, 12% have palpable nodules on physical examination. In patients with subacute thyroiditis, the thyroid is enlarged, firm, and tender to palpation. In patients with postpartum or painless thyroiditis, the thyroid usually is mildly enlarged but not tender. In patients with toxic nodules, the thyroid usually has irregular enlargement with palpable nodules.

Diagnosis

Thyrotoxicosis is diagnosed upon a finding of elevated thyroid hormones, usually both free T_4 and T_3, and a suppressed TSH concentration. Some patients will have an isolated elevation in free T_3 level—hence the name T_3 *thyrotoxicosis*. Elevations in total T_4 and T_3 levels can occur in euthyroid patients who have abnormalities or elevations in thyroid-binding globulins, as well as thyroid hormone resistance.

The serum TSH concentration will be undetectable in ultrasensitive assays (detection limits of 0.1 milli-international units/mL at most) in patients with primary hyperthyroidism. Patients with a low TSH concentration accompanied by an elevated free T_3 and free T_4 level have overt hyperthyroidism, whereas patients with normal free T_3 and free T_4 levels have subclinical disease. Subclinical hyperthyroidism increases the risk of osteoporosis and atrial tachyarrhythmias in the elderly.

The treatment of hyperthyroidism depends on the etiology of the disease. Therefore, it is essential to recognize the exact etiology before therapeutic interventions.

Therapy

Treatment of thyrotoxicosis in adults includes the use of thionamides (propylthiouracil or methimazole), radioactive iodine, β-blockers, and occasionally surgery. Thionamides primarily function by blocking thyroid hormone synthesis and immunomodulation. Propylthiouracil also blocks peripheral conversion of T_4 to T_3 to some extent. Euthyroidism typically is restored after 3–10 weeks of therapy, and treatment usually is continued for 6–24 months. Following the discontinuation of thionamide administration, remission continues in less than one half of patients. Lifelong monitoring is warranted in patients with thionamide-induced remission because of the risk of relapse, especially postpartum.

Iodine 131 often provides a permanent cure for hyperthyroidism due to Graves disease, toxic solitary nodule, and toxic multinodular goiter. Hyperthyroidism in as many as 75% of patients with Graves disease will be cured within 2–6 months of therapy. The radioactive iodine usually is administered after inducement of the euthyroid state with thionamides to reduce the risk of exacerbation of the thyrotoxicosis. After an ablative course of radioactive iodine, approximately 50% of patients will have permanent hypothyroidism, and another 3% per year will become hypothyroid. Replacement doses of levothyroxine should be administered to treat these patients with postablative hypothyroidism. The use of radioactive iodine is absolutely contraindicated in pregnant or breast-feeding women, and women should not attempt pregnancy for 6 months after treatment.

Other supplemental therapies that can be helpful in the treatment of thyroid diseases include β-adrenergic blocking agents to control sympathomimetic symptoms. In patients with subacute thyroiditis, the pain usually is controlled with aspirin or other nonsteroidal anti-inflammatory agents. In approximately 20% of patients, a course of corticosteroids will be necessary to control the symptoms of subacute thyroiditis. Removal of the offending tumor is necessary to control hyperthyroidism in patients with gestational trophoblastic disease, struma ovarii, or a TSH-secreting pituitary adenoma.

Pregnancy

The diagnosis of hyperthyroidism in pregnancy is more difficult because of the similarity of symptoms between thyrotoxicosis and normal pregnancy, as well as because of pregnancy-induced changes on thyroid function tests. One should suspect hyperthyroidism during pregnancy in a patient with *hyperemesis gravidarum*, no weight gain or weight loss, hyperdefecation, or tachycardia when arising from rest. Women should be advised to keep taking prescribed thyroid medications when they discover they are pregnant. For more information, see the current edition of *Precis: Obstetrics*.

Hypothyroidism

The clinical manifestations of hypothyroidism result from inadequate production and secretion of thyroid hormones to meet the metabolic demands of the body. The most frequent etiology for primary hypothyroidism is autoimmune (Hashimoto) thyroiditis. Hypothyroidism also may follow the surgical removal or radioactive iodine ablation of the thyroid gland. Hypothyroidism may develop in patients who receive therapeutic radiation therapy of the head and neck, so these patients should be monitored closely.

Patients with Hashimoto thyroiditis usually have a nontender, firm, diffusely enlarged goiter. Additionally, there is an atrophic form of the disease in which the thyroid cannot be palpated. Hashimoto thyroiditis can be associated with other autoimmune diseases, such as type 1 diabetes mellitus, premature ovarian failure, Addison disease, hypoparathyroidism, vitiligo, and pernicious anemia.

Clinical Features

The clinical signs and symptoms of hypothyroidism include fatigue, lethargy, cold intolerance, dry skin, hair loss, constipation, myalgia, carpal tunnel syndrome, and weight gain, which is typically less than 5–10 kg. Neuropsychiatric symptoms include impaired memory, depression, irritability, and dementia. Many of the classic findings of hypothyroidism are nonspecific and can be difficult to distinguish from findings of normal pregnancy. Menstrual dysfunction is common, with menorrhagia most frequent; however, amenorrhea can occur because of anovulation.

Diagnosis

Clinical findings suggestive of hypothyroidism require laboratory confirmation with thyroid function tests. Primary hypothyroidism—in which thyroid function is impaired directly, usually as a sequela of Hashimoto thyroiditis—is characterized by an elevated TSH level. In overt hypothyroidism the elevated TSH level is accompanied by a low serum free T_4 level, whereas in subclinical hypothyroidism the free T_4 level is normal.

Central hypothyroidism due to hypothalamic–pituitary dysfunction is typified by a low or low normal TSH level accompanied by a low or low normal free T_4 level. Central hypothyroidism is relatively uncommon but should be considered in patients with hypothalamic–pituitary disease. The presence of thyroid antibodies sometimes can help confirm the diagnosis of Hashimoto thyroiditis.

Therapy

Levothyroxine is the treatment of choice for patients with hypothyroidism. The usual replacement dose of levothyroxine is approximately 1.6 micrograms/kg per day and should be adjusted after an equilibration period of 4–6 weeks to maintain the TSH level in the lower half of the reference range (0.5–2.5 microunits/mL). Levothyroxine is well absorbed unless administered with ferrous sulfate, calcium carbonate, cholestyramine, aluminum hydroxide, or sucralfate. In women with suspected or known ischemic heart disease, levothyroxine should be initiated with a low dose (12.5–25 micrograms/d) and slowly titrated to therapeutic levels. The administration of excess levothyroxine as recognized by suppressed TSH should be avoided because it may result in bone loss and atrial fibrillation.

Pregnancy

In pregnancy, untreated overt hypothyroidism may result in an increased risk of preterm labor and delivery, low birth weight, placental abruption, preeclampsia, fetal death, and intellectual impairment (5). Patients already undergoing treatment should not discontinue therapy without consultation with their physician. The adverse pregnancy events resulting from maternal hypothyroidism have prompted some authors to advocate for universal screening of all pregnant women. A policy of universal screening has not been adopted; rather, women at moderate to high risk of hypothyroidism are screened (6). For more details on hypothyroidism and pregnancy, see the current edition of *Precis: Obstetrics*.

References

1. U.S. Preventive Services Task Force, Agency for Healthcare Research and Quality. Screening for thyroid disease, topic page. Rockville (MD): USPSTF AHRQ; 2004. Available at: http://www.ahrq.gov/clinic/uspstf/uspsthyr.htm. Retrieved November 14, 2008.

2. Saller B, Broda N, Heydarian R, Gorges R, Mann K. Utility of third generation thyrotropin assays in thyroid function testing. Exp Clin Endocrinol Diabetes 1998;106(suppl 4): S29–33.

3. Soldin OP, Tractenberg RE, Hollowell JG, Jonklaas J, Janicic N, Soldin SJ. Trimester-specific changes in maternal thyroid hormone, thyrotropin, and thyroglobulin con-

centrations during gestation: trends and associations across trimesters in iodine sufficiency. Thyroid 2004;14: 1084–90.

4. Mestman JH. Hyperthyroidism in pregnancy. Best Pract Res Clin Endocrinol Metab 2004;18:267–88.

5. Haddow JE, Palomaki GE, Allan WC, Williams JR, Knight GJ, Gagnon J, et al. Maternal thyroid deficiency during pregnancy and subsequent neuropsychological development of the child. N Engl J Med 1999;341:549–55.

6. Abalovich M, Amino N, Barbour LA, Cobin RH, De Groot LJ, Glinoer D, et al. Clinical Practice Guideline. Management of thyroid dysfunction during pregnancy and postpartum: an endocrine society clinical practice guideline. J Clin Endocrinol Metab 2007;92:S1–S47.

Coagulopathies

Nicole Marshall and D. Ware Branch

Venous Thromboembolism

Venous thromboembolism is an appreciable health issue. Each year, approximately 2 million people in the United States experience deep vein thrombosis (DVT); approximately 600,000 of these patients develop pulmonary embolism, and 60,000 die (1). Despite advances in diagnosis and treatment, thromboembolic disease continues to have an enormous effect on patient well-being and health care costs.

Diagnosis

The ability to diagnose DVT by history and physical examination is modest at best. A high index of suspicion will serve the physician and patient well (Box 55).

Pretest Probability and D-dimer Test

In nonpregnant patients without comorbidities, clinical prediction rules—eg, the Wells prediction rule—can be helpful in determining whether a patient requires imaging studies to rule out venous thromboembolism. For patients with a low pretest probability for DVT and pulmonary embolism (Tables 25 and 26), negative D-dimer test results indicate a low likelihood of venous thromboembolism (2), and no further studies are necessary. In patients with an intermediate to high pretest probability, imaging studies are recommended.

Ultrasound Techniques

Ultrasound techniques are commonly used as the first-line diagnostic tool in symptomatic individuals suspected of having a DVT in a lower extremity. Real-time ultrasonography may allow visualization of the clot in the proximal deep veins of the leg; visualization of the clot has virtually 100% positive predictive value for proximal DVT. The technique of determining whether the vein fails to collapse under gentle transducer pressure (compression ultrasonography) is exceedingly sensitive and has a positive predictive value of 84% for proximal DVT in nonpregnant patients.

Real-time ultrasonography commonly is supplemented with Doppler flow ultrasound imaging, a technique that identifies alterations in venous flow. The combination of real-time ultrasound imaging and Doppler flow studies is more than 90% sensitive and specific for the detection of proximal DVT in nonpregnant, symptomatic patients. In pregnant patients, the uterus should be displaced from the vena cava when imaging the lower-extremity venous system with Doppler flow ultrasound imaging.

Real-time and Doppler ultrasonography are less satisfactory for the evaluation of the lower leg (calf); each technique has a sensitivity of approximately 50% in

---

Box 55

American Academy of Family Physicians and the American College of Physicians Recommendations for the Diagnosis of Venous Thromboembolism in Primary Care

- Validated clinical prediction rules should be used to estimate pretest probability of venous thromboembolism, both deep vein thrombosis (DVT) and pulmonary embolism, and for the basis of interpretation of subsequent tests.

- In appropriately selected patients with low pretest probability of DVT or pulmonary embolism, obtaining a high-sensitivity D-dimer is a reasonable option, and a negative result indicates a low likelihood of venous thromboembolism.

- Ultrasonography is recommended for patients with intermediate to high pretest probability of DVT in the lower extremities.

- Patients with intermediate or high pretest probability of pulmonary embolism require diagnostic imaging studies.

Data from Qaseem A, Snow V, Barry P, Hornbake ER, Rodnick JE, Tobolic T, et al. Current diagnosis of venous thromboembolism in primary care: a clinical practice guideline from the American Academy of Family Physicians and the American College of Physicians. Joint American Academy of Family Physicians/American College of Physicians Panel on Deep Venous Thrombosis/Pulmonary Embolism. Ann Intern Med 2007;146:454–8.

Resources

Coagulopathies

American Association of Blood Banks
http://www.aabb.org

American Society of Hematology
http://www.hematology.org

National Alliance for Thrombosis and Thrombophilia
http://www.nattinfo.org

National Heart, Lung, and Blood Institute
http://www.nhlbi.nih.gov

National Hemophilia Foundation
http://www.hemophilia.org

Table 25. Wells Prediction Rule for Diagnosing Deep Vein Thrombosis: Clinical Evaluation Table for Predicting Pretest Probability of Deep Vein Thrombosis*

Clinical Characteristic	Score
Active cancer (treatment ongoing, within previous 6 months, or palliative)	+1
Paralysis, paresis, or recent plaster immobilization of the lower extremities	+1
Recently bedridden for more than 3 days or major surgery within 12 weeks requiring general or regional anesthesia	+1
Localized tenderness along the distribution of the deep venous system	+1
Entire leg swollen	+1
Calf swelling 3 cm larger than asymptomatic side (measured 10 cm below tibial tuberosity)	+1
Pitting edema confined to the symptomatic leg	+1
Collateral superficial veins (nonvaricose)	+1
Alternative diagnosis at least as likely as deep vein thrombosis	−2

*Clinical possibility: low, less or equal to 0; intermediate, 1–2; high, greater or equal to 3. In patients with symptoms in both legs, the more symptomatic leg is used.

Reprinted from The Lancet, Vol. 351, Wells PS, Anderson DR, Bormanis J, Guy F, Mitchell M, Gray L, et al, Value assessment of pretest probability of deep-vein thrombosis in clinical management, Pages 1795–8, copyright 1997, with permission from Elsevier.

Table 26. Wells Prediction Rule for Diagnosing Pulmonary Embolism: Clinical Evaluation Table for Predicting Pretest Probability of Pulmonary Embolism*

Clinical Characteristic	Score
Previous pulmonary embolism or deep vein thrombosis	+1.5
Heart rate greater than 100 beats per minute	+1.5
Recent surgery or immobilization	+1.5
Clinical signs of deep vein thrombosis	+3
Alternative diagnosis less likely than pulmonary embolism	+3
Hemoptysis	+1
Cancer	+1

*Clinical probability of pulmonary embolism: low, 0–1; intermediate, 2–6; high, greater than or equal to 7.

Reprinted from American Journal of Medicine, Chagnon I, Bounameaux H, Aujesky D, Roy PM, Gourdier AL, Cornuz J, et al. Vol 113, Comparison of two clinical prediction rules and implicit assessment among patients with suspected pulmonary embolism, pages 269–75, copyright 2002, with permission from Elsevier.

nonpregnant patients. Likewise, these ultrasound techniques have limited utility in the diagnosis of thrombosis above the inguinal ligament.

VENOGRAPHY

Venography (phlebography) is an excellent diagnostic tool for proximal and distal DVT, with high sensitivity, specificity, and predictive values. However, peripheral vein contrast injection venography commonly causes discomfort, and 2–3% of patients undergoing venography experience contrast-induced venous thrombosis. Because ultrasound techniques are reliable and noninvasive, venography is used infrequently except in special cases.

SPIRAL COMPUTED TOMOGRAPHY AND PULMONARY ANGIOGRAPHY

Spiral (or helical) computed tomography (CT) often is used as the initial test in patients suspected of having pulmonary embolism; it has replaced ventilation–perfusion scanning in many centers. Pulmonary angiography is extremely sensitive and specific for the diagnosis of pulmonary embolism, but its invasive nature, relatively high rate of serious side effects, and contraindications have prompted the development of less invasive alternatives. The major limitation of this modality has been concerns about sensitivity, although accuracy seems to improve with experience and improved technology. Spiral CT is 60–85% (90%) sensitive for segmental or larger pulmonary embolism but only approximately 20% sensitive for subsegmental pulmonary embolism (3, 4). Spiral CT has an overall specificity of 85–90% (95%) for pulmonary embolism. Thus, depending on the clinical circumstances, spiral CT may be used for the diagnosis of pulmonary embolism, but is somewhat less reliable for ruling it out. Patients with a high pretest probability but a negative finding on spiral CT should undergo pulmonary angiography or serial lower extremity ultrasonography (2).

Ventilation–perfusion lung scanning is the traditional imaging test in patients with suspected pulmonary embolism. A normal result on perfusion scan, which effectively excludes pulmonary embolism, is found in approximately 25% of symptomatic patients being investigated for the condition (1). Perfusion defects may have a variety of causes, including pulmonary embolism. The probability that perfusion defects result from pulmonary embolism is greater with increasing size and number of defects, with defects that are wedge shaped, and in the setting of a normal ventilation scan—ie, the perfusion defects are "mismatched" with regard to the ventilation scan. Segmental, mismatched defects are "highly probable" defects, representing pulmonary embolism in more than 90% of cases in which three or more such defects are seen (5).

The findings of many ventilation–perfusion studies in patients with suspected pulmonary embolism are neither negative nor highly probable, but have low or intermediate probability. Depending on the degree of clinical suspicion, many patients require additional testing to determine whether pulmonary embolism is present. Some clinicians initially perform noninvasive tests of the legs; if the results are positive, treatment is initiated. If the results are negative, pulmonary angiography or CT visualization of the pulmonary vasculature is indicated. Other clinicians favor moving directly to these diagnostic modalities when low- or intermediate-probability ventilation–perfusion scanning results are obtained, especially when the clinical suspicion is high.

Management

The treatment of acute venous thromboembolism is anticoagulation, preferably with low molecular weight LMW) heparin (Box 56) (6). Several formulations are available, all of which are composed of heparins of low molecular weight (mean molecular weight, 5,000 Da) formed by enzymatic or hydrolytic cleavage of unfractionated heparin (mean molecular weight, 15,000 Da). Depending on the specific depolymerization process used, pharmacologically distinct LMW heparins that are not interchangeable are formed (7). Like unfractionated heparin, LMW heparins exert their anticoagulant activity by binding antithrombin, thereby accelerating the inhibition of thrombin (factor IIa) and factor Xa. Because the ability to inactivate thrombin is related to molecular size, LMW have lower anti-factor IIa activity than anti-factor Xa activity and, thus, theoretically achieve a lower risk of bleeding at similar levels of anticoagulation. Also, because of decreased anti-factor IIa activity, monitoring the anticoagulant effect by measuring activated partial thromboplastin time (aPTT) is not possible; anti-factor Xa activity must be measured.

Low molecular weight heparins have several other distinct advantages compared with unfractionated heparin. They are administered subcutaneously and can be given on an outpatient basis (7). They have a longer half-life and less protein binding, resulting in greater bioavailability that does not change at different doses (4). The kidney excretes LMW heparin, and the pharmacokinetics are linear for antifactor Xa activity (8, 9). Thus, LMW heparin total body clearance and excretion increase as the injected dose increases. Consequently, LMW heparin can be used safely in nonpregnant patients with minimal laboratory monitoring. Animal and human studies suggest a lower risk of osteoporosis with LMW heparin than with unfractionated heparin (10, 11). Finally, LMW heparin is less likely than unfractionated heparin to be associated with heparin-induced thrombocytopenia, a major relative safety feature (12). The dosing regimens for the LMW heparin products available in the United States are shown in Table 27.

Treatment with unfractionated heparin is another clinical option. For patients with uncomplicated acute venous thromboembolism, a loading dose of 5,000 international units of unfractionated heparin (80 international units/kg) is administered intravenously. This dose is followed by a continuous infusion of heparin (40 international units/mL) at an hourly rate that achieves 30,000 international units in 24 hours. At 6 hours after the initial bolus of unfractionated heparin, the aPTT is measured, and the dosage of heparin is adjusted using a nomogram to maintain an aPTT of 1.5–2.5 times the control mean. Institutions with electronic order entry capabilities usually have standardized regimens.

Box 56

American Academy of Family Physicians and the American College of Physicians Recommendations for the Management of Venous Thromboembolism in Primary Care

- Low molecular weight (LMW) heparin rather than unfractionated heparin should be used whenever possible for the initial inpatient treatment of deep vein thrombosis (DVT). Either unfractionated heparin or LMW heparin is appropriate for the initial treatment of pulmonary embolism.

- Outpatient treatment of DVT and, possibly, pulmonary embolism with LMW heparin is safe and cost-effective for carefully selected patients and should be considered if the required support services are in place.

- Compression stockings should be used routinely to prevent postthrombotic syndrome, beginning within 1 month of diagnosis of proximal DVT and continuing for a minimum of 1 year after diagnosis.

- There is insufficient evidence to make specific recommendations for types of anticoagulation management of VTE in pregnant women.

- Anticoagulation should be maintained for 3–6 months for VTE secondary to transient risk factors and for more than 12 months for recurrent VTE. Although the appropriate duration of anticoagulation for idiopathic or recurrent VTE is not definitively known, there is evidence of substantial benefit for extended-duration therapy.

- Low molecular weight heparin is safe and efficacious for the long-term treatment of VTE in selected patients (and may be preferable for patients with cancer).

Data from Snow V, Qaseem A, Barry P, Hornbake ER, Rodnick JE, Tobolic T, et al. Management of venous thromboembolism: a clinical practice guideline from the American College of Physicians and the American Academy of Family Physicians. American College of Physicians; American Academy of Family Physicians Panel on Deep Venous Thrombosis/Pulmonary Embolism. Ann Intern Med 2007; 146:204-10.

Table 27. Low Molecular Weight Heparins Commercially Available in the United States

Low Molecular Weight Heparin	Prophylactic Dosage	Therapeutic Dosage
Enoxaparin sodium	40 mg once daily 30 mg twice daily	1 mg/kg twice daily or 1.5 mg/kg once daily
Dalteparin sodium	2,500–5,000 international units once daily; 2,500 international units twice daily	100 international units/kg twice daily
Tinzaparin sodium*		175 international units/kg once daily

*Approved for therapeutic use only.

Regardless of the heparin preparation used to manage acute DVT or pulmonary embolism, warfarin is started within 48 hours at a dosage of 2.5 mg or 5 mg once daily (in nonpregnant patients). Because the anticoagulant effect of warfarin is delayed up to 4 days, heparin and warfarin therapy should overlap for the first 4–5 days after an acute venous thromboembolism until an international normalized ratio of 2–3 has been achieved for 2 consecutive days.

Inherited and Acquired Thrombophilias

Inherited and acquired thrombophilias are associated with venous thromboembolism in obstetrics and gynecology. Depending on the population studied, as many as 70% of women experiencing a thrombotic event can be found to have a thrombophilia. In whites, the most common of the inherited thrombophilias are the factor V Leiden mutation and the prothrombin G20210A mutation. Elevated factor VIII levels, elevated factor IX levels, and hyperhomocysteinemia also are associated with an increased risk of thrombosis. Less common inherited thrombophilias include family-unique deficiencies of protein C, protein S, and antithrombin (Fig. 18).

Acquired thrombophilias include antiphospholipid syndrome, paroxysmal nocturnal hemoglobinuria, thrombocytosis, and cancer. Advancing age increases the likelihood of thrombosis—a 60-year-old individual has a 5–10-fold increased risk of thrombosis compared with that of a 20-year-old. Perhaps one of the most common risk factors for thrombophilias is overweight–obesity.

The utility of testing for inherited thrombophilias in a patient experiencing the first episode of vein thrombosis or venous embolism is debated because there is no clear evidence that modifying treatment based on the presence of an inherited thrombophilia alters outcome. Also, the incidence of inherited thrombophilias, such as a factor V Leiden mutation and the prothrombin mutation, varies according to race. Most experts, however, recommend testing for thrombophilias in an individual with recurrent thrombotic episodes or with thrombosis or embolism before age 50 years. One scheme for testing is shown in Box 57.

Factor V Leiden Mutation

Patients with the factor V Leiden mutation demonstrate a single-base transition in the gene that results in the substitution of arginine for glutamine at position 506 in the synthesized factor V protein. The mutated factor Va, therefore, is resistant to cleavage by activated protein C, which ultimately leads to an increased production of

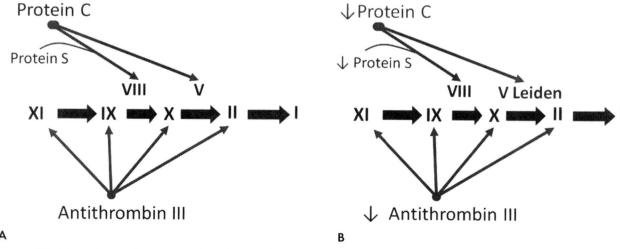

A

B

Figure 18. Normal coagulation cascade with natural occurring anticoagulants protein C, protein S, and antithrombin III. **A.** The inhibition of activated coagulation factors (denoted by the arrows). **B.** Thrombophilic disorders that increase the risk of thrombosis. (Courtesy of Thomas C. Peng, MD.)

thrombin and factor V Leiden mutation accounts for approximately 95% of all cases of activated protein C resistance. The prevalence of the gene mutation is race dependent; in the general population it ranges from 1% to 15%. In the United States, approximately 5–7% of whites carry the mutation.

Of patients presenting with venous thromboembolism, 10–50% carry the factor V Leiden mutation, depending on the population studied. It is estimated that individuals who are heterozygous for the mutation have an approximately fivefold greater risk of having venous thromboembolism compared with noncarriers. Individuals who are homozygous, who are uncommon, are estimated to have an initial venous thromboembolism risk that is 80-fold greater than that of noncarriers.

The diagnosis of factor V Leiden mutation is strongly suggested by demonstrating activated protein C resistance in the patient's plasma. The factor V Leiden mutation also may be diagnosed using a more expensive molecular genetic test that identifies the actual mutation.

Prothrombin G20210A Mutation

Prothrombin, also known as factor II, is the precursor to thrombin in the coagulation cascade; thrombin cleaves fibrinogen into fibrin. A G→A mutation at the 20210 position in the 3' untranslated region of the gene results in elevated plasma levels of prothrombin and increased thrombin generation, although the exact mechanism that results in a thrombophilic state is uncertain. In the United States, the heterozygosity for the prothrombin 20210 mutation occurs in 1–3% of the population and is more common in whites. Detection of this mutation is by a DNA-based test.

Protein C Deficiency

Protein C is a vitamin K–dependent glycoprotein synthesized in the liver and subsequently activated by the thrombin–thrombomodulin complex in plasma. Activated protein C exerts an anticoagulant effect by proteolytically degrading procoagulant factors Va and VIIIa. Any mutation that leads to decreased levels of protein C increases the patient's risk of thrombosis.

At present, more than 160 private mutations that affect protein C synthesis and function have been described. Protein C deficiency is inherited as an autosomal-dominant condition and is found in only 0.2–0.4% of the general population, making it significantly less common than the factor V Leiden or the prothrombin gene mutation. In turn, only 3–5% of patients with a history of vein thrombosis have protein C deficiency. Thus, the contribution of protein C deficiency to thrombosis is low.

Patients who are heterozygous for protein C deficiency are estimated to have an approximately 10-fold greater risk of vein thrombosis than does the general population. Homozygotes or double heterozygotes have a significantly more severe form of the disease and may present with neonatal purpura fulminans, a condition characterized by microthrombosis, bleeding, and tissue necrosis. Many authorities believe that patients with venous thromboembolism and protein C deficiency require anticoagulation for 12–24 months. It is important to note that patients with protein C deficiency are at risk for a rarely seen condition called *warfarin-induced skin necrosis*. It results from further suppression of protein C by warfarin before adequate anticoagulation has been achieved. This condition can be avoided by adequate anticoagulation with heparin followed by the slow initiation of warfarin.

Use of oral contraceptives may increase protein C levels. Acute thrombosis, liver disease, renal disease, heavy smoking, and disseminated intravascular coagulation may decrease protein C levels. Because protein C is a vitamin K–dependent factor, vitamin K deficiency and anticoagulation with warfarin may decrease its levels. Therefore, testing for protein C deficiency should be withheld until at least 2 weeks after discontinuing warfarin therapy. Because there are many family-specific mutations, genetic analysis is not a practical means of diagnosing protein C deficiency. Instead, one should perform a functional clotting-based test to diagnose the deficiency.

Protein S Deficiency

Protein S also is a vitamin K–dependent protein and functions as a cofactor of protein C in the degradation of the procoagulant factors Va and VIIIa. It also directly inactivates factors Va and Xa. Protein S is synthesized chiefly in vascular endothelium and the liver.

Like protein C, protein S has many known mutations that lead to an increased risk of thrombosis through decreased levels, decreased activity, or both. To date, more than 130 mutations have been identified in different families. Clinical protein S deficiency is an autosomal-dominant trait. The prevalence of protein S deficiency is 0.3–0.13%; among patients with a prior DVT, its prevalence is 1–5%. Like patients with protein C deficiency, patients with protein S deficiency may experience the rare condition of warfarin-induced skin necrosis. Patients who are homozygous for protein C deficiency or homozygous or double heterozygous for protein S deficiency present with neonatal *purpura fulminans* and extensive necrosis and are unlikely to be encountered during their pregnancies.

Because protein S levels can be decreased after acute thrombosis and anticoagulation therapy with warfarin, testing for the deficiency should not be performed until at least 2 weeks after the discontinuation of anticoagulation therapy. The use of oral contraceptives in inflammatory conditions, such as inflammatory bowel disease, lupus erythematosus, and rheumatoid arthritis, also can decrease protein S levels. In pregnancy, protein S levels normally are decreased, and the diagnosis of protein S deficiency is difficult.

The diagnosis of protein S deficiency should be made by a functional clotting assay or a free protein S assay rather than by a quantitative immunoassay of total protein S. Again, because of the large number of mutations, genetic analysis is not practical.

Antithrombin Deficiency

Antithrombin (formerly known as antithrombin III) is a glycoprotein that exerts its anticoagulation properties by inactivating thrombin and activated factors IX, X, XI, and XII. The overall result of its actions is a decrease in the production of thrombin and its half-life.

More than 120 mutations are known to decrease antithrombin levels or activity. Clinical antithrombin deficiency also is an autosomal-dominant inherited trait. Its penetrance is approximately 95%—much higher than for protein C and S deficiencies. The prevalence of antithrombin deficiency in the general population is only 0.02%, and only 1–3% of patients with a history of venous thromboembolism have the condition. Antithrombin deficiency is the most severe of the inherited thrombophilias; heterozygotes have a 10–20 times greater risk of thrombosis than do noncarriers. Homozygosity is rarely diagnosed; most homozygous mutations are probably incompatible with life.

A diagnosis of antithrombin deficiency is an indication for lifelong anticoagulation. Some patients with antithrombin deficiency do not respond well to heparin and may require high doses of heparin to achieve appropriate anticoagulation. In patients refractory to heparin, antithrombin concentrate may be administered with the goal of increasing the functional level of antithrombin to 120% of its normal level.

The diagnosis of antithrombin deficiency should be made by a functional clotting assay. Quantitative assays are available but are not clinically useful. Antithrombin levels are not affected by warfarin; however, levels may be decreased in patients with acute thrombosis or patients undergoing heparin anticoagulation.

Antiphospholipid Syndrome

Antiphospholipid antibodies are a family of autoantibodies (phospholipids, phospholipid-binding proteins, or phospholipid-binding protein complexes). Antiphospholipid syndrome is characterized by the presence of antiphospholipid antibodies and a syndrome of hypercoagulability (13). The most commonly detected antiphospholipid antibodies are anticardiolipin antibodies, lupus anticoagulant, and anti-β_2 glycoprotein-1 antibody. Deep vein thrombosis involving the lower extremities is one of the most common clinical manifestations of antiphospholipid syndrome, occurring in 30–55% of patients with the syndrome. Arterial thromboses, including myocardial infarction and stroke, may occur but are much less common than vein thromboses. Risk factors for thrombosis in patients with antiphospholipid syndrome include a history of thrombosis and persistently, moderately elevated titers of immunoglobulin G (IgG) anticardiolipin antibodies, each of which may increase a patient's risk of thrombosis fivefold.

Antiphospholipid antibodies also have been associated with pregnancy complications, particularly fetal death, severe placental insufficiency, preeclampsia, and recurrent miscarriage. These pregnancy associations were formalized in the 1999 International Consensus Criteria for the diagnosis of antiphospholipid syndrome (14) and were revised in 2005 (15).

Several mechanisms have been proposed to explain how antiphospholipid antibodies contribute to thrombosis (13). Endothelial cell activation and overexpression of adhesion molecules and cytokines have been implicated. Another theory focuses on an oxidant-mediated injury of vascular endothelium, because some anticardiolipin antibodies cross-react with oxidized low-density lipoprotein, which is a major contributor to atherosclerosis. It also has been proposed that antiphospholipid antibodies interfere with the function of the phospholipid-binding proteins that regulate coagulation, specifically prothrombin, protein C, annexin V, and tissue factor. Adverse pregnancy outcomes in patients with antiphospholipid syndrome also have been attributed to placental thrombosis. However, alternative mechanisms may be at play. For example, anticardiolipin antibodies impede trophoblast invasion in vitro, thereby further promoting placental insufficiency and pregnancy loss. Most recently, antiphospholipid antibodies have been shown to initiate a complement-dependent immune response at the maternal–fetal interface (16) in a murine model, and a similar mechanism seems to be important in antiphospholipid antibody-mediated thrombosis (17).

The diagnosis of antiphospholipid syndrome is based on clinical and laboratory criteria (Box 58). A patient must exhibit at least one of two clinical criteria (vascular thrombosis or pregnancy morbidity) and at least one of three laboratory criteria (a positive result on lupus anticoagulant testing; medium to high titers of IgG or IgM anticardiolipin antibodies; or anti-β_2 glycoprotein-I IgG, IgM antibody isotype, or both). Clinicians should recognize that antiphospholipid antibodies may be found in 1–5% of otherwise healthy individuals, though usually in low titers. Thus, the laboratory diagnosis of antiphospholipid syndrome requires positive laboratory results on two separate occasions at least 12 weeks apart. Classification of antiphospholipid syndrome should be avoided if less than 12 weeks or more than 5 years separates the positive antiphospholipid test and clinical manifestations (15).

Box 58

Revised Classification Criteria for Definite Antiphospholipid Syndrome

Antiphospholipid antibody syndrome (antiphospholipid syndrome) is present if at least one of the following clinical criteria and one of the following laboratory criteria that follow are met*:

Clinical Criteria

Vascular Thrombosis

One or more clinical episodes of arterial, vein, or small vessel thrombosis, in any tissue or organ. Thrombosis must be confirmed by objective validated criteria (ie, unequivocal findings of appropriate imaging studies or histopathology). For histopathologic confirmation, thrombosis should be present without significant evidence of inflammation in the vessel wall.

Pregnancy Morbidity

- One or more unexplained deaths of a morphologically normal fetus aged 10 or more weeks of gestation, confirmed by ultrasonography or direct examination
- One or more premature births of a morphologically normal neonate aged less than 34 weeks of gestation because of:

    —eclampsia or severe preeclampsia defined according to standard definitions, or

    —recognized features of placental insufficiency

- Three or more unexplained consecutive spontaneous abortions at less that 10 weeks of gestation, not associated with maternal anatomic or hormonal abnormalities and paternal and maternal chromosomal abnormalities.

Laboratory Criteria

Lupus Anticoagulant

Present in plasma, on two or more occasions at least 12 weeks apart, detected according to the guidelines of the International Society on Thrombosis and Haemostasis

Anticardiolipin Antibody IgG, IgM

Present in serum or plasma, medium or high titer (ie, greater than 40 IgG phospholipid units or IgM phospholipid units, or greater than the 99th percentile), on two or more occasions, at least 12 weeks apart, measured by a standardized ELISA

Anti-β_2 glycoprotein-I Antibody of IgG, or IgM, or Both

Present in serum or plasma (in titer greater than 99th percentile), on two or more occasions, at least 12 weeks apart, measured by a standardized ELISA, according to recommended procedures

*Classification of antiphospholipid syndrome should be avoided if less than 12 weeks or more than 5 years separate the positive antiphospholipid test result and the clinical manifestation. Coexisting inherited or acquired factors for thrombosis are not reasons for excluding patients from antiphospholipid syndrome trials. However, two subgroups of antiphospholipid syndrome patients should be recognized, according to:

   a. the presence and

   b. the absence of additional risk factors for thrombosis.

(continued)

Box 58

Revised Classification Criteria for Definite Antiphospholipid Syndrome *(continued)*

Indicative (but not exhaustive) manifestations of such cases include age (older than 55 years in men and older than 65 years in women) and the presence of any of the established risk factors for cardiovascular disease (hypertension, diabetes mellitus, elevated low-density lipoprotein or low high-density lipoprotein cholesterol levels, cigarette smoking, family history of premature cardiovascular disease, body mass index of 30 (expressed as weight in kilograms divided by height in meters squared), microalbuminuria, estimated glomerular filtration rate of less than 60 mL per minute), inherited thrombophilias, oral contraceptives use, nephrotic syndrome, malignancy, immobilization, and surgery. Thus, patients who fulfill criteria should be stratified according to contributing causes of thrombosis. A thrombotic episode in the past could be considered as a clinical criterion, provided that thrombosis is proved by appropriate diagnostic means and that no alternative diagnosis or cause of thrombosis is found. Superficial vein thrombosis is not included in the clinical criteria. Generally accepted features of placental insufficiency include:

- abnormal or non-reassuring fetal surveillance test(s); eg, a nonreactive nonstress test, suggestive of fetal hypoxemia
- abnormal Doppler flow velocimetry waveform analysis result suggestive of fetal hypoxemia; eg, absent end-diastolic flow in the umbilical artery
- oligohydramnios, eg, an amniotic fluid index of 5 cm or less
- a postnatal birth weight less than the 10th percentile for the gestational age

Investigators are strongly advised to classify antiphospholipid syndrome patients in studies into one of the following categories:

  I. more than one laboratory criteria present (any combination)

  IIa. lupus anticoagulant present alone

  IIb. anticoagulant antibody present alone

  IIc. anti-β_2 glycoprotein-I antibody present alone.

Abbreviation: IgG indicates immunoglobulin G; IgM, immunoglobulin M.

Miyakis S, Lockshin MD, Atsumi T, Branch DW, Brey RL, Cervera R, et al. International consensus statement on an update of the classification criteria for definite antiphospholipid syndrome (antiphospholipid syndrome). Journal of Thrombosis and Haemostasis 4 (2), 295–306. Copyright © 2006 Blackwell Publishing Ltd. Reproduced with permission of Blackwell Publishing Ltd.

Common Bleeding Disorders

Serious bleeding disorders occur infrequently in women. The two most common disorders encountered among women with active bleeding or a history of bleeding episodes are von Willebrand disease and autoimmune thrombocytopenic purpura.

Occasionally, an asymptomatic woman will be found to have thrombocytopenia or prolongation of the prothrombin time or partial thromboplastin time. Thrombocytopenia may be due to decreased platelet production or increased platelet destruction. The most common causes of decreased platelet production in otherwise asymptomatic women are infection (usually viral) and bone marrow disorders, including neoplastic disorders. The most common causes of increased platelet destruction are drug-induced thrombocytopenia and autoimmune disorders, including autoimmune thrombocytopenic purpura, systemic lupus erythematosus, and antiphospholipid syndrome.

In an asymptomatic woman, the causes of a prolonged prothrombin time are related to mishandling of the blood sample, liver disease, dysfibrinogenemia, or warfarin use. A prolonged partial thromboplastin time in an otherwise asymptomatic woman may result from mishandling of the blood sample; lupus anticoagulant; or deficiencies of factor VIII, factor IX, factor XI, factor XII, prekallikrein, or high-molecular-weight kininogen.

Von Willebrand Disease

Von Willebrand disease is the most common inherited bleeding disorder, occurring in up to 1.3% of individuals and without race or sex bias. The disease results from deficiencies or abnormalities of von Willebrand factor (vWF), a circulating glycoprotein synthesized by mega-karyocytes and endothelial cells. When released, vWF circulates in multimers complexed to clotting factor VIII (Figure 19). The vWF protein has two main functions. First, it binds to glycoprotein Ib on the platelet surface and also to specific targets, such as collagen and heparin-like substances in the subendothelial space. This binding allows vWF to facilitate platelet adhesion under conditions of high shear stress by forming a bridge between the platelet and the vascular endothelium. Second, vWF covalently binds to the N-terminus of factor VIII and promotes clotting. It is important to note that the binding of vWF to factor VIII protects factor VIII from proteolytic degradation. Hence, with decreased vWF levels, factor VIII levels also are decreased as a result of increased degradation.

There are three main subtypes of von Willebrand disease (Table 28), each with characteristic laboratory findings. The family history typically reveals mucocutaneous bleeding inherited in an autosomal-dominant fashion. The inheritance pattern is recessive in some subtypes (types 2A and 3). Additionally, penetrance is variable,

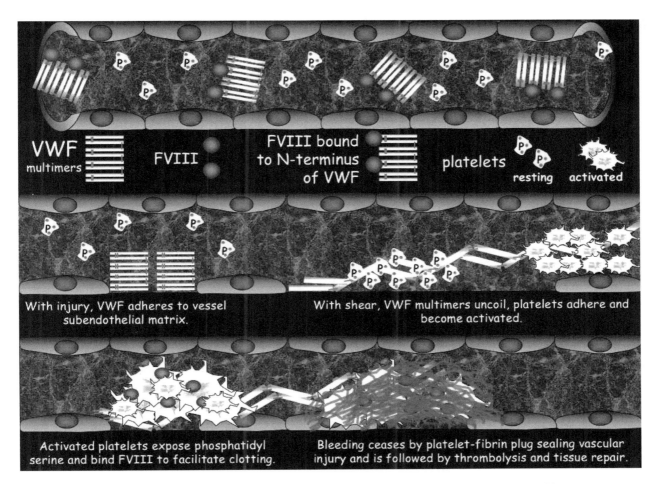

Figure 19. Mechanism of interaction between von Willebrand factor, factor VIII, and platelets in normal hemostasis. A cross-sectioned blood vessel shows stages of hemostasis. **Top.** Von Willebrand factor (vWF) is the carrier protein for blood clotting factor VIII. Under normal conditions vWF does not interact with platelets or the blood vessel wall that is covered with endothelial cells. **Middle left.** After vascular injury, vWF adheres to the exposed subendothelial matrix. **Middle right.** After vWF is uncoiled by local shear forces, the activated and aggregated platelets alter their membrane phospholipids exposing phosphatidylserine, and its activated platelet surface binds clotting factors from circulating blood and initiates blood clotting on this surface where fibrin is locally deposited. **Bottom right.** The combination of clotting and platelet aggregation and adhesion forms a platelet-fibrin plug, which results in the cessation of bleeding. The extent of clotting is carefully regulated by natural anticoagulants. Subsequently, thrombolysis initiates tissue repair and ultimately the vessel may be re-endothelialized and blood flow initiated. Abbreviations: FVIII indicates factor VIII; vWF, von Willebrand factor.
(National Heart, Lung, and Blood Institute [NHLBI]. The diagnosis, evaluation, and management of von Willebrand disease. Rockville [MD]: NHLBI; 2007. Available at: http://www.nhlbi.nih.gov/guidelines/vwd/vwd.pdf. Retrieved November 14, 2008. Used by permission of R. R. Montgomery.)

and patients from the same family with the same molecular defect may have a varied clinical course.

The patient's personal history usually includes a bleeding diathesis. Menorrhagia, epistaxis, or bleeding after tooth extraction are the most common symptoms. Studies of adolescent women with menorrhagia have found that up to 16% have von Willebrand disease (18).

Surgery for excessive menstrual bleeding should not be performed without the consideration of bleeding disorders in women younger than 30 years. The diagnosis of von Willebrand disease, however, can be difficult because of disease subtypes and because the presentation may vary, even in the same individual. Testing for

von Willebrand disease in a patient with a bleeding disorder is best accomplished as follows:

- Determine whether the patient has thrombocytopenia or coagulation cascade abnormalities by testing the platelet count, prothrombin time, and aPTT (the partial thromboplastin time may be prolonged in patients with moderate to severe von Willebrand disease)

- Perform a ristocetin cofactor activity assay. This test may need to be repeated if the suspicion is high and test results are equivocal or negative

- Perform a vWF antigen assay to quantify the degree of deficiency

Table 28. Von Willebrand Disease Subtypes

VWD Subtype	Frequency	Clinical Features	Inheritance	Factor VIII Response to Desmopressin
1	70% of VWD; 1–30/1,000	Mild to moderate bleeding	AD incomplete penetrance	Positive response
2A	10–15% of VWD	Mild to moderate bleeding	AD, and some AR	Less reliable response
2B	Less than 5% of VWD	Mild to moderate bleeding	AD more complete penetrance	Variable response
2M	Rare	Variable bleeding	AD	Heterogenous response
2N	Infrequent	Variable bleeding	AR	Probable response
3	Rare	Undetectable vWF, very low levels of FVIII, and severe bleeding	AR	Poor or no response

Abbreviations: AD indicates autosomal dominant; AR, autosomal recessive; FVIII, factor VIII; VWD, von Willebrand disease; vWF, von Willebrand factor.

- Perform a factor VIII function assay to quantify the degree of deficiency and help determine the disease subtype
- If any of the above tests are positive, which suggests von Willebrand disease, perform a vWF multimer assay to assess multimer structure and subtype the disease.

Treatment to prevent or control bleeding in women with von Willebrand disease includes therapy to increase endogenous vWF (desmopressin); supplementation of vWF by infusion of plasma vWF; and the use of agents that promote hemostasis, such as antifibrinolytics (eg, aminocaproic acid or tranexamic acid). For sources providing afull description of the management of von Willebrand disease, see Resources.

Autoimmune Thrombocytopenia Purpura

Autoimmune thrombocytopenic purpura, also known as idiopathic thrombocytopenic purpura, is the most common immune-mediated thrombocytopenic condition. The most common form of autoimmune thrombocytopenic purpura in adult women is a chronic condition. The condition results from increased platelet destruction due to autoantibodies directed against platelet surface antigens. Intravascular platelet survival is shortened, with most platelet destruction occurring in the spleen. The condition is diagnosed most often in women in the third and fourth decades of life.

The diagnosis of autoimmune thrombocytopenic purpura is one of exclusion in that none of the diagnostic features of the condition are specific. Thrombocytopenia is the hallmark of the condition and occurs without leukocyte abnormalities or nonhemorrhagic anemia. Easy bruising and petechiae are the typical early signs of thrombocytopenia; usually they do not appear until

the platelet counts fall below 50×10^9/L. In patients with platelet counts of less than $10–20 \times 10^9$/L, spontaneous epistaxis, gingival bleeding, and mucosal surface, hemorrhagic vesicles may appear. The most serious forms of bleeding are genitourinary, gastrointestinal, and intracranial. The gynecologic patient may present with menorrhagia.

Management of autoimmune thrombocytopenic purpura depends on the presence or absence of clinical bleeding, the degree of thrombocytopenia, and risks related to surgery or pregnancy. An otherwise asymptomatic, nonpregnant patient with autoimmune thrombocytopenic purpura and a platelet count of greater than $20–30 \times 10^9$/L does not require treatment. Patients with clinically important bleeding require medical therapy, and those with life-threatening hemorrhage require platelet transfusions and medical therapy. Asymptomatic women who are to undergo surgery are treated in order to increase and maintain the platelet count above 50×10^9/L. Women with recurrent episodes of bleeding or women whose platelet counts remain in the critical range (less than 20×10^9/L) may need splenectomy. Rarely, a woman with a life-threatening hemorrhage will require splenectomy as a last resort.

When treatment of autoimmune thrombocytopenic purpura is indicated, many experts prefer corticosteroids as the initial treatment, including during pregnancy. One regimen involves prednisone, started at a dosage of 1–1.5 mg/kg per day and continued until there is a clear response or for 4 weeks. Once a normal count is achieved, prednisone should be tapered. Up to 45% of patients with autoimmune thrombocytopenic purpura will respond favorably to corticosteroids; of these patients, most will have a normal platelet count within 4–6 weeks. Inadequate response to corticosteroids or relapse when the medication is tapered indicates that a favorable response to corticosteroids is unlikely and that other treatment should be considered. In pregnancy, corticosteroids are continued at the lowest dose that will maintain the platelet count above 50×10^9/L. Individuals will require "stress" doses of steroids while they are in labor or at the time of cesarean delivery.

Individuals who do not respond to corticosteroids or who relapse usually are treated with high-dose intravenous immune globulin (IVIG). Intravenous immune globulin also is preferred by some experts as a first-line treatment during pregnancy.

Splenectomy results in the highest cure rate in patients with autoimmune thrombocytopenic purpura; a complete response is seen in two thirds of patients undergoing the procedure. Pregnant women near term who are poorly responsive to corticosteroids or IVIG should undergo delivery and be reassessed thereafter. If the patient is remote from term, splenectomy may be required. The procedure may be done in the second trimester with good surgical exposure. After splenectomy, pneumococcal vaccination is indicated and may be given in pregnancy. The physician should be prepared for surgical or postpartum hemorrhage in all women with autoimmune thrombocytopenic purpura.

References

1. Stein PD, Henry JW, Gottschalk A. Mismatched vascular defects. An easy alternative to mismatched segmental equivalent defects for the interpretation of ventilation/perfusion lung scans in pulmonary embolism. Chest 1993;104:1468–71.

2. Qaseem A, Snow V, Barry P, Hornbake ER, Rodnick JE, Tobolic T, et al. Current diagnosis of venous thromboembolism in primary care: a clinical practice guideline from the American Academy of Family Physicians and the American College of Physicians. Joint American Academy of Family Physicians/American College of Physicians Panel on Deep Venous Thrombosis/Pulmonary Embolism. Ann Intern Med 2007;146:454–8.

3. Mullins MD, Becker DM, Hagspiel KD, Philbrick JT. The role of spiral volumetric computed tomography in the diagnosis of pulmonary embolism. Arch Intern Med 2000;160:293–8.

4. Fareed J, Jeske W, Hoppensteadt D, Clarizio R, Walenga JM. Are the available low-molecular-weight heparin preparations the same? Semin Thromb Hemost 1996;22(suppl 1):77–91.

5. de Monye W, Pattynama PM. Contrast-enhanced spiral computed tomography of the pulmonary arteries: an overview. Semin Thromb Hemost 2001;27:33–9.

6. Snow V, Qaseem A, Barry P, Hornbake ER, Rodnick JE, Tobolic T, et al. Management of venous thromboembolism: a clinical practice guideline from the American College of Physicians and the American Academy of Family Physicians. American College of Physicians; American Academy of Family Physicians Panel on Deep Venous Thrombosis/Pulmonary Embolism. Ann Intern Med 2007;146:204–10.

7. Prevention of deep vein thrombosis and pulmonary embolism. ACOG Practice Bulletin No. 84. American College of Obstetricians and Gynecologists. Obstet Gynecol 2007;110:429–40.

8. Harenberg J, Schneider D, Heilmann L, Wolf H. Lack of anti-factor Xa activity in umbilical cord vein samples after subcutaneous administration of heparin or low molecular mass heparin in pregnant women. Haemostasis 1993; 23:314–20.

9. Bratt G, Tornebohm E, Widlund L, Lockner D. Low molecular weight heparin (KABI 2165, Fragmin): pharmacokinetics after intravenous and subcutaneous administration in human volunteers. Thromb Res 1986;42:613–20.

10. Monreal M, Lafoz E, Olive A, del Rio L, Vedia C. Comparison of subcutaneous unfractionated heparin with a low molecular weight heparin (Fragmin) in patients with venous thromboembolism and contraindications to coumarin. Thromb Haemost 1994;71:7–11.

11. Muir JM, Hirsh J, Weitz JI, Andrew M, Young E, Shaughnessy SG. A histomorphometric comparison of the effects of heparin and low-molecular-weight heparin on cancellous bone in rats. Blood 1997;89:3236–42.

12. Warkentin TE, Levine MN, Hirsh J, Horsewood P, Roberts RS, Gent M, et al. Heparin-induced thrombocytopenia in patients treated with low-molecular-weight heparin or unfractionated heparin. N Engl J Med 1995;332:1330–5.

13. Levine JS, Branch DW, Rauch J. The antiphospholipid syndrome. N Engl J Med 2002;346:752–63.

14. Wilson WA, Gharavi AE, Koike T, Lockshin MD, Branch DW, Piette JC, et al. International consensus statement on preliminary classification criteria for definite antiphospholipid syndrome: report of an international workshop. Arthritis Rheum 1999;42:1309–11.

15. Miyakis S, Lockshin MD, Atsumi T, Branch DW, Brey RL, Cervera R, et al. International consensus statement on an update of the classification criteria for definite antiphospholipid syndrome (APS). J Thromb Haemost 2006;4: 295–306.

16. Salmon JE, Girardi G. Antiphospholipid antibodies and pregnancy loss: a disorder of inflammation. J Reprod Immunol 2008;77:51–6.

17. Pierangeli SS, Girardi G, Vega-Ostertag M, Liu X, Espinola RG, Salmon J. Requirement of activation of complement C3 and C5 for antiphospholipid antibody-mediated thrombophilia. Arthritis Rheum 2005;52:2120–4.

18. Claessens E, Cowell CA. Acute adolescent menorrhagia. Am J Obstet Gynecol 1981;139:277–80.

Index